D1408586

acute barbiturate poisoning

acute barbiturate poisoning

edited by

Henry Matthew

regional poisoning treatment centre,
the royal infirmary, edinburgh

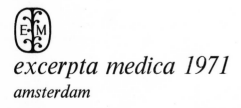

excerpta medica 1971
amsterdam

PUBLISHED JANUARY 1971

ISBN 90 219 2034 4

excerpta medica offices

Amsterdam	Herengracht 364
Buenos Aires	Florida 165, Galería Guëmes, 4° Piso, Esc. 454/461
London	Chandos House, 2 Queen Anne Street
Milan	Via San Senatore 6/2
New York	New York Academy of Medicine Building, 2 East 103rd Street
Tokyo	8th Floor, Sankaido Building, 1–9–13 Akasaka, Minato-ku

excerpta medica monograph

Printed in The Netherlands by Trio, The Hague
Set in 'Monotype' Times 10 pt 2 pt leaded
Bound by A. W. Sijthoff, Leyden
Cover Design Jean Paul Vroom

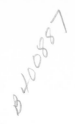

preface

The division of medicine into specialities has advantages when it comes to the treatment of the individual patient. This applies to the common condition of acute barbiturate poisoning. However, amongst the disadvantages is the difficulty in obtaining comprehensive information on the subject within the covers of one book. For example, a textbook on any aspect of acute poisoning can only provide limited information. As far as acute barbiturate poisoning is concerned, this has been remedied by the production of this monograph, which deals with all aspects of the subject.

No attempt has been made, in a book containing material by 26 contributors, to avoid overlap; nor has there been any endeavour to achieve uniformity of opinion. Conflicting views can therefore be expected, but it is hoped that the reader will be able to assess for himself the evidence on which opinions are based.

The editor expresses his gratitude to Dr. A. A. H. Lawson and Dr. A. T. Proudfoot for helpful advice in undertaking his pleasant duty of assembling such a team of experts from many countries, editing their manuscripts and reading the proofs.

January 1971   *Henry Matthew*

contents

addresses of first authors

R. C. B. Aitken   University Department of Psychiatry
(Royal Edinburgh Hospital)
Morningside Park
Edinburgh
U.K.

G. W. Beveridge   Department of Dermatology
The Royal Infirmary
Edinburgh
U.K.

H. A. Bloomer   Division of Kidney Disease
Department of Internal Medicine
University of Utah College of Medicine
Salt Lake City, Utah
U.S.A.

F. E. Camps   Department of Forensic Medicine
The London Hospital Medical College
London, E.1
U.K.

E. G. Comstock   American Academy of Clinical Toxicology
P.O. Box 2565
Houston, Texas
U.S.A.

A. K. Done   Department of Pediatrics
University of Utah Medical Center
Salt Lake City, Utah
U.S.A.

M. Govaerts-Lepicard   CNPTI Etablissement d'Utilité Publique
15, Rue Joseph Stallaert
Brussels 6
Belgium

I. Haider

Whitchurch Hospital
Whitchurch, Cardiff
U.K.

D. E. Hathway

Huntingdon Research Centre
Huntingdon
U.K.

N. Kessel

Department of Psychiatry
University of Manchester
Manchester
U.K.

A. A. H. Lawson

Regional Poisoning Treatment Centre
The Royal Infirmary
Edinburgh
U.K.

H. A. Lee

Saint Mary's General Hospital
Milton, Portsmouth
U.K.

C. McArdle

Pharmaceutical Department
The General Hospital
Birmingham
U.K.

J. W. McCulloch

Schools of Applied Social Studies
University of Bradford
Bradford
U.K.

L. C. Mark

Department of Anesthesiology
College of Physicians and Surgeons of
Columbia University
New York, N.Y.
U.S.A.

S. Moeschlin

Medizinische Klinik
Bürgerspital der Stadt Solothurn
4500 Solothurn
Switzerland

A. Myschetzky

Overlaegen ved Psykiatrisk Afd. E
Bispebjerg Hospital
Bispebjerg Bakke 23
2400 Copenhagen
Denmark

D. V. Parke Department of Biochemistry
University of Surrey
Guildford, Surrey
U.K.

H. Shubin Shock Research Unit
School of Medicine
University of Southern California
1322 North Vermont Avenue
Los Angeles, Calif.
U.S.A.

H. L. Verhulst Division of Poison Control BF-230
Food and Drug Administration
200 C Street, S.W.
Washington, D.C.
U.S.A.

H. Yatzidis 31 Acadimias Street
Athens 135
Greece

1. history of barbiturate poisoning

A. Myschetzky

In 1969, the centenary of chloral hydrate, the first real hypnotic drug, might have been celebrated. However, although barbituric acid had already been synthesized by von Baeyer in 1864, it was not until 1903 that the first barbituric acid compound with hypnotic qualities was introduced to therapy by Fischer and von Mering. The drug was diethyl-barbituric acid (barbitone).

During the following years the number of barbituric acid compounds with hypnotic effects increased considerably, more than 2,500 barbiturates being synthesized. The consumption of hypnotics of this kind steadily rose to enormous amounts in Europe and the United States. In 1968 in England and Wales over 17 million prescriptions, containing an average number of 80 tablets of barbiturate per prescription, were dispensed outside hospital.

Very soon after the introduction of hypnotic barbiturates, cases of fatal poisoning were reported. In many countries barbiturate poisoning has for a considerable period of time been the most common means of self-poisoning. In the poisoning treatment centre at Copenhagen 70% of all admissions during the years 1954–1956 were due to drugs of this sort. In 1965 barbiturate overdosage accounted for 50% of admissions to the Edinburgh poisoning treatment centre, but this figure had fallen to 30% by 1968.

Barbiturate poisoning is often a dangerous condition and 25 years ago the mortality rate of this form of poisoning was about 24% in Denmark (Clemmesen and Nilsson, 1961). In the best poisoning treatment centres the death rate from barbiturate poisoning has now been brought down to 1% or less (Matthew and Lawson, 1970).

At the beginning of the era of barbiturate overdosage the treatment of intoxication was either completely passive or limited to gastric lavage, administration of laxatives, and cardiac stimulants.

In the early thirties the administration of central analeptics like pentazole, nikethamide, and picrotoxin was very widely used, often in enormous doses. The popularity of this most unphysiological treatment was presumably due to the fact that slightly intoxicated patients would wake up immediately after the injection. Patients in a deeper state of coma might sometimes respond to energetic treatment with these drugs insofar that for a short time the patient might cough or sneeze only to relapse into deep coma. As repeated injections of large doses of the analeptic drug were given at short intervals, the patient would often become completely exhausted and 'shock', which so often accompanies severe barbiturate poisoning even when untreated, was aggravated. Cardiac arrhythmias were also frequently induced by these central analeptic drugs (Myschetzky, 1961).

The development of a more physiological procedure for the treatment of barbiturate poisoning must be mainly credited to Scandinavian doctors. Under the guidance of Carl Clemmesen at the Bispebjerg Hospital in Copenhagen, Kirkegaard (1951) showed that barbiturate-intoxicated rats had a longer survival time when treated with serum and artificial ventilation. His theory (developed by him together with G. C. Brun) was that circulatory shock was an important factor in the fatal course of these poisonings. Nilsson (1951) from Lund in Sweden, during his clinical studies in Carl Clemmesen's department, was able to demonstrate the paramount significance of ensuring a free airway. At the same time he showed that the use of central stimulants was unnecessary in milder cases of barbiturate intoxication and harmful in more severe cases.

A simple, reliable, and rapid spectrophotometric method for quantitative measurement of barbituric acid in serum was developed by Lous (1954), and later supplemented with a qualitative determination of the type of barbituric acid compound concerned by using thin-layer paper chromatography.

In 1949 Carl Clemmesen organized the first poisoning treatment centre in Scandinavia, especially for the treatment of narcotic poisoning, in his department of psychiatry in the Bispebjerg Hospital in Copenhagen. This centre has been a model for other centres throughout the world.

Carl Clemmesen's principles of treatment were:
1.   Centralization. This ensured sufficient experience for doctors and nurses in the treatment of severe narcotic poisoning as well as better and safer transport to the one unit in the area, serving a population of 1.3 million.
2.   Ensuring a free airway and sufficient ventilation by anaesthesiological measures.
3.   Close clinical control necessitating energetic combating of complications by anti-shock treatment, frequent change of the patient's position, regular suction of the airways, and regulation and maintenance of water and electrolyte balance.
4.   No stomach aspiration or lavage.
5.   No central stimulation.

Nowadays, with highly developed anaesthetic skills and advances in internal medicine, much of this seems obvious; in the late forties this was not the case. Most of the principles have been adopted and accepted generally. However, some of them, especially the last two, have given rise to considerable discussion.

The abandoning of stomach-washing was a consequence of the clinical experience that patients, treated by gastric lavage and instillation of charcoal and laxative, very often showed signs of aspiration to the bronchi and lungs. This was especially common when the stomach-washing had been performed before transport to the treatment centre. There was also, however, experimental evidence. Investigations by Harstad *et al.* (1942) had shown that, by the analytical methods then used, only insignificant amounts of barbiturate could be found in the aspirated washing-fluid. The reliability of these findings in 1942 has been questioned and to some degree disproved by Matthew *et al.* (1966), who recommend cautious gastric lavage up till four hours after the ingestion of an overdose of barbiturate. The development of a safe intubation technique and the availability of antibiotics have obviously diminished the risks from stomach washout in the unconscious patient and it is a natural and reasonable measure.

As far as the use of central stimulants is concerned, most clinicians have realised their dangers and inefficiency. This is especially the case in France, the United Kingdom and Scandinavia. In the United States of America and in German clinics, stimulation still has its advocates. In 1955 Shaw from Sidney developed what he thought to be a true antidote to barbituric acid hypnotics. This preparation, bemegride (Megimide), was eventually shown to be a simple central stimulant with the same liability to provoke convulsions and arrhythmias as other drugs of this sort.

During the last decade different methods aiming at an acceleration of the excretion of barbiturates have been developed. Treatment by artificial kidney is an effective but somewhat cumbersome procedure, which is usually restricted either to patients intoxicated by extremely high doses of barbiturate or to those cases, not very frequent, where severe renal damage already exists or has developed as a result of shock during the actual intoxication and necessitates such intervention. Peritoneal dialysis has had its advocates (Barbour, 1960) but is now very seldom used. Forced diuresis was originally introduced by Olsson (1949), using simple water load and mercury diuretics. In 1959 Mollaret *et al.* pointed out the significance of alkalinizing the urine, especially in phenobarbital poisoning due to the high pK of this drug. In 1960 Lassen developed an easily administrable and safe method of forced osmotic alkaline diuresis with urea as the diuretic agent. Similar methods have since been developed in many other places in Europe, using different diuretics.

As barbiturate poisoning of moderate severity responds readily to ordinary supportive treatment, forced diuresis should be restricted to the severest cases, *i.e.*, poisoning of such gravity that unconsciousness of more than 72 hours duration is to be expected. In poisoning with long-acting barbiturates the duration of coma can be diminished to 50% and even 33% by this measure (Myschetzky and Lassen, 1963). In elderly debilitated patients it seems reasonable to widen the indication for forced diuresis to some degree. In the Copenhagen centre, forced diuresis is used in about 6–8% of all cases of barbiturate poisoning.

It has become increasingly clear that barbiturate poisoning is not only a medical-anaesthesiological problem. Up to 95% of patients poisoned by drugs have taken the drug more or less deliberately. The majority of these patients require some sort of psychiatric care. True psychosis is the cause of self-poisoning in about 10% of patients. In most instances, acute affective disorders, often on the basis of a personality disorder, are responsible, but even these cases need psychiatric assessment.

As a natural consequence of the fact that the number of drugs suitable for attempted suicide or self-poisoning has been rapidly growing during the last fifteen years, the percentage of barbiturate poisoning is declining. This has led to increased problems of treatment, as many of the new drugs are more dangerous and the treatment of overdosage is more difficult.

A recent trend in the history of barbiturate poisoning is that, whereas until about ten years ago patients usually ingested one particular drug in an act of self-poisoning, now it is becoming increasingly common for more than one drug to be ingested at one and the same time. This may occur in as many as 30% of admissions to hospital of poisoned patients. It is therefore becoming less usual to encounter patients who have ingested only a barbiturate preparation.

A poisoning treatment centre has existed in Edinburgh, Scotland, for almost one hundred years, and during the last decade treatment centres have been established in several other places such as France (Paris, Lyon, Marseilles), Sweden, England, the Irish Republic, and The Netherlands. Poisons information services have been organized either in conjunction with treatment centres or, more frequently, independently of them. Information services exist in Europe in Belgium, Czechoslovakia, Denmark, France, the German Republics, the Netherlands, Norway, Portugal, Sweden, Switzerland and the United Kingdom. Such services are also available in Australia, Canada and the United States of America.

It is thus evident that over the past fifty years the incidence of acute barbiturate poisoning has steadily increased in the so-called developed countries. It is satisfactory to record that thanks to the enlightened lead of the Danish pioneers the mortality rate in hospital is usually less than 1%. It is less to the credit of the medical profession that many thousands of persons throughout the world die each year outside hospital from suicidal ingestion of barbiturates prescribed by doctors.

REFERENCES

BARBOUR, B. H. (1960), Peritoneal dialysis in the management of dialysable poisonings. *Clin. Res.*, 8, 114.
CLEMMESEN, C. and NILSSON, E. (1961), Therapeutic trends in the treatment of barbiturate poisoning. *Clin. Pharmacol.*, 2, 220.
FISCHER and VON MERING (1903), Therapie der Gegenwart. (Cit. Merck Index, 1968).
HARSTAD, E., MOLLER, K. and SIMESEN, M. (1942), Gastric aspiration. *Acta med. scand.*, 112, 478.
KIRKEGAARD, A. (1951), Severe acute barbiturate poisoning. Thesis, Copenhagen.
LASSEN, N. A. (1960), Treatment of severe acute barbiturate poisoning by forced diuresis and alkalinization of the urine. *Lancet*, 2, 338.
LOUS, P. (1954), Barbituric acid concentration in serum from patients with severe acute poisoning. *Acta pharmacol. (Kbh.)*, 10, 261.
MATTHEW, H. and LAWSON, A. A. H. (1970), *Treatment of common acute poisonings*. Livingstone, Edinburgh.
MATTHEW, H., MACKINTOSH, T. F., TOMPSETT, S. L. and CAMERON J. C. (1966), Gastric aspiration and lavage inacute poisoning. *Brit. med. J.*, 1, 1333.

MOLLARET, P., RAPIN, M., POCIDALO, J. and MONSALLIER, J. F. (1959), Treatment of acute barbiturate poisoning. *Presse méd.*, 67, 1435.

MYSCHETZKY, A. (1961), The significance of Megimide in the treatment of barbiturate poisoning. *Dan. med. Bull.*, 8, 33.

MYSCHETZKY, A. and Lassen, N. A. (1963), Osmotic diuresis and alkalinization of the urine in the treatment of severe acute barbiturate intoxication. *Dan. med. Bull.*, 10, 104.

NILSSON, S. E. H. (1951), Treatment of acute barbiturate poisoning. *Acta med. scand., Suppl.*, 253.

OLSSON, W. T. L. (1949), Blood lavage in barbiturate poisoning. *Nord. Med.*, 42, 1471.

SHAW, F. H. (1955), Further experiences with Megimide – a barbiturate antagonist. *Med. J. Aust.*, 2, 889.

2. biochemistry of the barbiturates

Dennis V. Parke

The duration and extent of pharmacological activity of a drug is often largely determined by the rate of its metabolic deactivation in the animal body. With no class of drugs is this more true than with the barbiturates, which have long been used as model systems for the study of the activities of the 'drug-metabolizing enzymes', both *in vivo* and *in vitro*. These enzymes, which are probably concerned primarily with the metabolism of endogenous steroids and anutrients of dietary origin, also metabolize synthetic drugs because these are, fortuitously, substrates also acceptable to the 'drug-metabolizing enzymes'. Furthermore, just as the metabolism of drugs is fortuitous, so indeed is any consequent loss of pharmacological activity. Metabolism of a drug may result in a decrease in pharmacological activity, or to an increase in activity, or to a change in the nature of the activity (Parke, 1968*a*). With the barbiturates, metabolism invariably leads to deactivation of the drug in the case of the oxobarbiturates, but in the case of N-methylbarbiturates and the thiobarbiturates, deactivation, activation, and change of character of the pharmacological activity may all occur, dependent upon the kinetics of the alternative pathways available for metabolism. In any study of the pharmacological activity or toxicity of barbiturates a knowledge of the metabolism is therefore of considerable importance.

Many of the investigations into the metabolism of barbiturates were undertaken during the 1940s and 1950s before the quantitative separatory techniques of thin-layer and gas-liquid chromatography became established. As a consequence, comprehensive accounts of the metabolic fate have been determined for relatively few barbiturates. The older classical techniques of solvent extraction of the urine obtained from animals and humans dosed with a barbiturate, followed by isolation, identification and semi-quantitation of the unchanged drug and its metabolites, have provided unequivocal evidence of the identity of the major metabolites. What is now needed is a quantitative reappraisal of the metabolic fate of barbiturates using the techniques of isotope dilution and gas-liquid chromatography (Martin and Driscoll, 1966) to determine a balance sheet for each drug, preferably in several different species. This might be supported by kinetic studies of metabolism both *in vivo* and *in vitro*, so that the sequence and relative significance of the alternative metabolic pathways could be ascertained. Such information would be of considerable value in understanding the duration and nature of pharmacological activity and the extent and mechanisms of toxicity.

As one might expect with a subject of such wide interest, reviews on the metabolism of barbiturates have appeared at regular intervals (Williams and Parke, 1964; Bush and Sanders, 1967), but in view of the wide quantitative differences demonstrated in different species the review of the metabolism of barbiturates in man (Mark, 1963) is of particular value.

SITES OF METABOLISM OF BARBITURATES

In all species of animal studied, the major site of metabolism of barbiturates is undoubtedly the liver. Early work showed that with pentobarbital, but not barbital, which is largely excreted unchanged, there was a prolongation of anaesthesia in animals with liver damage, the increase in the duration of pharmacological activity being proportional to the extent of impairment of hepatic function (Pratt, 1933; Pratt et al., 1932). Furthermore, anaesthesia due to pentobarbital (Scheifley and Higgins, 1940) or to thiopental (Shideman et al., 1947) was shown also to be prolonged in rats following partial hepatectomy. Other workers demonstrated that rat liver brei preparations were capable of metabolically deactivating barbiturates such as hexobarbital (Martin et al., 1940) and also thiobarbiturates such as thiopental (Shideman et al., 1947). Further evidence for the liver being the major site of metabolism was provided by the sophisticated surgical techniques of Kelly and Shideman (1949), Meyers and Peoples (1954) and others. The former workers showed that the rate of disappearance of thiopental in perfused heart-lung, heart-lung-kidney, and heart-lung-liver preparations of dog was slightly increased when the kidney was incorporated into the circuit and very greatly accelerated when the liver was included. The final proof of the role of the liver in the metabolism of barbiturates came with the demonstration by Brodie et al. (1955) that the enzymes responsible for catalysing these chemical changes are located within the endoplasmic reticulum (microsomes) of the liver cells. The enzymes that catalyse the biotransformations of the barbiturates were all shown to require reduced nicotinamide adenine dinucleotide phosphate (NADPH$_2$) together with molecular oxygen, and were subsequently shown to be mixed-function oxidases (oxygenases).

Another site of metabolism of barbiturates, but a minor one compared with the liver, is the kidney. Experiments with rats and rabbits dosed with thiopental or hexobarbital following bilateral nephrectomy, showed that the duration of anaesthesia was increased by the removal of the kidneys, particularly in the case of thiopental (Richards et al., 1953). Similar effects were, however, produced by ligation of the ureters and were found to be dependent more on the degree of uraemia than on the actual removal of kidney tissue, so that the role of the kidney as a site of metabolism was not unequivocally established. Studies with isolated kidney preparations *in vitro* were unanimous in showing that thiopental is metabolized by kidney tissue, but varied in the extents to which they found metabolism of pentobarbital and other oxybarbiturates to occur (Dorfman and Goldbaum, 1947; Gould and Shideman, 1952; Cooper and Brodie, 1957). It would seem, therefore, that thiopental and possibly other thiobarbiturates are metabolized in kidney, but at a much slower rate than in liver, and that oxybarbiturates are metabolized only very slowly, if at all, by the kidney.

Other tissues which have been shown to metabolize barbiturates include brain, heart, intestines, muscle and spleen (Martin *et al.*, 1940; Gould and Shideman, 1952). However, Cooper and Brodie (1957) have claimed that in the rabbit the oxybarbiturates, hexobarbital, pentobarbital and secobarbital, undergo biotransformation only in the liver, whereas the thiobarbiturates, thiopental and thiosecobarbital, undergo oxidative metabolism also in the kidneys and brain, although this is to a much lesser extent than occurs in the liver.

PATHWAYS OF METABOLISM OF BARBITURATES

The barbiturates are metabolized by reactions occurring at four different sites of the molecule (Williams, 1959):

1. C^5-Substituents may undergo oxygenation, oxidation, or complete removal.
2. N^1- and N^3-Alkyl groups may be removed, or unsubstituted N atoms may be methylated.
3. S^2 may be replaced by O, converting thiobarbiturates to the corresponding oxybarbiturates.
4. Scission of the barbiturate ring may occur, at the 1 : 6 bond, to give substituted malonylureas.

1. C^5-SUBSTITUENTS

All therapeutically useful barbiturates have two substituents at the C^5-atom, one or both of which may undergo metabolism by oxygenation to form an alcohol or a diol, followed possibly by oxidation to the corresponding ketone or carboxylic acid. Complete removal of a side chain may also occur, and has been reported in the case of the allyl substituent in secobarbital (Cochin and Daly, 1963), and with one of the ethyl groups in the case of barbital (Goldschmidt and Wehr, 1957). These oxygenated metabolites, derived from modification of the C^5-substituents, are almost invariably without pharmacological activity so that this mode of metabolism may be regarded as one of the most important in the deactivation and detoxication of the dialkyl barbiturates.

Oxygenation

Oxygenation of the C^5-substituent side chains appears to occur preferentially in the longest chain and at the ultimate (ω) or penultimate (ω-1) carbon atoms; oxygenation is however not restricted to the ω and (ω-1) carbon atoms, although these 2 positions do seem to bear the brunt of the attack (Maynert, 1965*b*). The product of ω-oxygenation would be a primary alcohol which would be expected to undergo subsequent rapid oxidation to give the corresponding aldehyde and carboxylic acid. This may indeed account for the extreme rarity of the occurrence of a primary alcohol as a metabolite of any barbiturate, although a primary alcohol has been demonstrated in the case of barbital, where 5-ethyl-5β-hydroxyethyl barbituric acid is a very minor metabolite (Goldschmidt and Wehr, 1957), and possibly also in the case of hexethal (5-ethyl-5-*n*-hexyl barbituric acid) where five alcoholic metabolites have been isolated (Maynert, 1965*b*). In a study of the metabolism of secobarbital by rabbit liver microsomal enzymes, Ide *et al.* (1967) were able to demonstrate the formation of the (ω-1)-hydroxysecobarbital but not the ω-hydroxysecobarbital, which could presumably be an intermediate in the formation of carboxysecobarbital (secobarbital acid), a known metabolite of secobarbital *in vivo*. However, as would be expected, synthetic ω-hydroxysecobarbital was found to be rapidly metabolized by the soluble enzymes of rabbit liver, to give carboxysecobarbital. ω-Carboxysecobarbital was formed quantitatively (99–101%) from ω-hydroxysecobarbital by incubation with rabbit-liver soluble-fraction, using either NAD or NADP as co-factor, but was obtained in only 22% yield from secobarbital with microsomes plus soluble fraction, and not at all with the soluble fraction alone. Moreover, the formation of ω-carboxysecobarbital by rabbit liver microsomes plus soluble fraction was inhibited by N_2, SKF–525A and chlorpromazine, and enhanced by addition of $NADPH_2$, to extents similar to those found for the formation of (ω-1)-hydroxysecobarbital.

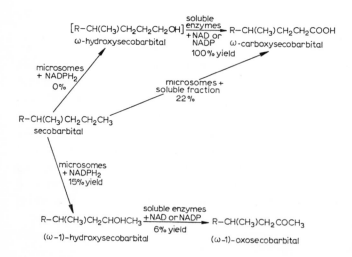

The facility with which ω-hydroxysecobarbital undergoes oxidation to give ω-carboxysecobarbital (100% yield), compared with the more difficult oxidation of (ω-1)-hydroxysecobarbital to the corresponding ketone (6% yield), may be the reason why ω-hydroxysecobarbital has not been demonstrated as a metabolite of secobarbital either *in vivo* or *in vitro*. This may also be the reason why primary alcohols formed by oxygenation of the ω-carbon atom are rarely found as metabolites of dialkylbarbiturates.

With the oxybarbiturates, oxygenation occurs to a greater extent at the (ω-1)-carbon atom than at the ω-carbon atom, although species differences may occur. In dog and man the (ω-1)-alcohol is the major metabolite of amobarbital (Frey and Magnussen, 1966), pentobarbital (Maynert, 1965a), secobarbital (Waddell, 1965) methohexital (Welles *et al.*, 1963) and hexethal (Maynert, 1965b), although with the last-named barbiturate the sum of the (ω-1)-oxygenated metabolites isolated from urine (alcohol plus ketone) was approximately 25% of the dose while the sum of the ω-oxygenated metabolites (carboxylic acids) was equal to 20%. In contrast, with the thiobarbiturates, oxygenation would seem to occur preferentially at the ω-carbon atom, for with thiopental and thiamylal the ω-carboxythiobarbiturates are major metabolites whereas the (ω-1)-hydroxythiobarbiturates are only minor products (Tsukamoto *et al.*, 1963b; Mark *et al.*, 1965).

Where oxygenation gives rise to a new asymmetric centre, as for example with pentobarbital and hexobarbital, optically isomeric forms of the hydroxybarbiturates are formed. Evidence has been obtained that this may occur in a stereo-selective manner, and in the case of pentobarbital the 1-isomer is preferentially formed with only this isomer undergoing subsequent oxidation to the corresponding ketone (Kuntzman *et al.*, 1967). Stereoselection of the substrate may also occur, and the d-enantiomer of hexobarbital has been shown to be more rapidly metabolized in the rat than the 1-enantiomer (Furner *et al.*, 1969b).

Oxygenation may also take place at a double bond of an allyl group, as is seen in the metabolism of secobarbital to secobarbital diol (Waddell, 1965), but this is a minor pathway and has not been observed in the *in vitro* metabolism of secobarbital by rat liver preparation (Ide *et al.*, 1967), nor with other allyl substituted barbiturates.

With cyclic substituents at the C^5 position, oxygenation occurs primarily at the 4'-position of a benzene ring, but possibly also to a minor extent at the 2'-position, so that phenobarbital is metabolized principally to p-hydroxyphenobarbital, but traces of o-hydroxyphenobarbital have also been detected (Glasson and Benakis, 1961). With 5-(1'-cyclohexyl) barbiturates, such as hexobarbital and cyclobarbital, oxygenation occurs at the 3'-position. Toki *et al.* (1963), using rabbit liver preparations, have shown that hexobarbital is first metabolized by oxygenation in the presence of microsomal enzymes, $NADPH_2$ and O_2, to yield 3'-hydroxyhexobarbital, which is then subsequently oxidized to 3'-ketohexobarbital by soluble enzymes. Presumably a similar mechanism operates in the metabolism of cyclobarbital to ketocyclobarbital. The new barbiturate, 5-(bicyclo-3,2,1-oct-2-en-2-yl)-5 ethyl barbituric acid (Reposal), a hypnotic with a bicyclic substituent at C^5, is also metabolized by oxygenation of this substituent, at a carbon atom adjacent to the double bond (Nielsen and Tarding, 1968).

Reposal   Metabolite

With barbiturates that contain a thioether group in the 5-alkyl substituent the sulphur atom also may undergo oxygenation, to give a sulphoxide group. The thio-barbiturate, methitural (5-(2'-methylthioethyl)-5-(1'-methylbutyl)-2-thiobarbituric acid), is metabolized in this way to give methitural sulphoxide (Dietz and Soehring, 1957).

Methitural   Methitural sulphoxide

Oxidation

Oxidation of the primary and secondary alcohols, the products of ω- and (ω-1)-oxygenation of the 5-alkyl and -cyclohexenyl substituents, gives rise to ω-carboxylic acids and (ω-1)-ketones, which are known metabolites of many barbiturates. ω-Carboxylic acids have been shown to be metabolites of pentobarbital, seconal, hexethal, thiopental, and thiamylal, but not of barbital, nor of phenobarbital, hexobarbital, and cyclobarbital–barbiturates containing cyclic substituents and in which the cyclic sub-stituent is oxygenated in preference to the alkyl substituent. (ω-1)-Ketones are formed in the metabolism of pentobarbital, seconal, hexethal, and with barbiturates con-taining alicyclic substituents such as hexobarbital, cyclobarbital, and heptabarbital; but they are not formed with barbital nor phenobarbital – where the aromatic substi-tuent is oxygenated to give a phenol, not an alcohol, nor to any extent with thiopental and thiamylal – thiobarbiturates in which (ω-1)-oxygenated metabolites are only minor metabolites.

Heptabarbital   Ketoheptabarbital

The major metabolite of amobarbital is a tertiary alcohol, 5-ethyl-5(3'-hydroxy-3'-methylbutyl)barbituric acid, which would be expected to be resistant to subsequent oxidation (see Williams, 1959, p. 67). This metabolite is found to be excreted in the urine unchanged, and possibly also as conjugates.

Ketones are also the major metabolites of the 2-bromoalkyl barbiturates, propallyl-onal (5-(2'-bromallyl)-5-isopropyl barbituric acid; Nostal) and butallylonal (5-(2'-bromallyl-5-secbutyl barbituric acid; Pernoston) (Williams, 1959).

Propallylonal   Ketopropallylonal

It has been shown with secobarbital (Ide et $al.$, 1967) and hexobarbital (Toki et $al.$, 1963) that the ketone metabolites are formed by oxidation of the corresponding secondary alcohols by enzymes of the soluble fraction of liver, and it might be presumed that this is a general enzymic mechanism involved in the formation of all ketone metabolites of barbiturates.

2. N^1- AND N^3-DEALKYLATION AND ALKYLATION

A number of clinically useful barbiturates have substituents, usually methyl groups, attached to the nitrogen atoms at positions 1 and 3 of the barbiturate ring. As these N-methyl barbiturates generally have similar pharmacological activity to the parent unsubstituted barbiturates, N-demethylation, unlike oxidation of the 5-substituents, does not result in marked loss of activity.

N-Dealkylation and the oxygenation of C^5-substituents are competing metabolic reactions. In the case of hexobarbital, N-demethylation would appear to be less important than oxygenation (Bush and Sanders, 1967), and in dogs, rats, and rabbits the oxygenated metabolites, hydroxyhexobarbital and ketohexobarbital, are more readily demethylated than is hexobarbital (Okui and Kuroiwa, 1963; Williams and Parke, 1964). In contrast, mephobarbital (5-ethyl-1-methyl-5-phenylbarbituric acid, Prominal) is quite rapidly demethylated, both in dogs, in which about 75% of a dose is demethylated to phenobarbital in 24 hours, and in man, where the plasma concentration of phenobarbital is always many times that of mephobarbital (Butler, 1952). However, rats demethylate only about half of an administered dose of mephobarbital (Butler et $al.$, 1952), so that there may be considerable species differences in the relative importances of these alternative metabolic pathways.

N-Methylbarbital and N^1, N^3-dimethylbarbital are both demethylated to barbital in the dog, and with N-methylbarbital this is extensive, as only traces of the unchanged drug are excreted (Butler and Bush, 1939). The metabolic removal of other N-alkyl groups may also occur, but the extent of dealkylation decreases markedly with increasing length of the alkyl chain. For example, the dealkylation in dogs of various N-alkyl derivatives of barbital occurs to the following extents: N-methylbarbital, 98%; N-ethylbarbital, 60–70%; N-propylbarbital, 10% (Butler, 1953). Methylbarbital, dimethylbarbital, mephobarbital, hexobarbital, and methohexital have been shown to undergo demethylation when incubated with liver microsomal enzymes, the rate of demethylation being many times greater with dimethylbarbital than with the other barbiturates (Smith *et al.*, 1963; McMahon, 1963).

Rates of N-demethylation of barbiturates by liver microsomes (from McMahon, 1963)

Barbiturate	Rate of N-demethylation (μmolesHCHO/g liver/hr)	
	Rat	Rabbit
N^1, N^3-Dimethylbarbital	0.78	1.57
N-Methylbarbital	0.14	0.32
Hexobarbital	0.06	0.12
Methohexital	0.00	0.24

The biological methylation of heterocyclic nitrogen atoms is well known, *e.g.* the N-methylation of pyridine, piperidine, and histamine, but evidence for the N-methylation of barbiturates is inconclusive and conflicting. Frey *et al.* (1959) have tentatively reported finding N-methyl derivatives in the urines of humans dosed with barbital, cyclobarbital, and butabarbital, and Deininger (1956) has shown that, to a small extent, norhexobarbital is methylated in mice to hexobarbital, a result that has not been confirmed, however, by subsequent investigators (Bush and Parrish, 1963).

S-Demethylation

A new type of dealkylation reaction, namely the S-demethylation of the 5-methylthioethyl side chain of methitural (5-(2-methylthioethyl)-5-(1-methylbutyl)-2-thiobarbituric acid), has been demonstrated *in vitro* (Mazel *et al.*, 1964). This reaction is catalysed by microsomal enzymes of rat liver in the presence of $NADPH_2$ and O_2 and was shown to differ from N-dealkylation and other oxygenase reactions in that it was not inhibited by SKF–525A (β-diethylaminoethyl diphenylpropylacetate), nor stimulated by pre-treatment of the animals with phenobarbitone (Mazel and Henderson, 1963).

Methitural

Desmethylmethitural

3. S²-DESULPHURATION

The replacement of the 2-sulphur atom by oxygen is a general reaction of the 2-thiobarbiturates. Unlike the metabolic oxygenation and oxidation of the C^5-substituents, desulphuration is a form of biotransformation that does not lead to the deactivation of barbiturates, for the oxygen analogues of all known 2-thiobarbiturates are pharmacologically active. For example, thiopental, a hypnotic with a short duration of activity, is metabolized to give pentobarbital, which has a longer duration of action.

The metabolic conversion of thiobarbiturates to their oxygen analogues has been shown to occur with thiobarbital (Bush *et al.*, 1961), thiophenobarbital (Raventos, 1954), thiobutobarbital (Dietz and Soehring, 1957), thiopental (Soehring and Dietz, 1956), thiamylal (Tsukamoto *et al.*, 1963*b*), thialbarbital (Tsukamoto *et al.*, 1963*b*), and methitural (Dietz and Soehring, 1957). The extent of desulphuration varies with the thiobarbiturate and with the animal species; it is not generally the major pathway of metabolism but 10–40% of most thiobarbiturates are converted to the corresponding oxybarbiturates and their metabolites. Thiobarbital injected into rabbits is excreted in the urine as barbital to an extent of 10% of the administered dose, and thiophenobarbital is similarly metabolized to give 35% of the dose as phenobarbital (Raventos, 1954). Thiopental, labelled with ^{35}S, has been shown to be desulphurated in rats and monkeys, and nearly 40% of the dose is excreted as the oxygen analogue, pentobarbital, and its metabolites (Taylor *et al.*, 1952). Rat liver homogenates have also been shown to extensively metabolize thiopental into pentobarbital (Winters *et al.*, 1955).

The desulphuration of thiopental and other thiobarbiturates has been the subject of some controversy because the oxygen analogues may also be formed as artefacts during the extraction of the metabolites from the urine with ether. However, chloroform and ethyl acetate do not have this effect and in experiments in which these solvents were used in place of ether, smaller but significant amounts of the oxybarbiturate were isolated, showing that the oxygen analogues were true metabolites of thiobarbiturates.

4. RING SCISSION

The barbiturate ring is considered to be relatively stable *in vivo* (Williams, 1959) but with the use of isotopically labelled barbiturates scission of the heterocyclic molecule has been demonstrated to occur, to a minor extent. The scission of the ring system is probably a hydrolytic process and occurs at the 1,6-position to give substituted malonylurea derivatives.

Amobarbital labelled with ^{15}N is metabolized in dogs to give as much as 10% of the dose as urea and other ring scission products (Maynert and Van Dyke, 1950*b*), and 2-^{14}C-pentobarbital in dogs similarly gives some 2–3% as urea (Titus and Weiss, 1955). Hexobarbital would also appear to undergo scission for it is metabolized in the rabbit to yield traces of cyclohexenyl methylacetyl-N'-methylurea (0.5% dose) (Tsukamoto *et al.*, 1958), and secobarbital is metabolized by rabbits to give an unidentified scission product (Tsukamoto *et al.*, 1963*a*). With the thiobarbiturates, thiopental is metabolized in rats to give 3% of the dose as thiourea (Taylor *et al.*, 1952), and thialbarbital in rabbits is metabolized to give 0.5–2% as thiourea and another neutral substance (Raventos, 1954).

Scission of the barbiturate ring does not appear to occur to any significant extent in the metabolism of barbital or phenobarbital. With 2-^{14}C-barbital, no ^{14}CO$_2$ was detected in the expired air of rats dosed with the barbiturate (Goldschmidt and Wehr, 1957), although this finding would not unequivocally exclude ring scission. With 2-^{14}C-phenobarbital administered to rats, isotopically labelled compounds such as urea or oxaluric or parabanic acid, which would be expected to be formed if ring scission occurred, were not detected in the urine (Glasson and Benakis, 1961).

Hexobarbital — Substituted malonylurea — CycloHexenyl-methylacetyl-N'-methyl urea

Thiopental — Substituted malonylthiourea — Substituted malonic acid

QUANTITATIVE ASPECTS OF THE METABOLISM OF BARBITURATES

BARBITAL
(Veronal; 5,5-diethylbarbituric acid)

In man and other mammals this long-acting barbiturate is excreted almost entirely unchanged in the urine over a period of several days. In chickens and turtles excretion is very much slower and the drug may be retained in the tissues for several weeks. Although it had been previously assumed that barbital was not metabolized, it has been shown with ^{14}C-barbital that metabolism does occur to a slight extent, and that this results in the hydroxylation, or in the elimination, of one of the ethyl substituent groups. Following administration to rats, 95% of the dose of ^{14}C-barbital is excreted in the urine unchanged, but hydroxy-barbital (5-ethyl-5β-hydroxyethylbarbituric acid) (0.8% of the dose) and its glucuro-nide conjugate (2%) together with 5-ethylbarbituric acid (2.5%) are also excreted in trace amounts (Goldschmidt and Wehr, 1957). No ^{14}CO$_2$ was detected in the expired air, from which it may be inferred that the barbituric acid ring in barbital is quite stable. Other workers (Ebert *et al.*, 1964) have shown that the total excretion of metabolites of ^{14}C-barbital in normal rats is 3.7% of dose, but that this increases to

Barbital	Hydroxybarbital	5-Ethylbarbituric acid

6.1% in barbital-tolerant rats, indicating that barbital, like so many other barbiturates, stimulates its own metabolism. It has been suggested that 5-ethyl-5-vinylbarbituric acid is an intermediate in the metabolism of barbital since 2-^{14}C-(5-ethyl-5-vinylbarbit-uric acid) is metabolized in the rat to hydroxybarbital and 5-ethylbarbituric acid, but this occurs to only a minor extent.

Pentobarbital
(Nembutal; 5-ethyl-5-(1′-methylbutyl)barbituric acid)

The major metabolites of pentobarbital in dog and man are the two optical isomers of 5-ethyl-5-(3′-hydroxy-1′-methylbutyl)barbituric acid (hydroxypentobarbital or pentobarbital alcohol). Both isomers have been isolated from the urine of dogs treated with pentobarbital (Maynert and Dawson, 1952; Titus and Weiss, 1955), and from the urine of human subjects (Maynert, 1965a). Using 2-^{14}C-pentobarbital, Titus and Weiss (1955) have shown that more than 70% of a dose of pentobarbital administered to dogs is excreted in the urine as the optical isomers of hydroxypentobarbital. A num-ber of other metabolites were detected, including a small amount (4–5%) of pento-barbital carboxylic acid(5-ethyl-5-(3′-carboxy-1′-methylpropyl) barbituric acid) traces (1%) of the unchanged drug, and a small amount of urea (2–3%) which results from the scission of the barbiturate ring. Pentobarbital carboxylic acid, together with hydroxypentobarbital, was also identified, by paper chromatography, in the urine of human subjects dosed with pentobarbital (Frey *et al.*, 1959).

Pentobarbital is more rapidly metabolized in the dog than in man (Brodie *et al.*, 1953), and the ratios of the two stereo-isomeric alcohol metabolites formed in the two species differ (Maynert, 1965a). Using ^{15}N-labelled pentobarbital, it has been shown that with human subjects 40–50% of a 500-mg dose was excreted in the urine in the first 2 days with 83% in 4 days. Hydroxypentobarbital accounted for 21% of the dose in 2 days and 40% in 4 days, and the ratio of the levorotatory alcohol to the dextro-

rotatory alcohol was 5:4. The remainder of the isotopic material present in the urine (about 40% of the dose) was not identified but could possibly be accounted for as glucuronide conjugates of the alcohols, together with ketopentobarbitone and carboxylic acid derivatives. Only a trace amount (1% of dose) was excreted in the urine as urea plus ammonia. With dogs, 80–85% of a 50 mg/kg dose of ^{15}N-pentobarbital was excreted in the urine in 24 hours, 40–55% of the dose being present as hydroxypentobarbital, with a ratio of the l-isomer to d-isomer of 2:3 (Maynert, 1965a).

Using a quantitative method for the determination of metabolites of pentobarbital, based on paper chromatography, it has been shown that pentobarbital is metabolized by rat liver homogenates into the l- and d-isomers of hydroxypentobarbital, which are produced in the ratio of approximately 3:1. A minor metabolite, which it is suggested is the corresponding ketone, is also produced. The isomers of hydroxypentobarbital are formed by enzymes of the hepatic microsomal fraction in the presence of NADPH$_2$ and O$_2$, and the ketopentobarbital is formed from the l-alcohol, but not the d-isomer, by the soluble fraction of the liver in the presence of NAD (Kuntzman et al., 1967).

AMOBARBITAL

(amylobarbitone; Amytal; 5-ethyl-5-isopentylbarbituric acid)

The major metabolite of amobarbital is the tertiary alcohol 5-ethyl-5-(3'-hydroxy-3'-methylbutyl)barbituric acid (hydroxyamobarbital), and in the dog some 65% of a dose of amobarbital appears in the urine as this metabolite (Maynert and Van Dyke, 1950b; Maynert et al., 1952). In a study in mice, rats, rabbits, guinea-pigs, and one human subject (a suicidal attempt with high dosage of amobarbital), only hydroxyamobarbital and other metabolites were shown to be present in the urine, and no unchanged drug was detected even during the first few hours after dosage (Irrgang, 1965). The author concluded from these experiments that amobarbital is very rapidly metabolized and in consequence has only a very short initial hypnotic action of its own; the continued pharmacological activity being due to the metabolite, hydroxyamobarbital, which, it was suggested, had weaker but more prolonged hypnotic activity than the parent drug. Subsequently, Frey and Magnussen (1966) showed that in dog and man there is no evidence that amobarbital is very rapidly metabolized, nor that hydroxyamobarbital has hypnotic activity; unchanged amobarbital was still present in the serum of dogs 24 hours after oral administration, and was detected in the urine of dogs and human subjects for several days after oral dosage. Two human male subjects who each received a 500 mg dose of ^{15}N-labelled amobarbital, excreted a total of 70% and 100% of the dose (51% and 73% respectively was ether-extractable) in the urine over 5 days; both excreted 51% of the dose as hydroxyamobarbital, and this accounted for all the ether-soluble material present in the urine of one subject,

Amobarbital   Hydroxyamobarbital

but only 70% of the ether-soluble material of the second subject (Maynert, 1965a).

Using ^{15}N-labelled amobarbital, it has been shown that the barbiturate ring may undergo scission and (in dogs) some 10% of the dose is metabolized into urea and other products (Maynert and Van Dyke, 1950b).

HEXETHAL
(Ortal; 5-ethyl-5-hexylbarbituric acid)

In a study of the metabolic fate of hexethal in dogs ten different metabolites, equivalent to 53% of the dose, were isolated from the urine by counter-current distribution of ethereal extracts (Maynert, 1965b). Four of these compounds were reasonably fully identified, three others were shown to be hydroxylated derivatives, and the remaining three were shown to be a ketone, an ester, and a hydroxy acid. With all of the metabolites it was generally assumed that it was the hexyl side chain that had undergone chemical change. No unchanged hexethal was isolated from the urine and only traces (about 1 % of dose) of glucuronide conjugates were excreted.

The identities of the metabolites and the amounts of each present in the urine are shown in Table 1, and tentative pathways for metabolism are given below:

TABLE I

Metabolites of Hexethal excreted in dog urine (from Maynert, 1965*b*).

Metabolite	Modified hexyl side chain	Yield* (% dose)
A. 5-ethyl-5-(5′-ketohexyl) barbituric acid	$-CH_2CH_2CH_2CH_2COCH_2$	9.1 (7–11)
B. 5-ethyl-5-(5′-hydroxyhexyl) barbituric acid	$-CH_2CH_2CH_2CH_2CHOHCH_3$	14.9 (14–16)
C. 5-ethyl-5-(5′-carboxyamyl) barbituric acid	$-CH_2CH_2CH_2CH_2CH_2COOH$	3.8 (3.–4)
D. 5-ethyl-5-(3′-carboxypropyl) barbituric acid	$-CH_2CH_2CH_2COOH$	15.7 (14–18)
E. a hydroxy acid	$-(C_4H_8)$ (CHOH) (COOH)	2.0 (1.3–2.6)
F. 5-ethyl-5-(3′- or 4′-ketohexyl) barbituric acid	$-CH_2CH_2COCH_2CH_2CH_3$ or $-CH_2CH_2CH_2COCH_2CH_3$	2.3 (2.0–2.8)
G. an alcohol		2.2 (1.6–2.5)
H. an alcohol		1.6 (1.5–2.8)
I. an ester		0.7 (0.4–1.0)
J. an alcohol		0.7 (0.6–0.8)

* The mean and the range (in parentheses) of 4 animals.

PHENOBARBITAL
(Luminal; 5-ethyl-5-phenylbarbituric acid)

The major pathway for the metabolism and deactivation of phenobarbital is the oxidation of the aromatic ring to give p-hydroxyphenobarbital (5-ethyl-5(4'-hydroxyphenyl)barbituric acid). This is the main metabolite in dog and man and has been found, together with the unchanged drug, in the urines of humans poisoned with phenobarbital (Curry, 1955; Algeri and McBay, 1956). In dogs it is excreted in the urine almost entirely as a conjugate with glucuronic acid (Butler, 1954). In man it is only partly conjugated but the conjugate is the sulphate and not the glucuronide (Butler, 1956). This metabolite of phenobarbital is formed only slowly, for after a single dose of phenobarbital (300 mg) to human subjects the unchanged drug and the metabolite, p-hydroxyphenobarbital, were detectable in the urine for a period of 2–4 weeks after dosage (Frey et al., 1959). Metabolites other than p-hydroxyphenobarbital may also be formed, for Cochin and Daly (1963), using a thin-layer chromatographic technique to examine the urine of patients dosed with phenobarbital, detected another metabolite, but this was not identified.

When 2-^{14}C-phenobarbital was administered intravenously (90 mg/kg) to rats, 45% of the dose was excreted in the urine in 24 hours and 7 radioactive metabolites were detected (Glasson and Benakis, 1961). These comprised unchanged phenobarbital (13% of the dose), p-hydroxyphenobarbital (9%) and its glucuronide (12%), and possibly o-hydroxyphenobarbital (1%), together with a trace of another conjugate of a hydroxyphenobarbital. Two other metabolites (a total of 9%), one being a conjugate of the other, remained unidentified but were shown not to be parabanic acid,

Phenobarbital   p-Hydroxyphenobarbital   o-Hydroxyphenobarbital

oxaluric acid, or urea, which are possible metabolites if the barbiturate ring were to undergo scission. When 2-^{14}C-phenobarbital was administered intravenously to rabbits, most of the radioactivity was excreted in the urine as the glucuronide conjugate of p-hydroxyphenobarbital, only a trace occurred as free p-hydroxyphenobarbital, but 40% of the dose was present as unchanged phenobarbital (Fujimoto et al., 1968).

PRIMACLONE

(Primidone; Mysoline; 5-ethyl-dihydro-5-phenyl-4, 6(2H,5H)-pyrimidinedione)

This is a derivative, not of barbituric acid, but of the 2-deoxy analogue, 4,6(2H, 5H)-pyrimidinedione, which may be prepared by the electrolytic reduction of phenobarbitone. In both dog and man this anti-convulsant drug, which is used in the treatment of epilepsy, is converted partly into its oxidation product, phenobarbital, and is excreted in the urine as unchanged primidone, phenobarbital, and p-hydroxypheno-

Ethylphenylmalondiamide

barbital. The extent of the oxidation in man is approximately 15% of the dose, but in the dog it is only 5% (Butler and Waddell, 1956; Plaa *et al.*, 1958). Primidone also undergoes scission of the pyrimidine ring to give ethylphenylmalondiamide (Thorp, 1955; Swineyard *et al.*, 1954).

A recent study of the metabolism of primidone in rabbits has shown that the major metabolite, in this species at least, is the ring scission product, ethylphenylmalondiamide (Fujimoto *et al.*, 1968). Using thin-layer chromatography techniques, these workers have shown that after an oral dose of primidone (400 mg/kg) rabbits excrete in their urine unchanged primidone (20% of dose), ethylphenylmalondiamide (48%), phenobarbital (4%), and *p*-hydroxyphenobarbital and its glucuronide (about 6%). Further evidence that the scission of the hexahydropyrimidine ring occurs more readily than its oxidation to a barbituric acid is shown by the periods of maximum excretion of these two metabolites, for the highest excretion of ethylphenylmalondiamide occurs at 25–40 hours after dosing whereas that of phenobarbital does not occur until 40–56 hours afterwards (Fujimoto *et al.*, 1968).

CYCLOBARBITAL
(Cyclodorm; Phanodorn; 5-(1′-cyclohexen-1′-yl)-5-ethylbarbituric acid)

Cyclobarbital is metabolized by rabbits, and rabbit liver homogenates, to a cyclohexenone derivative, ketocyclobarbital (5-ethyl-5-(3′-oxo-1′-*cyclo*hexenyl)barbituric acid), which is pharmacologically inactive (Tsukamoto *et al.*, 1955). In the rabbit, 44% of a dose (0.1–0.2 g/kg) is excreted in the urine as ketocyclobarbital in 1–2 days and none of the drug is excreted unchanged. There is evidence that, in rabbits, ketocyclobarbital undergoes further metabolism to a considerable extent (Tsukamoto *et al.*, 1955). In man, metabolism of cyclobarbital is perhaps not as extensive as in the rabbit and 18–22% of a dose of cyclobarbital is excreted in the urine as ketocyclobarbital together with 2–7% as the unchanged drug (Fretwurst *et al.*, 1932). Meta-

Cyclobarbital   Ketocyclobarbital

bolism in man is slow, for ketocyclobarbital has been detected in human urine even 5 or 6 days after a dose of cyclobarbital (Frey *et al.*, 1959).

SECOBARBITAL
(Seconal; 5-allyl-5-(1′-methylbutyl)barbituric acid)

Very little work has been published on quantitative aspects of the metabolism of secobarbital. The first studies on the metabolism of this barbiturate were carried out by Tsukamoto *et al.* (1963*a*), who showed that rabbits metabolized secobarbital by ω- and (ω-1)-oxidation, with the latter predominating. Hydroxysecobarbital (5-allyl-5-[3′-hydroxy-1′-methylbutyl]barbituric acid), the major product, and secobarbital acid (5-allyl-5-[3′-carboxy-1′-methylpropyl]barbituric acid) were isolated from the urine, which was shown also to contain unchanged secobarbital and an unidentified ring-scission product. Further work has shown that the major metabolites of seco-barbital in man and dog are the two diastereoisomers of hydroxysecobarbital, and secodiol (5-[2′,3′-dihydroxypropyl]-5-[1′-methylbutyl]barbituric acid), which have been isolated from human urine to account for about 50% of the dose (Waddell, 1962, 1963 and 1965). Only 5% of the dose of secobarbital was excreted unchanged by human subjects (Waddell, 1965).

A fourth metabolite, 5-(1′-methylbutyl)barbituric acid, and also 5-hydroxy-5-(1′-methylbutyl)barbituric acid, which is formed by the spontaneous atmospheric oxida-tion of 5-(1′methylbutyl)barbituric acid, were also found in the urine of human patients (Cochin and Daly, 1963). These substances could be formed by the removal of the allyl group and, although it has been suggested that they may be artefacts present as impurities in the original secobarbital (Bush and Sanders, 1967), a similar allyl-substituted heterocyclic compound, diallylmelamine, has been shown to undergo metabolic de-allylation and di-hydroxylation of the allyl group (Zins, 1965).

When secobarbital was incubated with rat liver microsomal preparations, the two diastereoisomers of hydroxysecobarbital were formed in the same relative proportions as were found in rat urine (Waddell, 1965). Using a gas chromatographic technique for the identification of metabolites, Ide *et al.*, (1967) have shown that, on incubation with the 9000 g supernatant fraction of rabbit liver, secobarbital is metabolized by (ω-1)-oxidation to hydroxysecobarbital and by ω-oxidation to secobarbital acid. The oxygenation to (ω-1)-hydroxysecobarbital is catalysed by $NADPH_2$-dependent micro-somal enzymes, which do not, however, give rise to the formation of ω-hydroxyseco-barbital, the probable intermediate in the formation of secobarbital acid. (ω-1)- and ω-hydroxysecobarbital are oxidized to ketosecobarbital and secobarbital acid respectively by the soluble fraction of rabbit liver (100,000 g supernatant) in the presence of either NAD or NADP. In these *in vitro* studies of the metabolism of secobarbital by rat liver the allyl group was found to remain unchanged in all of the metabolites (Ide *et al.*, 1967). Nevertheless, secodiol has been shown to be present as a metabolite of secobarbital in intact rats (Niyogi, 1964).

METHOHEXITAL
(Brevital; 5-allyl-1-methyl-5(1′-methyl-2′,3′-pentynyl)barbituric acid)

Of the three likely sites of metabolism in this short-acting anaesthetic, namely the N^1-methyl group, and the two C^5-substituents, it is the 5-methylpentynyl substituent which is most readily attacked. When (1-methyl-^{14}C)-methohexital was injected into rats, 83% of the radioactivity was excreted in the faeces and 19% in the urine in 48 hours, whereas with dogs 30% was excreted in the faeces and 60% in the urine (Welles *et al.*, 1963). In the rat there is rapid biliary excretion of the drug, for more than 50% of the radioactivity is excreted in the bile in one hour, with a total of 78% in 24 hours. The major metabolite present in the urines of rats and dogs, and probably also the major product excreted in the bile, was shown to be hydroxymethohexital (1-methyl-5-allyl-5-[4′-hydroxy-1′-methyl-2′,3′-pentynyl]barbituric acid). The deme-

Methohexital   Hydroxymethohexital

thylation of methohexital is only a minor pathway of metabolism (about 1% of dose) in both the rat and the dog (Welles *et al.*, 1963).

HEXOBARBITAL

(Evipal; Cyclonal; 5-(1′-*cyclo*hexen-1′-yl)-1,5-dimethylbarbituric acid)

This barbiturate is metabolized by oxidation of the cyclohexenyl ring, by N-deme-thylation and, to a minor extent, by ring scission. In the dog, four metabolites were isolated from the urine: 3′-ketohexobarbital (1% of the dose); another isomeric ketohexobarbital, possibly 6-ketohexobarbital (0.5%); the N-demethylated products norhexobarbital (0.2%); and 3′-ketonorhexobarbital (5%). Only 0.2% of the dose was excreted in the urine unchanged (Bush *et al.*, 1953). In rabbits, the metabolites present in the urine were found to be 3′-hydroxyhexobarbital (16% dose), 3′-ketohexobarbital (4.5%), 3′-ketonorhexobarbital (5%), and a ring scission product, *cyclo*hexenylmethyl-N′-methylacetylurea (0.5%) (Tsukamoto *et al.*, 1958). In man, ketohexobarbital, nor-hexobarbital, and ketonorhexobarbital have been demonstrated by paper chromato-graphy of the urine from subjects taking hexobarbital (Frey *et al.*, 1959). From the work of Bush *et al.* (1953), it has been concluded that hexobarbital in the dog is not directly demethylated to any extent, but that the relatively large amount of ketonor-hexobarbital isolated from the urine is produced by demethylation of 3′-ketohexo-barbital. Oxidation to ketohexobarbital also precedes demethylation in the meta-bolism of hexobarbital in rats and rabbits.

Hexobarbital   3′-Hydroxyhexobarbital   3′-Ketohexobarbital

*cyclo*Hexenylmethyl-acetyl-N′-methylurea   3′-Hydroxynorhexobarbital   3′-Ketonor hexobarbital

The hydroxylation of hexobarbital to 3'-hydroxyhexobarbital by rabbit liver has been shown to be catalysed by an $NADPH_2$-dependent microsomal enzyme system, and the oxidation to 3'-ketohexobarbital is effected by a soluble liver enzyme (Toki et al., 1963). Both hydroxy- and keto-hexobarbital are demethylated more rapidly than is hexobarbital in vitro (Okui and Kuroiwa, 1963).

THIOPENTAL
(Pentothal; 5-ethyl-5-(1'-methylbutyl)-2-thiobarbituric acid)

Thiopental is the 2-sulphur analogue of pentobarbital and is only slowly metabolized, at a rate of about 15% per hour in man, 10% per hour in rat, and even more slowly in dog (Brodie et al., 1950, 1951). Contrary to previous belief, it has now been shown that metabolism of thiopental is of major importance in the rapid reduction of circulating levels of the drug, and consequently it plays a considerable role in limiting the duration of action of thiopental. In man, it is almost completely metabolized, by oxidation of the 5-substituent, to give thiopentalcarboxylic acid (5-ethyl-5-(3'-carboxy-1'-methylpropyl)thiobarbituric acid), and, to a lesser extent, by desulphuration to give pentobarbital and its metabolites, all of which are excreted in the urine. Only traces of the drug (0.3% dose in 24 hours) are excreted unchanged. This metabolism of thiopental has been shown to occur in the liver, at the rate of about 17 µg/g liver/hr in vitro (Mark et al., 1965). Although the major metabolite in man is thiopentalcarboxylic acid, which accounts for 10–25% for the dose, this appears to be only a minor metabolite in the dog (Brodie et al., 1950). With rabbit liver homogenates the major metabolite is again thiopentalcarboxylic acid, but a small amount of a (ω-1)-hydroxylated product, hydroxythiopental (5-ethyl-5-(3'-hydroxy-1'-methylpropyl)thiobarbituric acid, is also formed (Cooper and Brodie, 1957).

The desulphuration of ^{35}S-thiopental has been studied in rats, and over four days nearly 90% of the isotope is excreted in the urine, with some 27% as inorganic sulphate, 8% as sulphate esters, and 3% as thiourea (Taylor *et al.*, 1952). Thiopental is also largely desulphurated by rat liver homogenates to give pentobarbital and its metabolites (Winters *et al.*, 1955). The desulphuration of thiopental is, however, a minor pathway of metabolism in man (Bush *et al.*, 1961), and Furano and Greene (1963), using a gas-chromatographic method, were unable to detect pentobarbital in human blood 15 minutes after administration of thiopental; but in view of the slow rate of metabolism of thiopental, and the minor role of the desulphuration pathway in man, this is not surprising.

It has been suggested that the desulphuration of thiopental may occur spontaneously during the extraction of urine if ether is used, but other workers using different solvents have shown that desulphuration is also a biological reaction (Frey *et al.*, 1961).

THIAMYLAL

(thioseconal; Surital; 5-allyl-5-(1'-methylbutyl)-2-thiobarbituric acid)

As with other thiobarbiturates, thiamylal is metabolized by simultaneous desulphuration and oxidation of the 5-alkyl substituents. A study of the metabolic fate in rabbits, using ethyl acetate extraction of the urine to avoid spontaneous desulphuration, has resulted in the isolation and characterization of six compounds from the urine (Tsukamoto *et al.*, 1963*b*). These six products, which together accounted for only 13% of the dose of thiamylal, were identified as: 5-allyl-5-(3'-carboxy-1'-methylpropyl)-2-thiobarbituric acid (carboxythiamylal) (8% of the dose); 5-allyl-5-(3'-hydroxy-1'-methylbutyl)-2-thiobarbituric acid (hydroxythiamylal) (0.2%); unchanged thiamylal (4%); and the desulphurated products – secobarbital (1%); carboxysecobarbital (0.1%); and hydroxysecobarbital (0.01%). When the major metabolite, car-

Thiamylal   ω-1 and (ω-1)- oxidation   Hydroxythiamylal   Carboxythiamylal

desulphuration

Secobarbital   ω-and (ω-1)- oxidation   Hydroxysecobarbital   Carboxysecobarbital boxythiamylal, was re-administered to a rabbit it was excreted unchanged in the urine and was re-isolated, in 64% yield, together with only a trace of the desulphurated analogue (Tsukamoto *et al.*, 1963*b*).

THIALBARBITAL
(Intranarcon; Kemithal; 5-allyl-5-(2'-cyclohexen-1'-yl)-2-thiobarbituric acid)

Thialbarbital is metabolized by desulphuration to give the 2-oxygen analogue, 5-allyl-5-(2'-cyclohexenyl)barbituric acid, and by oxidation to give ketothialbarbital, which was presumed to be 5-allyl-5-(4'-oxo-2'-cyclohexenyl)-2-thiobarbituric acid. On administration to rabbits, thialbarbital is slowly excreted in the urine as a mixture of the unchanged thiobarbiturate (2% of dose was isolated), the desulphurated product (allylcyclohexenyl barbituric acid) (2.7% isolated), ketothialbarbital, and ring scission products such as thiourea (0.5–2% isolated) (Raventos, 1954; Carrington and Raventos, 1946).

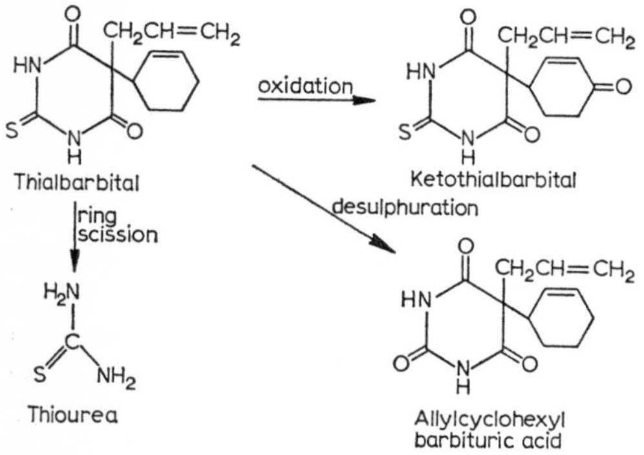

Thialbarbital — oxidation → Ketothialbarbital — desulphuration → Allylcyclohexyl barbituric acid; ring scission → Thiourea

RATES OF METABOLISM AND DURATION OF ACTION OF BARBITURATES

Barbiturates vary considerably in the duration of their hypnotic or anaesthetic activities (see Table 2) and have been classified on the basis of these differences into four groups (Williams, 1959):

1.   Long duration of action (8–12 hours), *e.g.*, barbital, phenobarbital, allobarbital.
2.   Moderate duration of action (2–8 hours), *e.g.*, amobarbital, pentobarbital, cyclobarbital, hexethal.
3.   Short duration of action (1–4 hours), *e.g.*, secobarbital, methylbarbital.
4.   Ultra-short-acting (5–30 minutes), *e.g.*, hexobarbital, methohexital and the thiobarbiturates.

The duration of action of barbiturates of Groups 1–3 is largely dependent on the rate of metabolic deactivation of the barbiturate and on the rate of its excretion in the urine. With the ultra-short-acting, Group 4, duration of action is determined by metabolic deactivation and, in the case of the thiobarbiturates at least, by sequestration into the depot fat, thus effectively removing much of the drug from the circulation, preventing its pharmacological action, and delaying its metabolic deactivation. From the list of plasma half-life periods of various barbiturates in man, given in Table 2, it may be seen that the thiobarbiturates generally have a much shorter half-life ($t_{0.5}$) than the corresponding oxybarbiturates. For example, for thiopental, $t_{0.5} = 8$ hr, whereas for the oxygen analogue, pentobarbital, $t_{0.5} = 1.8$ day; and methitural, which has a methylthioethyl group at C-5 in place of the ethyl group of thiopental, has a plasma half-life period even shorter than that of thiopental, with $t_{0.5} = 3$ hr. Similarly, a methyl group at N-1 shortens the plasma half-life period, and methohexital ($t_{0.5} = 3.5$ hr) and hexobarbital ($t_{0.5} = 5$ hr) have much shorter periods of activity than secobarbital ($t_{0.5} = 1.2$ day) and cyclobarbital ($t_{0.5} = 1.5$ day) which have similar C-5 substituents but no N-methyl group. Furthermore, N-methylbarbital has a much shorter plasma half-life than barbital and is much more quickly metabolized.

TABLE 2

Half-life periods of barbiturates in human plasma

Barbiturate		Plasma half-life period	Reference
Phenobarbital	(Group 1)*	3.4 day	Brilmayer and Loennecken, 1962
Allobarbital		2.0 day	Lous, 1954
Pentobarbital	(Group 2)*	1.8 day	Fazekas et al., 1956
Cyclobarbital		1.5 day	Brilmayer and Loennecken, 1962
Secobarbital	(Group 3)*	1.2 day	Fazekas et al., 1956
Thiopental		8 hr	Brodie, 1952
Thialbarbital		7 hr	Brodie, 1952
Hexobarbital	(Group 4)*	5 hr	Brodie, 1952
Methohexital		3.5 hr	Brand et al., 1963
Methitural		3 hr	Brand et al., 1959

* The grouping according to Williams, 1959.

LOCATION OF BARBITURATE-METABOLIZING ENZYMES

The enzymes which catalyse the oxygenation of the C-5 side chains, to form alcohols and phenols, are located in the microsomal fraction of liver homogenates, require reduced nicotinamide adenine dinucleotide phosphate ($NADPH_2$) and molecular oxygen for activity, and are inhibited by carbon monoxide. They are therefore typical of the mixed function oxidase activities that have been associated with the cytochrome P-450 of the hepatic endoplasmic reticulum. The components of this oxygenating (hydroxylating) system are $NADPH_2$, the phospholipid-protohaeme-sulphide-protein complex–cytochrome P-450, and a linking electron transport system containing cyto-chrome P-450 reductase and probably $NADPH_2$-cytochrome reductase. The mechan-ism of oxygenation of a drug is postulated as follows:

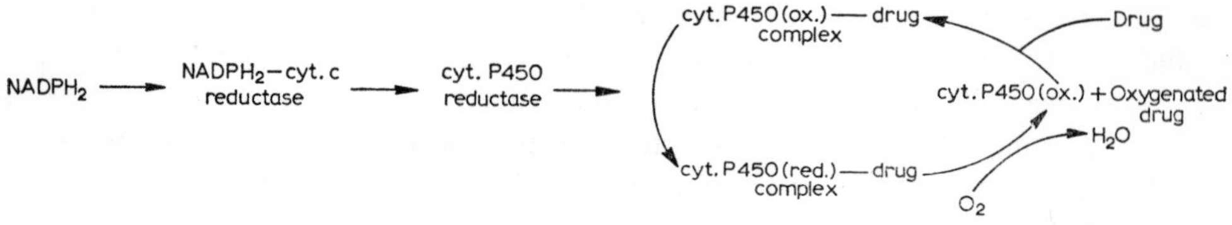

The same enzyme system is probably also responsible for the demethylation of N-1 methyl groups, the desulphuration of the 2-sulphur atoms, and the sulphoxidation of thioether groups:

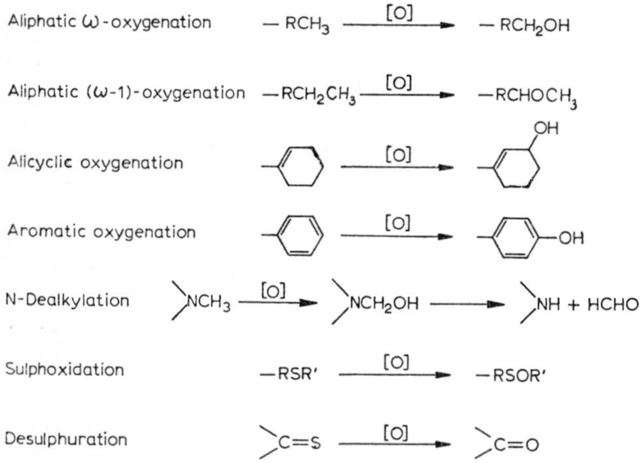

The subsequent oxidation of the C-5 alcohol substituents to carboxylic acids and ketones is catalysed by enzymes of the soluble fraction (100,000 g supernatant) of liver homogenates, which require either NAD or NADP as co-enzyme. The enzymic mechanisms of the oxidative metabolism of C-5 substituents have been studied with hexobarbital (Toki *et al.*, 1963), pentobarbital (Kuntzman *et al.*, 1967), and seco-barbital (Ide *et al.*, 1967). The carboxylic acids formed by oxidation of C-5 substi-tuents may be further metabolized by β-oxidation, *e.g.*, hexethal is metabolized first to the 5'-carboxyamyl derivative and then to the 3'-carboxypropyl derivative, and presumably these enzymes would be mitochondrial in origin.

The nature and location of the enzymes involved in the scission of the barbiturate ring have not been studied, and it has not been ascertained that they are even mammalian enzymes. This hydrolytic scission could, of course, be due to enzymes of the gastrointestinal microflora acting upon orally-administered barbiturates before absorption, or upon metabolites of orally or parenterally administered barbiturates that are excreted in the bile.

A number of metabolites of barbiturates are excreted as glucuronide conjugates. The enzymes, glucuronyl transferases, which effect these particular conjugations with glucuronic acid have not been especially studied, but it would be expected that, like other glucuronyl transferase activity, this would be located in the endoplasmic reticulum of the liver.

FACTORS AFFECTING METABOLISM OF BARBITURATES

Many factors are known to affect the metabolism of barbiturates and other drugs, and these have been shown to include the following (Parke, 1968b):

Genetic factors: species and strain differences;

Physiological factors: age, diet, hormones, sex, pregnancy, intestinal microflora, and disease;

Pharmacodynamic factors: tissue distribution and body composition, binding to plasma proteins, competitive inhibition of the biotransformation, and excretion by other drugs;

Environmental factors: induction and inhibition of drug-metabolizing enzymes by anutrients of the environment, e.g., dietary anutrients, food additives, pesticides, carbon monoxide, and by stress.

GENETIC FACTORS

It is well known that the hepatic drug-metabolizing enzymes in different animal species may catalyse the same biotransformation reactions at markedly different rates. The rates of metabolism of hexobarbital by microsomal preparations from rats, rabbits, and mice vary considerably with the period of incubation, and indicate that the enzyme is less stable in the rat liver preparation, although the cytochrome P-450 content remains constant (see Table 3; Gram and Fouts, 1966).

Differences in the hexobarbital-induced sleeping times of different strains of mice have been described (Jay, 1955), and differences in the rates of metabolism of hexobarbital have been demonstrated in different strains both of rats (Furner et al., 1969) and rabbits (Cram et al., 1965a). The basal levels of metabolism of hexobarbital in rabbits (see Table 4) range from 20 μmole/g microsomal nitrogen/hour for Cottontail rabbits to 250 for Californian and New Zealand rabbits, but after pretreatment with phenobarbital are approximately of the same order of activity. The variation in the metabolism of hexobarbital is not necessarily paralleled by a similar variation in the metabolism of other drugs.

TABLE 3

Species differences in rates of metabolism of hexobarbital (from Gram and Fouts, 1966)

Species	Hexobarbital metabolism by liver 9000 xg supernatant μmole metabolized/g N in:			
	15 min	30 min	60 min	90 min
Rat	75	95	125	125
Mouse	30	75	150	210
Rabbit	40	75	170	230

TABLE 4

Metabolism of hexobarbital by different strains of rabbits (from Cram et al., 1965a).

Strain of rabbit	Rate of metabolism of hexobarbital *in vitro* μmole/g hepatic microsomal N/hr	
	Basal levels	Phenobarbital induced
California	250	490
Dutch	140	330
English	170	340
New Zealand	250	520
Wild Jacks	220	540
Cottontails	20	490

The effects of genetics, sex, age and pretreatment with drugs on the metabolism of hexobarbital by rats are shown in Table 5, and it is readily apparent that there is an interdependence of these factors which makes it difficult to formulate generalities for

TABLE 5

Metabolism of hexobarbital by different strains of rats (from Furner et al., 1969a).

Strain of rat	Sex	Rate of metabolism of hexobarbital *in vitro* (μmole/g liver/15 min)			
		30-day-old		100-day-old	
		Basal	Phenobarbital-induced	Basal	Phenobarbital-induced
Holtzman	M	0.8	2.1	0.9	2.4
	F	0.2	1.5	0.5	1.2
Long Evans	M	1.0	2.6	1.3	3.4
	F	0.9	2.2	0.3	2.2
Sprague-Dawley	M	1.0	2.0	1.4	2.3
	F	0.5	2.1	0.4	1.6
Wistar	M	0.8	2.3	1.9	2.4
	F	0.5	2.0	1.0	2.2

any one factor in isolation from the others. The increase in the rate of the basal metabolism of hexobarbital with increase of age, which is exhibited by the Wistar strain (see also Table 8) and has often been assumed to be of general application, is not exhibited to the same extent by the other strains, and actually decreases in female rats of the Long Evans strain. Moreover, this difference in the Wistar rats largely disappears after phenobarbital pretreatment. The sex difference, which results in male rats metabolizing drugs at a much faster rate than females, can also be seen to be dependent on age and genetic strain, and is annulled or greatly reduced by phenobarbital pretreatment.

PHYSIOLOGICAL FACTORS

Although there is considerable interdependence of the factors which affect drug metabolism, generalities concerning certain factors do have validity. This is true of the development of these enzymes with the age of the animal. Newborn animals and humans metabolize barbiturates less readily than adults and consequently barbiturates are more toxic to the neonates. For example, the oral LD_{50} of phenobarbital for adult rats is 320 mg/kg but for 1–3-day-old rats is only 120 mg/kg (Yeary et al., 1966). On the other hand, the effects of the nutrition of the animal seem to be highly interdependent on species, strain, sex, and the nature of the drug, for in the rat, hexobarbital, but not all drugs, is metabolized faster by the male than by the female. After starvation of the male rat the metabolism of barbiturates, and other drugs which show sex dependence, is impaired, whereas the metabolism of drugs which show no sex dependence is enhanced; in contrast, the metabolism of all drugs by female rat liver is enhanced by starvation (Kato and Gillette, 1965).

The effect of sex on the metabolism of barbiturates is well known in rats, but has not been similarly observed in other species, save perhaps mice. The oxidative metabolism of hexobarbital and phenobarbital is generally much greater in male than in female rats, and consequently the hypnotic effect for the same level of dose is much less in the male animals. The difference becomes manifest only at puberty and is abolished by castration. Administration of testosterone to female rats results in an increase of the metabolism of hexobarbital to a level comparable with that of male animals, and administration of estrogens to male animals brings about the opposite effect (Quinn et al., 1958). Androgens also enhance drug metabolism in mice and administration of 19-nortestosterone derivatives (anabolic) to male mice has been shown to increase the hepatic microsomal metabolism of hexobarbital, although testosterone and methyltestosterone (androgenic) have the opposite effect (Novick et al., 1966). It is likely that in both rats and mice the stimulation of the drug-metabolizing enzymes and the metabolism of barbiturates is due to the anabolic activity rather than to the androgenic activity of the male steroid hormones.

The metabolism of barbiturates may also be affected by estrogenic and progestational steroids. Chronic administration of the progestogen norethynodrel has been shown to enhance the hepatic microsomal metabolism of hexobarbital, whereas chronic administration of progesterone has no significant effect and chronic administration of norethynodrel plus the estrogen, mestranol (Enovid), inhibits hexobarbital metabolism (Juchau and Fouts, 1966). The progestogen lynestrenol, when administered to mice 48 hours before dosage with barbiturates, accelerates the elimination of phenobarbital from the plasma, slightly increases the hepatic microsomal metabolism of hexobarbital, and reduces the hexobarbital sleeping time (Rümke and Noordhoek, 1969). Lynestrol has also been shown to reduce, and mestranol to increase, the sleeping times of phenobarbital and hexobarbital in female and male mice, but neither steroids have any effect on the sleeping time of barbital, a barbiturate which is not greatly metabolized (Blackham and Spencer, 1969).

The pituitary-adrenal system has a regulatory function in the control of drug metabolism. Adrenalectomy generally reduces the ability of rats to metabolize barbiturates but normal activity is restored by prednisolone or cortisone (Remmer, 1958). Moreover, the durations of pharmacological activity of pentobarbital and hexobarbital have been shown to be reduced in stressed animals. The duration of activity of barbitone, whose action is terminated more by excretion than metabolism, is unaffected by stress (Driever and Bousquet, 1965). This stimulation of the metabolism of barbiturates was not observed if the stressed animals were adrenalectomized or hypophysectomized.

Administration of thyroxine to male rats decreases the rate of hexobarbital metabolism by 50%, but in female rats increases the metabolism by a similar amount. Thyroidectomy reduces the rate of hexobarbital metabolism in rats of both sexes but this is restored in only the female rats by administration of triodothyronine (Kato and Takahashi, 1968).

Liver disease, such as obstructive jaundice, results in a decreased rate of metabolism of hexobarbital and other drugs, and leads to a prolongation of hexobarbital sleeping time (McLuen and Fouts, 1961). It has also been suggested that the functional state of the reticulo-endothelial system may affect the duration of action of barbiturates. Stimulation of this system in mice by zymosan increased the sleeping times of hexobarbital, pentobarbital, and barbital by approximately 100%. This is unlikely to be due to impaired metabolism and may be the result of inactivation of corticosterone by the stimulated reticuloendothelial system (Wooles and Borzelleca, 1966).

INDUCTION OF BARBITURATE METABOLISM

The activities of the hepatic drug-metabolizing enzymes have been shown to be markedly increased as the result of pretreatment of animals with a wide variety of chemicals including drugs, polycyclic hydrocarbons, pesticides, food additives, naturally-occurring anutrients of the diet, and steroids (Conney, 1967). As a result of this increased enzyme activity, the rates of biotransformation of barbiturates and, of course, other drugs, are substantially increased. Since the pharmacological activities of barbiturates are generally removed by biotransformation, the intensities and durations of their pharmacological activities are correspondingly reduced.

Inducers of the drug-metabolizing enzymes fall into several different categories according to their mode of action and the nature of the enzymes that are induced. For example, although the hydroxylation of hexobarbital and phenobarbital is increased by pretreatment with phenobarbital and other barbiturates and drugs, it is not similarly increased by carcinogenic polycyclic hydrocarbons, although these compounds do increase the aromatic hydroxylation of acetanilide and zoxazolamine, the 0-dealkylation of phenacetin, and many other pathways of drug metabolism (Conney, 1967). Moreover, the individual inductive effects of phenobarbital and carcinogenic polycyclic hydrocarbons, such as 3-methylcholanthrene, are additive when animals are pretreated with both of these compounds (Gillette, 1963a).

Pretreatment of an animal with a drug or other inducing agent usually results in the activation of those particular enzymes that are concerned in the metabolism of that compound, and this may be considered as substrate-induction of these enzymes. It would therefore be expected that any drug that was also an enzyme inducer would, on repeated administration, lead to a progressive increase in its own metabolism and, where that metabolism resulted in deactivation, would consequently lead to a progressive loss of intensity and duration of pharmacological activity. Therefore on repeated administration tolerance to the drug becomes manifest and it is necessary to administer progressively larger doses to obtain the same pharmacological response. This phenomenon of drug tolerance due to the stimulation by drugs of their own metabolic deactivation has been widely studied in barbiturates and has been observed for example with hexobarbital, pentobarbital, and phenobarbital in rats, rabbits, and dogs (Remmer, 1962, 1964b; Remmer and Siegert, 1962, 1964; Ernster and Orrenius, 1965). However, tolerance to barbital is not attributed to enzyme induction since this barbiturate is not metabolized to any appreciable extent.

The list of drugs which are known to accelerate the rate of metabolic deactivation of barbiturates is very extensive and quite independent of the nature of their pharmacological activity. Hypnotics (barbiturates, glutethimide), tranquillizers (meprobamate), muscle relaxants (carisoprodol), anticonvulsants (diphenylhydantoin), anaesthetics (nitrous oxide), antipsychotics (chlorpromazine), central nervous system stimulants (nikethamide), hypoglycaemic agents (tolbutamide), anti-inflammatory agents (phenylbutazone), antihistamines (chlorcyclizine), and alkaloids (nicotine) are but a few among the wide range of drugs that have been shown to induce the hepatic drug-metabolizing enzymes which metabolize barbiturates. Nevertheless, not all drugs possess this ability to potentiate the metabolism of barbiturates, and substances such as aspirin, amphetamine, sulphanilamide, and thalidomide are quite devoid of such activity, while morphine and certain related alkaloids actually lead to a decrease in the rate of metabolism. In these extensive studies of the enzyme-inductive effects of drugs the rates of metabolism of barbiturates, particularly hexobarbital, have been widely used as standard tests for the evaluation of the induction.

The metabolism of barbiturates is also markedly stimulated by the chlorinated hydrocarbon insecticides. The metabolism of hexobarbital in rats, and in primates such as the squirrel monkey, has been shown to be increased by pretreatment with DDT (Hart and Fouts, 1963; Juchau *et al.*, 1966), or chlordane (Hart *et al.*, 1963; Cram *et al.*, 1965*b*). Oxidation of hexobarbital is also increased by pretreatment with benzene hexachloride, and a reduction of the normal narcotic effect of this barbiturate was observed to last for a period of two weeks after pretreatment of rats with the γ-isomer, for four weeks after the α-isomer, and for eight weeks following the β-isomer (Koransky *et al.*, 1964*b*). The metabolism of hexobarbital and phenobarbital by rats is also increased by pretreatment with *o, p'*-DDD (2,2-(*o*-chlorophenyl, *p*-chlorophenyl)-1, 1-dichloroethane) (Kupfer and Peets, 1966; Straw *et al.*, 1965). On the other hand, certain organophosphate insecticides appear to have more of an inhibitory effect on the metabolism of hexobarbital (Welch *et al.*, 1959).

Carcinogenic polycyclic hydrocarbons such as 3-methylcholanthrene and 3,4-benzpyrene, which stimulate the metabolism of many drugs, particularly those which involve aromatic hydroxylation, do not appear to enhance the metabolism of barbiturates such as hexobarbital and pentobarbital, which are metabolized by aliphatic oxygenation, or N-methylbarbital, which is metabolized by N-demethylation (Conney, 1967). Furthermore, pretreatment of rats with the carcinogen N-hydroxy-N-2-fluorenylacetamide results in an increase of the narcosis produced by pentobarbital, the result no doubt of the hepatocellular damage caused by the carcinogen and a reduction in the activity of the drug-metabolizing enzymes (Weisburger *et al.*, 1965).

INHIBITION OF BARBITURATE METABOLISM

The metabolism of barbiturates is inhibited by the simultaneous administration of other drugs, steroids and anutrient chemicals which compete with the barbiturates for the same drug-metabolizing enzymes. Subsequent to this initial phase of competitive inhibition there may follow, usually after an interval of 12 hours or so, a period of increased metabolic activity due to the induction of the drug-metabolizing enzymes. Inhibition and induction are therefore often relative terms determined by the time interval between pretreatment of the animal with other drugs and the administration of the barbiturate (see Fig. 1). With potent inhibitors of the drug-metabolizing enzymes, like SKF 525A (2-diethylaminoethyl 2,2-diphenylvalerate hydrochloride) and chlorcyclizine, reversal of the inhibition of the enzymes metabolizing pentobarbital occurs after about 12 hours, but with potent enzyme-inducing agents like glutethimide reversal occurs after a shorter period (Kato *et al.*, 1964). A similar biphasic pattern of inhibition followed by stimulation is seen in the metabolism of hexobarbital by liver homogenates from rats pretreated with SKF 525-A (Rogers *et al.*, 1963).

The inhibitory effects of the secondary and primary amine analogues of SKF 525-A (tertiary amine) on the rate of metabolism of hexobarbital in the intact rat and in the isolated perfused rat liver have also been studied. When hexobarbital was administered to rats 45 minutes after the SKF inhibitors, all three compounds prolonged the sleeping times to similar extents, but when administered 5 hours after the inhibitors the sleeping times were less and decreased in the order tertiary amine (SKF 525-A) > secondary amine > primary amine, suggesting that the N-dealkylation of SKF 525-A competes with hexobarbital side-chain oxygenation for the same enzyme system (Stitzel et al., 1966).

Microsomal N-demethylation and C-oxygenation have been shown to be reversibly inhibited in rat liver by the administration of ethanol (Schüppel, 1969) which would therefore be expected to inhibit the metabolism of barbiturates and give rise to a potentiation of their pharmacological activity, a view supported by the observations of Wiberg et al., (1969).

THE INDUCTION OF ENZYMES BY BARBITURATES

The ability of various drugs and foreign compounds to induce marked increases in activity of the drug-metabolizing enzymes is now well known (Conney, 1967), and although the list of such compounds is extensive the drug most often used as the model inducing-agent is phenobarbital. Many other barbiturates also manifest this property and barbital, cyclobarbital, hexobarbital, heptobarbital, pentobarbital, phenobarbital, and thiopental have all been shown to increase the activities of these hepatic enzymes and to diminish markedly the pharmacological effects of barbiturates, anticoagulants and other drugs (Mark, 1963). The inductive effect appears to be a property of the barbiturate molecule and not of its metabolites, for p-hydroxyphenobarbital, the major metabolite of phenobarbital, does not exhibit any significant induction of the drug-metabolizing enzymes (Minegishi et al., 1968).

Most of the known pathways of drug metabolism have been shown to be stimulated by pretreatment with phenobarbital (see Table 6), but of the hepatic enzymes concerned in the metabolism of nutrients only glucose-6-phosphate dehydrogenase is similarly stimulated (see Table 7). This induction of the hepatic drug-metabolizing enzymes is an example of substrate-induction of an enzyme system, and one might therefore expect all lipid-soluble compounds which are metabolized by these particular microsomal enzymes to be inducers. Furthermore, the enzyme system which is responsible for the oxygenation of drugs and anutrients is unusual in that it is able to catalyse the metabolism of a vast number of different compounds, yet it exhibits a high degree of specificity for both the substrate and the nature of the reaction catalysed. Such specificity for a diversity of substrates and reactions could result from substrate-induced changes in the conformation of the enzyme protein or in its configurational relationship with respect to its prosthetic group or its membrane environment, which would effect suitable modification of the active site. Induction of such an enzyme

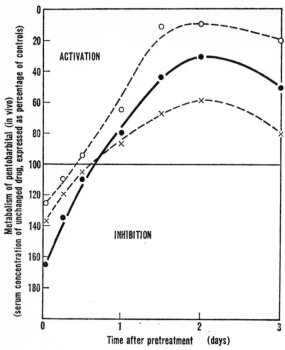

Fig. 1. Activation and inhibition of the metabolism of pentobarbital by pretreatment with foreign compounds. Pentobarbital (20 mg/kg) was administered intraperitoneally to female rats at various time intervals after pretreatment with a single dose of glutethimide (40 mg/kg) o---o, SKF 525A (50 mg/kg) ●—●, or chlorcyclizine (25 mg/kg) x---x. The serum concentrations of pentobarbital were determined 1 hour later (Kato *et al.*, (1964).

TABLE 6

Pathways of drug metabolism stimulated by phenobarbital

Metabolic pathway	Substrate metabolized	Reference
Aromatic oxygenation	Aniline	Kato and Takanaka (1968)
	3,4-Benzpyrene	Conney *et al.* (1960)
	Biphenyl	Creaven and Parke (1966)
	Ethylaniline	Lange (1967)
	Methylaniline	Uehleke and Greim (1968)
	Warfarin	Ikeda *et al.* (1968)
	Zoxazolamine	Conney *et al.* (1960)
Aliphatic oxygenation	Androgens	Conney and Klutch (1963)
	Cortisol	Burnstein (1968)
	Carisoprodol	Kato and Takayanaghi (1966)
	Ethylbenzene	McMahon and Sullivan (1966)
	Hexobarbital	Conney *et al.* (1960)
	Meprobamate	Kato *et al.* (1964)
	Pentobarbital	Conney *et al.* (1961)
	Trichloroethylene	Leibman and McAllister (1967)

Metabolic pathway	Substrate metabolized	Reference
N-oxygenation	Aniline	Lange (1967)
	4-Aminobiphenyl	Uehleke and Greim (1968)
	4-Chloroaniline	Uehleke (1967)
	2-Naphthylamine	Uehleke (1968)
	4-Phenetidine	Uehleke (1969)
S-oxygenation	Chlorpromazine	Rubin *et al.* (1964)
O-dealkylation	Alkoxybiphenyls	Davies and Creaven (1967)
	Methoxyflurane	Van Dyke (1966)
	2-Nitroanisole	Uehleke (1967)
	4-Nitroanisole	Netter and Seidel (1964)
	Phenacetin	Gillette (1963*b*)
N-dealkylation	Amidopyrine	Conney *et al.* (1960)
	Butynamine	Kato and Takayanaghi (1966)
	Diphenhydramine	Kato and Takayanaghi (1966)
	Meperidine	Remmer and Alsleben (1958)
	Methylaniline	Uehleke and Greim (1968)
	Methylbarbital	Henderson and Mazel (1964)
	3-Methyl-4-monoethyl-aminoazo-benzene	Conney *et al.* (1960)
	Morphine	Kato and Takayanaghi (1966)
Desulphuration	Parathion	Alary and Brodeur (1969)
Dehalogenation	Methoxyflurane	Van Dyke (1966)
	Halothane	Van Dyke (1966)
	Thyroxine	Schwartz *et al.* (1969)
Nitro reduction	p-Nitrobenzoic acid	Cram *et al.* (1965*a*)
	Chloramphenicol	Remmer and Merker (1963)
Azo reduction	Neoprontosil	Kato and Takayanaghi (1966)
Hydrolysis	Procaine	Remmer and Merker (1963)
	Methyl butyrate	Brodeur (1967)
	Parathion	Alary and Brodeur (1969)
Glucuronide formation	Sulphadimethoxine	Remmer (1964*a*)
	Bilirubin	Yaffe *et al.* (1966)
	Salicylamide	Yaffe *et al.* (1966)
	p-Nitrophenol	Zeidenberg *et al.* (1967)

system, whether resulting from decreased degradation of enzyme protein or from increased synthesis, should consequently result in a stimulation of all of the diverse enzymic activities usually manifested by the enzyme. Hence, pretreatment with one substrate, phenobarbital, may result in the enhancement of a whole range of drug-metabolizing enzyme activities.

MODE OF ACTION

Stimulation of the hepatic microsomal drug-metabolizing enzymes occurs only as

TABLE 7

Effect of phenobarbital and barbital on rat liver enzymes (from Platt and Cockrill, 1967).

Enzyme	Percentage of control activity after pretreatment with:	
	Barbital	Phenobarbital
Glucose-6-phosphate dehydrogenase	147	161
6-Phosphogluconate dehydrogenase	95	133
Glutamate dehydrogenase	82	62
Lactate dehydrogenase	52	55
Phosphohexose isomerase	95	119
Glutamate-pyruvate transaminase	80	95
Glucose-6-phosphatase	91	68

the result of treating live animals with the inducing agent, and addition to enzyme preparations *in vitro* produces no effect. Induction occurs even after adrenalectomy, hypophysectomy, or thyroidectomy so that stimulation of the hypophyseal-adreno-cortical system, or of the thyroid, is not involved.

This stimulation of drug-metabolizing activity may be due to:

1. increased rate of synthesis of enzyme proteins by induction at either the nuclear or ribosomal levels.

2. decreased rate of degradation of enzyme proteins, or possibly RNA concerned in their biosynthesis.

3. increased rate of synthesis of co-enzymes such as $NADPH_2$.

4. alteration of the conformation or of the membrane environment of the enzymes.

The time interval between administration of the phenobarbital and the appearance of increased enzyme activities, a period of 12–24 hours, tends to exclude the possibility that the increased activities are due to *in vivo* changes in the conformation or environment of the enzyme. Furthermore, the increased activity resulting from phenobarbital pretreatment has been shown to be located in the microsomal fraction of the liver and is not due to stimulation of the $NADPH_2$–generating system that is present in the soluble fraction. Phenobarbital pretreatment gives rise to an increase in liver weight and a marked increase in microsomal protein, which results from both a decreased rate of breakdown and an increased rate of synthesis of microsomal protein (Shuster and Jick, 1966). Phenobarbital also induces an increase of cytochrome P-450 (Ernster and Orrenius, 1965), cytochrome P-450 reductase activity, and $NADPH_2$ – cytochrome c reductase activity (Jick and Shuster, 1966); it increases the rate of amino-acid incorporation, the messenger-RNA content, the number of microsomal binding sites for messenger-RNA (Kato *et al.*, 1966), and the DNA-dependent RNA-polymerase activity (Gelboin *et al.*, 1967). Other workers have shown that the chromatin is modified, increasing its ability to function as a template for RNA synthesis (Piper and Bousquet, 1968). These accumulated cytochemical data, together with the fact that the increased protein synthesis and much of the increased enzyme activity are abolished by actinomycin D, an inhibitor of messenger-RNA synthesis (Orrenius et al., 1965), support the hypothesis that stimulation of the synthesis of the microsomal enzymes, and a large proportion of the enhanced enzyme activity, is mediated through an activation of DNA-dependent RNA synthesis. Phenobarbital also increases the phospholipid content of the hepatic microsomal fraction, but this is attributed to a decreased rate of catabolism rather than to an increased rate of synthesis (Holtzman and Gillette, 1966).

In kinetic studies of the effects of phenobarbital induction it has been shown that with type I substrates (most drugs and anutrients) the V_{max} values are increased but the Michaelis constants (K_m) are not significantly changed (Rubin et al., 1964; Gram et al., 1968b). However with aniline, a type II substrate (amines and certain N-containing compounds which probably form ligand complexes with cytochrome P-450), both the K_m value and the binding constant (K_s) are increased by phenobarbital treatment (Guarino et al., 1969).

Phenobarbital, like chlordane and other drugs and insecticides, stimulates a variety of hepatic microsomal drug-metabolizing enzymes and causes a marked proliferation of the smooth-surfaced endoplasmic reticulum of the hepatic cell, whereas carcinogenic polycyclic hydrocarbons stimulate only a few drug-metabolizing enzymes and do not cause any pronounced increase in the smooth endoplasmic reticulum (Fouts and Rogers, 1965). The phenobarbital-induced increase in the content of phospholipid, microsomal protein, cytochrome P-450, as well as the increased activities of the $NADPH_2$–cytochrome c reductase and drug-metabolizing activity, have been correlated with the morphological changes of the endoplasmic reticulum (Staübli et al., 1969).

Phenobarbital and other substances that induce the drug-metabolizing enzymes and increase the size of the liver, such as α-benzene hexachloride, have been shown also to increase, in normal physiological proportions, the liver content of proteins, lipids, glycogen and water, and do not produce any hepatocellular damage. The content of DNA of the liver and the rate of incorporation of labelled thymidine into DNA are both increased, from which it has been concluded that phenobarbital initiates growth processes in the liver which are accompanied by de novo synthesis of DNA (Schlicht et al., 1968). Regenerating liver following partial hepatectomy, like the hepatic tissue of foetuses or neonates, is characterized by rapid proliferation of hepatocytes and low levels of activity of drug-metabolizing enzymes. In all of these cases the livers have the capacity to respond to the action of inducing agents like phenobarbital, producing increased activity of the drug-metabolizing enzyme systems and an increase in the content of cytochrome P-450 (Gram et al., 1968a).

Phenobarbital has also been shown to increase the cytochrome P-450 content and the activities of several oxidative drug-metabolizing enzymes in the kidney tissue of rabbits but not of rats (Uehleke and Greim, 1968).

When the pretreatment with phenobarbital, or other barbiturates or drugs, is terminated, regression of this enhanced enzymic activity occurs and the levels of enzyme proteins slowly return to normal. If, however, actinomycin D is administered at the termination of pretreatment, this regression of enzyme synthesis and enzymic activity does not immediately occur (Ernster and Orrenius, 1965).

EFFECT OF SEX, GENETICS AND AGE ON INDUCTION

The induction of the hepatic microsomal drug-metabolizing enzyme systems by phenobarbital and other drugs is a fundamental biochemical effect that has been shown to occur in many different animal species including rat, mouse, guinea pig, rabbit, dog, and man. The degree of response may however be quantitatively affected by sex, genetic characteristics, and the age of the animal. In a study of the pheno-barbital induction of hexobarbital metabolism carried out in different strains of rats (Furner *et al.*, 1969a), only modest differences in the magnitude of response to pheno-barbital were attributable directly to genetic variation, but much greater differences were observed to be due to sex (see Table 5). The rate of metabolism of hexobarbital was increased 2- to 7-fold in female rats, but only 1.5- to 3-fold in male rats, thereby considerably reducing the sex difference that is manifest in the unstimulated animals. The different magnitude of response to phenobarbital that may be obtained with different strains of a given species is perhaps better illustrated by the work of Cram *et al.* (1965a) with different strains of rabbits. These workers showed that phenobar-bital produces a stimulation of hexobarbital metabolism of 2.0- to 2.4-fold in Cali-fornia, Dutch, English, New Zealand and Wild Jack rabbits, but results in a 25-fold increase in Cottontail rabbits, which normally have a very low level of hexobarbital metabolism and are restored to a level comparable to other strains of rabbit by the phenobarbital treatment (see Table 4). The magnitude of response to phenobarbital

TABLE 8

Effect of phenobarbital pretreatment on some parameters of hepatic drug-metabolism in Wistar rats of different ages (from Kato and Takanaka, 1968).

Parameter	Phenobarbital-induced increase (%) Age of rats: (days)			
	40	100	300	600
Liver weight	24	11	9	4
Microsomal protein	23	12	8	6
NADPH$_2$ oxidase	180	84	46	20
NADPH$_2$-cytochrome c reductase	250	115	52	22
Cytochrome P-450	260	130	60	37
Amidopyrine N-demethylation	710	395	175	36
Hexobarbital hydroxylation	490	295	135	34
Aniline hydroxylation	165	94	40	31
p-Nitrobenzoic acid reduction	255	105	45	32

induction is markedly diminished with increasing age of the animal, and Kato and Takanaka (1968) have shown that the phenobarbital-induced increase in a number of enzyme parameters ranges from 4% to 37% for 600-day-old rats to 23% to 710% in 40-day-old animals (see Table 8). Treatment of pregnant rats and rabbits with phenobarbital during late pregnancy considerably stimulated the drug-metabolizing enzymes of the liver of the newborn animals (Pantuck et al., 1968).

INDUCTION OF OTHER ENZYME SYSTEMS

The NADPH$_2$-dependent microsomal oxygenases of the liver metabolize not only drugs and anutrient chemicals but also numerous other substrates of the body, e.g., fatty acids, cholesterol, steroid hormones, and thyroxine. Induction of these enzymes might therefore be expected to result in increased metabolism of these other substrates. The biosynthesis of cholesterol has been shown to be enhanced by pretreatment with phenobarbitone which results in an increase in the incorporation of ^{14}C-acetate into cholesterol but does not increase the incorporation of ^{14}C-mevalonate into cholesterol nor the plasma cholesterol levels (Mitoma et al., 1968). Pretreatment with phenobarbital also increases the microsomal hydroxylation of cortisol (Conney et al., 1965; Burstein et al., 1967), testosterone and Δ^4-androstene-3, 17-dione (Conney and Klutch, 1963) and estradiol (Levin et al., 1968); and N-phenylbarbital increases the hydroxylation of cortisol in man (Kuntzman et al., 1968). The administration of barbiturates may therefore lead to changes in the biosynthesis and degradation of cholesterol and in the steroid hormones, which could have considerable physiological consequences.

Phenobarbital treatment of rats also increases the microsomal deiodination of thyroxine, the hepatocellular binding of the hormone, and its biliary excretion (Schwartz et al., 1969). Similarly, the liver microsomal esterase activity of rat, but not the kidney esterase activity, is induced by pretreatment with phenobarbital (Schwark and Ecobichon, 1968).

Mitochondrial enzymes may also be induced, and phenobarbital increases the activity of the hepatic mitochondrial enzyme, δ-aminolevulinic acid synthetase, with a concomitant increase in porphyrin synthesis. The activity of this enzyme induced by phenobarbital does not however reach the high levels induced by allylisopropylacetamide, hexachlorobenzene, or griseofulvin, substances which are known to precipitate attacks of human hepatic porphyria (Wada et al., 1968). Enzymes involved in mitochondrial oxidations are also induced by pretreatment with phenobarbital but there is a characteristic 2-day lag period before this effect becomes manifest (Zeidenberg et al., 1967).

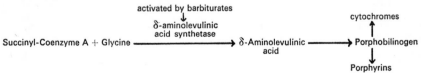

Barbiturates also increase het biosynthesis of ascorbic acid, which in rats leads to an increased excretion of ascorbic acid and glucuronic acid. This may be the result of an increase in activity of uridine diphosphate glucose (UDPG) dehydrogenase, an enzyme present in the cytoplasm of the liver cell, for pretreatment with phenobarbital has been shown to elicit an increase in the activity of rat liver UDPG dehydrogenase and also an increase in microsomal glucuronyl transferase activity (Zeidenberg *et al.*, 1967).

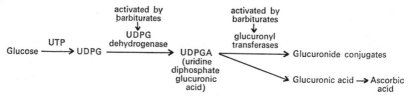

EFFECTS OF ENZYME INDUCTION ON PHARMACOLOGICAL ACTIVITY

The induction of the hepatic microsomal drug-metabolizing enzymes by pretreatment with barbiturates gives rise to an increased rate of metabolism of other drugs, pesticides, and toxic chemicals. When metabolism results in deactivation of the drug or chemical, enzyme induction will reduce the pharmacological or toxicological response, but where the opposite occurs (that is, metabolism gives rise to compounds of greater activity), enzyme induction will give rise to an increase in pharmacological activity or toxicity.

As examples of the former case, phenobarbital and other barbiturates are known to increase the metabolism and decrease the toxicity of the following: strychnine (Kato *et al.*, 1962), parathion (Alary and Brodeur, 1969), malathion (Brodeur, 1967), benzene hexachloride (Koransky *et al.*, 1964a), phenacetin and paracetamol (Büch *et al.*, 1967), and bishydroxycoumarin (Lucas, 1967). Phenobarbital stimulates the hydroxylation of warfarin in the 6-, 7- and 8-positions of the aromatic ring, decreasing its therapeutic anticoagulant effect in man (Ikeda *et al.*, 1968); heptabarbital (Aggeler and O'Reilly, 1969) and phenobarbital (Cucinell *et al.*, 1965) produce similar effects with bishydroxycoumarin (Dicumarol). The volatile anaesthetics, trichloroethylene (Leibman and McAllister, 1967), halothane and methoxyflurane (Van Dyke, 1966) are similarly more rapidly metabolized and deactivated after phenobarbital treatment. With the combination of phenobarbital and diphenylhydantoin used in the treatment of epilepsy, chronic administration causes the phenobarbital to accelerate the metabolism of the diphenylhydantoin and as a consequence reduces its anticonvulsant effect (Cucinell *et al.*, 1964).

Examples of barbiturate treatment resulting in increased toxicity through increased metabolism include the greater susceptibility to the hepatotoxic effects of carbon tetrachloride (Garner and McLean, 1969), the increased toxicity of acetylsalicylic acid (Coldwell and Solomonraj, 1968), and the increased toxicity of Schradan and a number of other organophosphate insecticides (Vardanis, 1966), as the result of phenobarbital treatment. Phenobarbital also enhances the activity of the microsomal oxyge-nase, which brings about N-oxygenation, and increases the N-hydroxylation of the carcinogens 2-naphthylamine (Uehleke and Brill, 1968) and 4-aminobiphenyl (Uehe-leke and Nestel, 1967), with a possible increase in carcinogenic activity. It also en-hances the N-hydroxylation of p-phenetidine, a minor metabolite of phenacetin, and consequently increases the tendency of this compound to convert haemoglobin into methaemoglobin, with the increased possibilities of haemolysis and cyanosis resulting from the metabolism of phenacetin (Uehleke, 1969).

THERAPEUTIC USAGE OF BARBITURATE INDUCTION

Pretreatment of rats with phenobarbital increases the glucuronyl transferase activity of liver slices and increases their capacity to conjugate bilirubin (Adlard et al., 1969). This particular enzymic induction has been utilized therapeutically in the treatment of adults and infants suffering from congenital, non-haemolytic, unconjugated hyper-bilirubinaemia. Administration of phenobarbital to these subjects resulted in a marked decrease in the serum bilirubin concentration and in the bilirubin half-life period (Crigler and Gold, 1969; Kreek and Sleisenger, 1968).

No doubt these profound effects that barbiturates have upon the activities of the drug-metabolizing enzymes will lead to the innovation of further applications in therapeutics.

REFERENCES

ADLARD, B. P. F., LESTER, R. G. and LATHE, G. H. (1969), The effect of phenobarbitone treatment of rats and of protein deprivation on the capacity of liver slices to conjugate bilirubin. *Biochem. Pharma-col.*, 18, 59.

AGGELER, P. M. and O'REILLY, R. A. (1969), Effect of heptabarbital on the response to bishydroxy-coumarin in man. *J. Lab. clin. Med.*, 74, 229.

ALARY, J. G. and BRODEUR, J. (1969), Studies on the mechanism of phenobarbital-induced protection against parathion in adult female rats. *J. Pharmacol. exp. Ther.*, 169, 159.

ALGERI, E. J. and McBAY, A. J. (1956), Metabolite of phenobarbital in human urine. *Science*, 123, 183.

BLACKHAM, A. and SPENCER, P. S. J. (1969), The effects of oestrogens and progestins on the response of mice to barbiturates. *Brit. J. Pharmacol.*, 37, 129.

BRAND, L., MARK, L. C., BURNS, J. J., DAYTON, P. G., TALLER, D. and PAPPER, E. M. (1959), Physio-logical disposition of methitural in man. *Med. exp. (Basel)*, 1, 339.

BRAND, L., MARK, L. C., SNELL, M. Mc. M., VRINDTEN, P. and DAYTON, P. G. (1963), Physiologic disposition of methohexital in man. *Anesthesiology*, 24, 331.

BRILMAYER, H. and LOENNECKEN, S. J. (1962), Die Eliminationsgeschwindigkeit von Barbiturat aus dem Blut akut intoxizierter Patienten. *Arch. int. Pharmacodyn.*, 136, 137.

BRODEUR, J. (1967), Studies on the mechanism of phenobarbital-induced protection against malathion and EPN. *Canad. J. Physiol.*, 45, 1061.

BRODIE, B. B., MARK, L. C., PAPPER, E. M., LIEF, P. A., BERNSTEIN, E. and ROVENSTEIN, E. A. (1950), The fate of thiopental in man and a method for its estimation in biological material. *J. Pharmacol. exp. Ther.*, 98, 85.

BRODIE, B. B., MARK, C. C., LIEF, P. A., BERNSTEIN, E. and PAPPER, E. M. (1951), Acute tolerance to thiopental. *J. Pharmacol. exp. Ther.*, 102, 215.

BRODIE, B. B. (1952), Physiological disposition and chemical fate of thiobarbiturates in the body. *Fed. Proc.*, 11, 632.

BRODIE, B. B., BURNS, J. J., MARK, L. C., LIEF, P. A., BERNSTEIN, E. and PAPPER, E. M. (1953), The fate of pentobarbital in man and dog and a method for its estimation in biological material. *J. Pharmacol. exp. Ther.*, 109, 26.

BRODIE, B. B., AXELROD, J., COOPER, J. R., GAUDETTE, L., LADU, B. N., MITOMA, C. and UDENFRIEND, S. (1955), Detoxication of drugs and other foreign compounds by liver microsomes. *Science*, 121, 603.

BÜCH, H., GERHARDS, W., PFLEGER, K., RÜDIGER, W. and RUMMEL, W. (1967), Metabolische Umwandlung von Phenacetin und N-Acetyl-p-Aminophenol nach Vorbehandlung mit Phenobarbital. *Biochem. Pharmacol.*, 16, 1585.

BURNSTEIN, S. (1968), Determination of initial rates of cortisol 2α- and 6β-hydroxylation by hepatic microsomal preparations in guinea pigs: effect of phenobarbital in two genetic types. *Endocrinology*, 82, 547.

BURSTEIN, S., KIMBALL, H. L., KLAIBER, E. L. and GUT, M. (1967), Metabolism of 2α- and 6β-hydroxycortisol in man: determination of production rates of 6β-hydroxycortisol with and without phenobarbital administration. *J. clin. Endocr.*, 27, 491.

BUSH, M. T., BUTLER, T. C. and DICKINSON, H. L. (1953), The metabolic fate of 5-(1-cyclohexen-1-yl)-1,5-dimethylbarbituric acid (hexobarbital, Evipal) and of 5-(1-cyclohexen-1-yl)-5-methylbarbituric acid ('nor-Evipal'). *J. Pharmacol. exp. Ther.*, 108, 104.

BUSH, M. T., MAZEL, P. and CHAMBERS, J. (1961), The metabolic fate of thiobarbiturates: thiobarbital in man. *J. Pharmacol. exp. Ther.*, 134, 110.

BUSH, M. T. and PARRISH, H. (1963), Methylation of barbiturates *in vivo*. *Fed. Proc.*, 22, 480.

BUSH, M. T. and SANDERS, E. (1967), Metabolic fate of drugs: barbiturates and closely related compounds. *Ann. Rev. Pharmacol.*, 7, 57.

BUTLER, T. C. and BUSH, M. T. (1939), The metabolic fate of N-methyl-barbituric acids. *J. Pharmacol. exp. Ther.*, 65, 205.

BUTLER, T. C. (1952), Quantitative studies of the metabolic fate of mephobarbital (N-methyl phenobarbital). *J. Pharmacol. exp. Ther.*, 106, 235.

BUTLER, T. C., MAHAFFEE, D. and MAHAFFEE, C. (1952), The role of the liver in the metabolic disposition of mephobarbital. *J. Pharmacol. exp. Ther.*, 106, 364.

BUTLER, T. C. (1953), Further studies of metabolic removal of alkyl groups from nitrogen in barbituric acid derivatives. *Proc. Soc. exp. Biol. (N.Y.).*, 84, 105.

BUTLER, T. C. (1954), Metabolic oxidation of phenobarbital to p-hydroxyphenobarbital. *Science*, 120, 494.

BUTLER, T. C. (1956), The metabolic hydroxylation of phenobarbital. *J. Amer. pharm. Ass., sci. Ed.*, 116, 326.

BUTLER, T. C. and WADDELL, W. J. (1956), Metabolic conversion of primidone (Mysoline) to phenobarbital. *Proc. Soc. exp. Biol. (N.Y.)*, 93, 544.

CARRINGTON, H. C. and RAVENTOS, J. (1946), Kemithal, a new intravenous anaesthetic. *Brit. J. Pharmacol.*, 1, 215.

COCHIN, J. and DALY, J. W. (1963), The use of thin-layer chromatography for the analysis of drugs. II. Isolation and identification of barbiturates and non-bartiburate hypnotics from urine, blood, and tissue. *J. Pharmacol. exp. Ther.*, 139, 154.

COLDWELL, B. B. and SOLOMONRAJ, G. (1968), The effect of barbiturates on salicylate metabolism in the rat. *Clin. Toxicol.*, 1, 431.

CONNEY, A. H., DAVISON, C., GASTEL, R. and BURNS, J. J. (1960), Adaptive increases in drug-metabolizing enzymes induced by phenobarbital and other drugs. *J. Pharmacol. exp. Ther.*, 130, 1.

CONNEY, A. H., MICHAELSON, I. A. and BURNS, J. J. (1961), Stimulatory effect of chlorcyclizine on barbiturate metabolism. *J. Pharmacol. exp. Ther.*, 132, 202.

CONNEY, A. H. and KLUTCH, A. (1963), Increased activity of androgen hydroxylases in liver microsomes of rats pretreated with phenobarbital and other drugs. *J. biol. Chem.*, 238, 1611.

CONNEY, A. H., JACOBSON, M., SCHNEIDMAN, K. and KUNTZMAN, R. (1965), Induction of liver microsomal 6-β-hydroxylase by diphenylhydantoin or phenobarbital. An explanation for the increased excretion of 6-hydrocortisol in humans treated with these drugs. *Life Sci.*, 4, 1091.

CONNEY, A. H. (1967), Pharmacological implications of microsomal enzyme induction. *Pharmacol., Rev.*, 19, 317.

COOPER, J. R. and BRODIE, B. B. (1957), Enzymatic oxidation of pentobarbital and thiopental. *J. Pharmacol. exp. Ther.*, 120, 75.

CRAM, R. L., JUCHAU, M. R. and FOUTS, J. R. (1965a), Differences in hepatic drug metabolism in various rabbit strains before and after pretreatment with phenobarbital. *Proc. Soc. exp. Biol. (N.Y.)*, 118, 872.

CRAM, R. L., JUCHAU, M. R. and FOUTS, J. R. (1965b), Stimulation by chlordane of hepatic drug metabolism in the squirrel monkey. *J. Lab. clin. Med.*, 66, 906.

CREAVEN, P. J. and PARKE, D. V. (1966). The stimulation of hydroxylation by carcinogenic and non-carcinogenic compounds. *Biochem. Pharmacol.*, 15, 7.

CRIGLER, J. F. JR. and GOLD, N. I. (1969), Effect of sodium phenobarbital on bilirubin metabolism in an infant with congenital, non-haemolytic, unconjugated hyperbilirubinemia and kernicterus. *J. clin. Invest.*, 48, 42.

CUCINELL, S. A., KOSTER, R., CONNEY, A. H. and BURNS, J. J. (1964), Stimulatory effect of phenobarbital on the metabolism of diphenylhydantoin. *J. Pharmacol. exp. Ther.*, 141, 157.

CUCINELL, S. A., CONNEY, A. H., SANSUR, M. and BURNS, J. J. (1965), Drug interactions in man. I. Lowering effect of phenobarbital on plasma levels of bishydroxycoumarin (Dicumarol) and diphenyl-hydantoin (Dilantin). *Clin. Pharmacol. Ther.*, 6, 420.

CURRY, A. S. (1955), A note on a urinary metabolite of phenobarbitone. *J. Pharm. Pharmacol.*, 7, 1072.

DAVIES, W. H. and CREAVEN, P. J. (1967), The effect of carcinogenic and non-carcinogenic compounds on the O-dealkylating activity of the hepatic microsomal enzyme system of the rat. *Biochem. Pharmacol.*, 16, 1839.

DEININGER, R. (1956), Über Wirkungsänderungen der Barbitursäuren durch Beeinflussung der Methylierungsvorgänge am Stickstoff *in vivo. Naunyn-Schmiedeberg's Arch. exp. Path. Pharmak.*, 227, 316.

DIETZ, W. and SOEHRING, K. (1957), Experimentelle Beiträge zum Nachweiss von Thiobarbitursauren aus dem Harn mit Hilfe der Papierchromatographie. *Arch. Pharm. (Weinheim)*, 290, 80.

DORFMAN, A. and GOLDBAUM, L. R. (1947), Detoxication of barbiturates. *J. Pharmacol. exp. Ther.*, 90, 330.

DRIEVER, C. W. and BOUSQUET, W. F. (1965), Stress-drug interactions: evidence for rapid enzyme induction. *Life Sci.*, 4, 1449.

EBERT, A. G., YIM, G. K. W. and MIYA, T. S. (1964), Distribution and metabolism of barbital-^{14}C in tolerant and non-tolerant rats. *Biochem. Pharmacol.*, 13, 1267.

ERNSTER, L. and ORRENIUS, S. (1965), Substrate-induced synthesis of the hydroxylating enzyme system of liver microsomes. *Fed. Proc.*, 24, 1190.

FAZEKAS, J. F., GOLDBAUM, L. R., KOPPANYI, T. and SHEA, J. G. (1956), Study on the effect of over-doses of pentylenetetrazol and barbiturate combinations in human volunteers. *Amer. J. med. Sci.*, 231, 531.

FOUTS, J. R. and ROGERS, L. A. (1965), Morphological changes in the liver accompanying stimulation of microsomal drug metabolizing activity by phenobarbital, chlordane, benzpyrene or methylcholan-threne in rats. *J. Pharmacol. exp. Ther.*, 147, 112.

FRETWURST, F., HALBERKANN, J. and REICHE, F. (1932), Phanodorm und seine Wiederausscheidung mit dem Harn. *Münch. med. Wschr.*, 79, 1429.

FREY, H. H., SUDENDEY, F. and KRAUSE, D. (1959), Vergleichende Untersuchungen über Stoffwechsel, Ausscheidung und Nachweis von Schlafmitteln aus der Barbitursäure-Reihe. *Arzneimittel-Forsch.*, 9, 294.

FREY, H. H., DOENICKE, A. and JÄGER, G. (1961), Quantitative Bedeutung der Desulfurierung im Stoffwechsel von Thiobarbituraten. *Med. exp. (Basel)*, 4, 243.

FREY, H. H. and MAGNUSSEN, M. P. (1966), Contribution to the metabolism of amobarbital and the pharmacological significance of its main metabolite, 5-ethyl-5-(3-hydroxyisopentyl)barbituric acid. *Arzneimittel-Forsch.*, 16, 612.

FUJIMOTO, J. M., MASON, W. H. and MURPHY, M. (1968), Urinary excretion of primidone and its metabolites in rabbits. *J. Pharmacol. exp. Ther.*, 159, 379.

FURANO, E. S. and GREENE, N. M. (1963), Metabolic breakdown of thiopental in man determined by gas-chromatographic analysis of serum barbiturate levels. *Anesthesiology*, 24, 796.

FURNER, R. L., GRAM, T. E. and STITZEL, R. E. (1969a), Factors affecting the metabolism and response to hexobarbital. *Pharmacology*, 2, 181.

FURNER, R. L., McCARTHY, J. S., STITZEL, R. E. and ANDERS, M. W. (1969b), Stereoselective metabolism of the enantiomers of hexobarbital. *J. Pharmacol. exp. Ther.*, 169, 153.

GARNER, R. C. and McLEAN, A. E. M. (1969), Increased susceptibility to carbon tetrachloride poisoning in the rat after pretreatment with oral phenobarbitone. *Biochem. Pharmacol.*, 18, 645.

GELBOIN, H. V., WORTHAM, J. S. and WILSON, R. G. (1967), 3-Methylcholanthrene and phenobarbital stimulation of rat liver RNA polymerase. *Nature (Lond.)*, 214, 281.

GILLETTE, J. R. (1963a), Factors that affect the stimulation of the microsomal drug enzymes induced by foreign compounds. *Advanc. Enzyme Reg.*, 1, 215.

GILLETTE, J. R. (1963b), Metabolism of drugs and other foreign compounds by enzymatic mechanisms. *Prog. Drug Res.*, 6, 11.

GLASSON, B. and BENAKIS, A. (1961), Étude du phenobarbital C–14 dans l'organisme du rat. (2nd communication). *Helv. physiol. pharmacol. Acta*, 19, 323.

GOLDSCHMIDT, S. and WEHR, R. (1957), Ueber Barbiturate III. Mitteilung. Der Metabolisms von Veronal. *Hoppe-Seylers Z. physiol. Chem.*, 308, 9.

GOULD, T. C. and SHIDEMAN, F. E. (1952), The *in vitro* metabolism of thiopental by a fortified cell-free tissue preparation of the rat. *J. Pharmacol. exp. Ther.*, 104, 427.

GRAM, T. E. and FOUTS, J. L. (1966), Time course difference in the metabolism of drugs by hepatic microsomes from rats, rabbits, and mice. *J. Pharmacol. exp. Ther.*, 152, 363.

GRAM, T. E., GUARINO, A. M., GREENE, F. E., GIGON, P. L. and GILLETTE, J. R. (1968a), Effect of partial hepatectomy on the responsiveness of microsomal enzymes and cytochrome P-450 to phenobarbital or 3-methyl-cholanthrene. *Biochem. Pharmacol.*, 17, 1769.

GRAM, T. E., WILSON, J. T. and FOUTS, J. R. (1968b), Some characteristics of hepatic microsomal systems which metabolize aminopyrine in the rat and rabbit. *J. Pharmacol. exp. Ther.*, 159, 172.

GUARINO, A. M., GRAM, T. E., GIGON, P. L., GREENE, F. E. and GILLETTE, J. R. (1969), Changes in Michaelis and spectral constants for aniline in hepatic microsomes from phenobarbital-treated rats. *Molec. Pharmacol. (N.Y.)*, 5, 131.

HART, L. G. and FOUTS, J. R. (1963), Effects of acute and chronic DDT administration on hepatic microsomal drug metabolism in the rat. *Proc. Soc. exp. Biol. (N.Y.)*, 114, 388.

HART, L. G., SHULTICE, R. W. and FOUTS, J. R. (1963), Stimulatory effects of chlordane on hepatic microsomal drug metabolism in the rat. *Toxicol. appl. Pharmacol.*, 5, 371.

HENDERSON, J. F. and MAZEL, P. (1964), Studies of the induction of microsomal S-, N-, and O-demethylases. *Biochem. Pharmacol.*, 13, 1471.

HOLTZMAN, J. L. and GILLETTE, J. R. (1966), The effect of phenobarbital on the synthesis of microsomal phospholipid in female and male rats. *Biochem. biophys. Res. Commun.*, 24, 639.

IDE, H., YOSHIMURA, H. and TSUKAMOTO, H. (1967), Metabolism of drugs, LII. Enzymatic study on secobarbital metabolism. *Chem. pharm. Bull.*, 15, 411.

IKEDA, M., CONNEY, A. H. and BURNS, J. J. (1968), Stimulatory effect of phenobarbital and insecticides on warfarin metabolism in the rat. *J. Pharmacol. exp. Ther.*, 162, 338.

IRRGANG, K. (1965), Pharmacological investigation of 5-ethyl-5-(3-hydroxyisoamyl)-barbituric acid, a metabolite of 5-ethyl-5-isoamylbarbituric acid. *Arzneimittel-Forsch.*, 15, 688.

JAY, G. (1955), Variation in response of various mouse strains to hexobarbital (Evipal). *Proc. Soc. exp. Biol. (N.Y.)*, 90, 378.

JICK, H. and SHUSTER, L. (1966), The turnover of microsomal reduced nicotinamide adenine dinucleotide phosphate-cytochrome C reductase in the livers of mice treated with phenobarbital. *J. biol. Chem.*, 241, 5366.

JUCHAU, M. R. and FOUTS, J. R. (1966), Effects of norethynodrel and progesterone on hepatic microsomal drug-metabolizing enzyme systems. *Biochem. Pharmacol.*, 15, 891.

JUCHAU, M. R., GRAM, T. E. and FOUTS, J. R. (1966), Stimulation of hepatic microsomal drug-metabolizing enzyme systems in primates by DDT. *Gastroenterology*, 51, 213.

KATO, R., CHIESARA, E. and VASSANELLI, P. (1962), Increased activity of microsomal strychnine-metabolizing enzyme induced by phenobarbital and other drugs. *Biochem. Pharmacol.*, 11, 913.

KATO, R., CHIESARA, E. and VASSANELLI, P. (1964), Further studies on the inhibition and stimulation of microsomal drug-metabolizing enzymes of rat liver by various compounds. *Biochem. Pharmacol.*, 13, 69.

KATO, R. and GILLETTE, J. R. (1965), Effect of starvation on NADPH-dependent enzymes in liver microsomes of male and female rats. *J. Pharmacol. exp. Ther.*, 150, 279.

KATO, R. and TAKAYANAGHI, M. (1966), Differences among the action of phenobarbital, methylcholanthrene and male sex hormone on microsomal drug-metabolizing enzyme systems of rat liver. *Jap. J. Pharmacol.*, 16, 381.

KATO, R., JONDORF, W. R., LOEB, L. A., BEN, T. and GELBOIN, H. V. (1966), Studies on the mechanism of drug-induced microsomal enzyme activities. V. Phenobarbital stimulation of endogenous messenger RNA and polyuridylic-acid-directed L-(^{14}C)-phenylalanine incorporation. *Molec. Pharmacol. (N.Y.)*, 2, 171.

KATO, R. and TAKAHASHI, A. (1968), Thyroid hormone and activities of drug-metabolizing enzymes and electron transport systems of rat liver microsomes. *Molec. Pharmacol. (N.Y.)*, 4, 109.

KATO, R. and TAKANAKA, A. (1968), Effect of phenobarbital on electron transport system, oxidation and reduction of drugs in liver microsomes of rats of different age. *J. Biochem. (Tokyo)*, 63, 406.

KELLY, A. R. and SHIDEMAN, F. E. (1949), Liver as major organ involved in detoxification of thiopental by dog. *Fed. Proc.*, 8, 306.

KORANSKY, W., PORTIG, J., VOHLAND, H. W. and KLEMPAU, I. (1964a), Die Elimination von α- und γ-Hexachlorcyclohexan und ihre Beeinflussung durch Enzyme der Lebermikrosomen. *Naunyn-Schmiedeberg's Arch. exp. Path. Pharmak.*, 247, 49.

KORANSKY, W., PORTIG, J., VOHLAND, H. W. and KLEMPAU, I. (1964b), Aktivierung von Mikrosomenenzymen durch Hexachlorcyclohexan-Isomere. Ihr Einfluss auf die Scillirosidvergiftung der Ratte. *Naunyn-Schmiedeberg's Arch. exp. Path. Pharmak.*, 247, 61.

KREEK, M. J. and SLEISENGER, M. H. (1968), Reduction of serum-unconjugated-bilirubin with phenobarbitone in adult congenital non-haemolytic unconjugated hyperbilirubinaemia. *Lancet II*, 73.

KUNTZMAN, R., IKEDA, M., JACOBSON, M. and CONNEY, A. H. (1967), A sensitive method for the determination and isolation of pentobarbital-C^{14} metabolites and its application to *in vitro* studies of drug metabolism. *J. Pharmacol. exp. Ther.*, 157, 220.

KUNTZMAN, R., JACOBSON, M., LEVIN, W. and CONNEY, A. H. (1968), Stimulatory effect of N-phenylbarbital (phetharbital) on cortisol hydroxylation in man. *Biochem. Pharmacol.*, 17, 565.

KUPFER, D. and PEETS, L. (1966), The effect of o,p–DDD on cortisol and hexobarbital metabolism. *Biochem. Pharmac.*, 15, 573.

LANGE, G. (1967), Verschiedene Induktion der mikrosomalen N- und p- Hydroxylierung von Anilin und N-Äthylanilin bei Kaninchen. *Naunyn-Schmiedeberg's Arch. exp. Path. Pharmak.*, 257, 230.

LEIBMAN, K. C. and McALLISTER, W. J. JR. (1967), Metabolism of trichloroethylene in liver micro. somes. III. Induction of the enzymic activity and its effect on excretion of metabolites. *J. Pharmacol. exp. Ther.*, 157, 574.

LEVIN, W., WELCH, R. M. and CONNEY, A. H. (1968), Effect of phenobarbital and other drugs on the metabolism and uterotropic action of estradiol -17β and estrone. *J. Pharmacol. exp. Ther.*, 159, 362.

LOUS, P. (1954), Plasma levels and urinary excretion of three barbituric acids after oral administration to man. *Acta pharmacol. (Kbh.)*, 10, 147.

LUCAS, O. N. (1967), Study of the interaction of barbiturates and dicumarol and their effect upon prothrombin activity, haemorrhage, and sleeping time in rats. *Canad. J. Physiol.* 45, 905.

McLUEN, E. F. and FOUTS, J. R. (1961), The effect of obstructive jaundice on drug metabolism in rabbits. *J. Pharmacol. exp. Ther.*, 131, 7.

McMAHON, R. E. (1963), The demethylation *in vitro* of N-methyl barbiturates and related compounds by mammalian liver microsomes. *Biochem. Pharmacol.*, 12, 1225.

McMAHON, R. E. and SULLIVAN, H. R. (1966), Microsomal hydroxylation of ethylbenzene. Stereospecificity and the effect of phenobarbital induction. *Life Sci.*, 5, 921.

MARK, L. C. (1963), Metabolism of barbiturates in man. *Clin. Pharmacol. Ther.*, 4, 504.

MARK, L. C., BRAND, L., KAMVYSSI, S., BRITTON, R. C., PEREL, J. M., LANDRAU, M. A. and DAYTON, P. G. (1965), Thiopental metabolism by human liver *in vivo* and *in vitro*. *Nature (Lond.)*, 206, 1117.

MARTIN, S. J., HERRLICH, H. C. and CLARK, B. B. (1940), The effect of various tissues on the detoxication of Evipal in the dog. *Anesthesiology*, 1, 153.

MARTIN, H. F. and DRISCOLL, J. C. (1966), Gas-chromatographic identification and determination of barbiturates. *Analyt. Chem.*, 38, 345.

MAYNERT, E. W. and VAN DYKE, H. B. (1950a), The metabolic fate of pentobarbital. Isotope dilution experiments with urine after administration of labelled pentobarbital. *J. Pharmacol. exp. Ther.*, 98, 174.

MAYNERT, E. W. and VAN DYKE, H. B. (1950b), The metabolism of Amytal labelled with N^{15} in dogs. *J. Pharmacol. exp. Ther.*, 98, 180.

MAYNERT, E. W. and DAWSON, J. M. (1952), Ethyl(3-hydroxy-1-methylbutyl)barbituric acids as metabolites of pentobarbital. *J. biol. Chem.*, 195, 389.

MAYNERT, E. W., DAWSON, J. M. and WASHBURN, E. (1952), Ethyl(3-hydroxyisoamyl)barbituric acid as the principal metabolite of amytal. *J. biol. Chem.*, 195, 397.

MAYNERT, E. W. (1965a), The alcoholic metabolites of pentobarbital and amobarbital in man. *J. Pharmacol. exp. Ther.*, 150, 118.

MAYNERT, E. W. (1965b), On the specificity of penultimate oxidation. *J. Pharmacol. exp. Ther.*, 150, 476.

MAZEL, P. and HENDERSON, J. F. (1963), Enzymatic S-demethylation. *Pharmacologist*, 5, 241.

MAZEL, P., HENDERSON, J. F. and AXELROD, J. (1964), S-Demethylation by microsomal enzymes. *J. Pharmacol. exp. Ther.*, 143, 1.

MEYERS, F. H. and PEOPLES, D. (1954), The positive role of the liver in the rapid metabolism of thiopental. *Anesthesiology*, 15, 146.

MINEGISHI, K., KUROIWA, Y. and OKUI, S. (1968), Studies on the metabolic N-demethylation. VII. Effect of p-hydroxyphenobarbital on the oxidative demethylation in rat liver. *Chem. pharm. Bull.*, 16, 1829.

MITOMA, C., YASUDA, D., TAGGS, J. S., NEUBAUER, S. E., CALDERONI, F. J. and TANABE, M. (1968), Effects of various chemical agents on drug metabolism and cholesterol biosynthesis. *Biochem. Pharmacol.*, 17, 1377.

NETTER, K. J. and SEIDEL, G. (1964), An adaptively stimulated O-demethylating system in rat liver microsomes and its kinetic properties. *J. Pharmacol. exp. Ther.*, 146, 61.

NIELSEN, P. and TARDING, F. (1968), The metabolic fate of 5-(bicyclo-3,2,1-oct-2-en-2-yl)-5-ethyl barbituric acid (Reposal). *Acta pharmacol. (Kbh.)*, 26, 521.

NIYOGI, S. K. (1964), Detection of secobarbital metabolite in the urine of rat. *Nature (Lond.)*, 202, 1225.

NOVICK, W. J., STOHLER, C. M. and SWAGZDIS, J. (1966), The influence of steroids on drug metabolism in the mouse. *J. Pharmacol. exp. Ther.*, 151, 139.

OKUI, S. and KUROIWA, Y. (1963), Metabolic N-demethylation. II. Barbiturate-induced acceleration of N-methylbarbiturate metabolism. *Chem. pharm. Bull.*, 11, 163.

ORRENIUS, S., ERICSSON, J. L. E. and ERNSTER, L. (1965), Phenobarbital-induced synthesis of the microsomal drug-metabolizing enzyme system and its relationship to the proliferation of endoplasmic membranes: a morphological and biochemical study. *J. Cell Biol.*, 25, 627.

PANTUCK, E., CONNEY, A. H. and KUNTZMAN, R. (1968), Effect of phenobarbital on the metabolism of pentobarbital and meperidine in fetal rabbits and rats. *Biochem. Pharmacol.*, 17, 1441.

PARKE, D. V. (1968a), The metabolism of drugs. In: J. M. Robson and R. S. Stacey (Ed) *Recent Advances in Pharmacology*, 4th ed., 29. Churchill, London.

PARKE, D. V. (1968b), Factors which affect the metabolism of drugs. In: J. M. Robson and R. S. Stacey (Ed) *Recent Advances in Pharmacology*, 4th ed., 75. Churchill, London.

PIPER, W. N. and BOUSQUET, W. F. (1968), Phenobarbital and methylcholanthrene stimulation of rat liver chromatin template activity. *Biochem. biophys. Res. Commun.*, 33, 602.

PLAA, G. L., FUJIMOTO, J. M. and HINE, C. H. (1958), Intoxication from primidone due to its biotransformation to phenobarbitone. *J. Amer. med. Ass.*, 168, 1769.

PLATT, D. S. and COCKRILL, B. L. (1967), Liver enlargement and hepatoxicity: an investigation into the effects of several agents on rat liver enzyme activities. *Biochem. Pharmacol.*, 16, 2257.

PRATT, T. W., VANLANDINGHAM, H. W., TALLEY, E. E., NELSON, J. M. and JOHNSON, E. O. (1932), Studies of the liver function of dogs. *Amer. J. Physiol.*, 102, 148.

PRATT, T. W. (1933), A comparison of the action of phenobarbital (Nembutal) and sodium barbitain rabbits as related to the detoxicating powers of the liver. *J. Pharmacol. exp. Ther.*, 48, 285.

QUINN, G. P., AXELROD, J. and BRODIE, B. B. (1958), Species, strain, and sex differences in metabolism of hexobarbitone, amidopyrine, antipyrine, and aniline. *Biochem. Pharmacol.*, 1, 152.

RAVENTOS, J. (1954), The distribution in the body and metabolic fate of barbiturates. *J. Pharm. Pharmacol.*, 6, 217.

REMMER, H. (1958), Die Verstärkung der Abbaugeschwindigkeit von Evipan durch Glykocorticoide. *Naunyn-Schmiedeberg's Arch. exp. Path. Pharmak.*, 233, 184.

REMMER, H. and ALSLEBEN, B. (1958), Die Aktivierung der Entgiftung in den Lebermikrosomen während der Gewohnung. *Klin. Wschr.*, 36, 332.

REMMER, H. (1962), Drug tolerance. In: J. L. Mongar and A. V. S. De Reuck (Ed) Ciba Foundation Symposium on *Enzymes and Drug Action*, 276, Little, Brown, Boston.

REMMER, H. and SIEGERT, M. (1962), Kumulation und Elimination von Phenobarbital. *Naunyn-Schmiedeberg's Arch. exp. Path. Pharmak.*, 243, 479.

REMMER, H. and MERKER, H. J. (1963), Drug-induced changes in the liver endoplasmic reticulum: association with drug-metabolizing enzymes. *Science*, 142, 1657.

REMMER, H. (1964a), Vermehrte Glukuronidierung von Sulfadimethoxin während und nach Phenobarbitalbehandlung bei Ratten. *Naunyn-Schmiedeberg's Arch. exp. Path. Pharmak.*, 247, 461.

REMMER, H. (1964b), Gewöhnung an Hexobarbital durch beschleunigten Abbau. *Arch. int. Pharmacodyn.*, 152, 346.

REMMER, H. and SIEGERT, M. (1964), Beschleunigter Arzneimittelabbau durch Enzyminduktion beim Hunde nach Behandlung mit Phenobarbital. *Naunyn-Schmiedeberg's Arch. exp. Path. Pharmak.*, 247, 522.

RICHARDS, R. K., TAYLOR, J. D. and KUETER, K. E. (1953), Effect of nephrectomy on the duration of sleep following administration of thiopental and hexobarbital. *J. Pharmacol. exp. Ther.*, 108, 461.

ROGERS, L. A., DIXON, R. L. and FOUTS, J. R. (1963), The effects of SKF 525-A on hepatic glycogen and rate of hepatic drug metabolism. *Biochem. Pharmacol.*, 12, 341.

RUBIN, A., TEPHLY, T. R. and MANNERING, G. J. (1964), Kinetics of drug metabolism by hepatic microsomes. *Biochem. Pharmacol.*, 13, 1007.

RÜMKE, C. L. and NOORDHOEK, J. (1969), The influence of lynestrenol on the rate of metabolism of phenobarbital, phenytoin, and hexobarbital in mice. *Europ. J. Pharmacol.*, 6, 163.

SAIDMAN, L. J. and EGER, E. I. (1966), The effect of thiopental metabolism on duration of anesthesia. *Anesthesiology*, 27, 118.

SCHEIFLEY, C. H. and HIGGINS, G. M. (1940), The effect of partial hepatectomy on the action of certain barbiturate derivatives and a phenylurea derivative. *Amer. J. med. Sci.*, 200, 264.

SCHLICHT, I., KORANSKY, W., MAGOUR, S. and SCHULTZE-HERMANN, R. (1968), Grosse und DNS-Synthese der Leber unter dem Einfluss körperfremder Stoffe. *Naunyn-Schmiedeberg's Arch. exp. Path. Pharmak.*, 261, 26.

SCHÜPPEL, R. (1969), Hemmung der Hydroxylierung von Arzneimitteln *in vivo* unter Äthanolbelastung. *Naunyn-Schmiedeberg's Arch. exp. Path. Pharmak.*, 265, 156.

SCHWARK, W. S. and ECOBICHON, D. J. (1968), Subcellular localization and drug-induced changes of rat liver and kidney esterases. *Canad. J. Physiol.*, 46, 207.

SCHWARTZ, H. L., KOZYREFF, V., SURKS, M. I. and OPPENHEIMER, J. H. (1969), Increased deiodination of L-thyroxine and L-triiodothyronine by liver microsomes from rats treated with phenobarbital. *Nature, (Lond.)*, 221, 1262.

SHIDEMAN, F. E., KELLY, A. R. and ADAMS, B. J. (1947), The role of the liver in the detoxication of thiopental (Pentothal) and two other thiobarbiturates. *J. Pharmacol. exp. Ther.*, 91, 331.

SHUSTER, L. and JICK, H. (1966), The turnover of microsomal protein in the liver of phenobarbital-treated mice. *J. biol. Chem.*, 241, 5361.

SMITH, J. A., WADDELL, W. J. and BUTLER, T. C. (1963), Demethylation of N-methyl derivatives of barbituric acid, hydantoin, and 2,4-oxazolidinedione by rat liver microsomes. *Life Sci.*, 2, 486.

SOEHRING, K. and DIETZ, W. (1956), Pentobarbital – ein Abbauprodukt von thiopental. *Klin. Wschr.*, 34, 705.

STÄUBLI, W., HESS, R. and WEIBEL, E. R. (1969), Correlated morphometric and biochemical studies on the liver cell. II. Effects of phenobarbital on rat hepatocytes. *J. Cell Biol.*, 42, 1.

STITZEL, R. E., ANDERS, M. W. and MANNERING, G. J. (1966), Inhibition of drug metabolism. III. Inhibition of hexobarbital metabolism in the intact rat and in the isolated perfused liver by 2-diethylaminoethyl 2,2-diphenyl-valerate HCl (SKF 525-A) and its N-de-ethylated derivatives. *Molec. Pharmacol. (N.Y.)*, 2, 335.

STRAW, J. A., WATERS, I. W. and FREGLY, M. J. (1965), Effect of *o,p*-DDD on hepatic metabolism of pentobarbital in rats. *Proc. Soc. exp. Biol. Med. (N.Y.)*, 118, 391.

SWINEYARD, E. A., TEDESCHI, D. H. and GOODMAN, L. S. (1954), Effects of liver damage and nephrectomy on anticonvulsant activity of Mysoline and phenobarbital. *J. Amer. pharm. Ass.*, 43, 114.

TAYLOR, J. D., RICHARDS, R. K. and TABERN, D. L. (1952), Metabolism of ^{35}S thiopental (Pentothal). Chemical and paper chromatographic studies of ^{35}S excretion by the rat and monkey. *J. Pharmacol. exp. Ther.*, 104, 93.

THORP, J. M. (1955), Physiological disposition of the anticonvulsant 'Mysoline'. In: *Congrès International de Biochimie*, 3e Congrès, Brussels, 1955. Résumés des Communications, Vol. 1, 132. Academic Press, New York.

TITUS, E. and WEISS, H. (1955), The use of biologically prepared radioactive indicators in metabolic studies: metabolism of pentobarbital. *J. biol. Chem.*, 214, 807.

TOKI, K., TOKI, S. and TSUKAMOTO, H. (1963), Metabolism of drugs. XXXVIII. Enzymic oxidation of methylhexabital. 2. Reversible oxidation of 3-hydroxymethylhexabital. *J. Biochem.*, 53, 43.

TSUKAMOTO, H., TAKABATAKE, E. and ARIYOSHI, T. (1955), Metabolism of drugs. V. Excretion rate of a metabolite of ethylhexabital. *Pharm. Bull. (Tokyo)*, 3, 459.

TSUKAMOTO, H., YOSHIMURA, H. and TOKI, S. (1958), Metabolism of drugs. XVIII. The metabolic fate of methylhexabital (5-cyclohexenyl-3, 5-dimethylbarbituric acid). 8. The quantitative determination of main biotransformation products of methylhexabital in the urine of rabbits by ultraviolet spectrophotometry. *Chem. pharm. Bull.*, 6, 88.

TSUKAMOTO, H., YOSHIMURA, H. and IDE, H. (1963a), Metabolism of drugs. XXXII. The metabolic fate of secobarbital [5-allyl-5-(1-methylbutyl) barbituric acid]. *Chem. pharm. Bull.*, 11, 9.

TSUKAMOTO, H., YOSHIMURA, H., IDE, H. and MITSUI, S. (1963b), Metabolism of drugs. XXXVI. Metabolic fate of thiamylal [5-allyl-5-(1-methylbutyl)-2-thiobarbituric acid]. *Chem. pharm. Bull.*, 11, 427.

UEHLEKE, H. (1967), Stimulierung einiger mikrosomaler Fremdstoff-Oxydationen durch Phenobarbital, Methylcholanthren und Chlorphenothan linzeln und in Kombinationen. *Naunyn-Schmiedeberg's Arch. exp. Path. Pharmak.*, 259, 66.

UEHLEKE, H. and NESTEL, K. (1967), Hydroxyaminobiphenyl and nitrosobiphenyl: biological oxidation products of 4-aminobiphenyl and reduction products of 4-nitrobiphenyl. *Naunyn-Schmiedeberg's Arch. exp. Path. Pharmak.*, 257, 151.

UEHLEKE, H. and BRILL, E. (1958), Increased metabolic N-oxidation of 2-naphthylamine in dogs after phenobarbital pretreatment. *Biochem. Pharmacol.*, 17, 1459.

UEHLEKE, H. and GREIM, H. (1968), Stimulation of drug oxidation in kidney microsomes by phenobarbital. *Naunyn-Schmiedeberg's Arch. exp. Path. Pharmak.*, 261, 152.

UEHLEKE, H. (1969), N-Hydroxylierung von p-Phenetidin *in vivo* und durch isolierte Mikrosomen aus Lebern und Nieren: Stimulierung durch Phenobarbital-Vorbehandlung. *Naunyn-Schmiedeberg's Arch. exp. Path. Pharmak.*, 264, 434.

VAN DYKE, R. A. (1966), Metabolism of volatile anaesthetics. III. Induction of microsomal dechlorinating and ether-cleaving enzymes. *J. Pharmacol. exp. Ther.*, 154, 364.

VARDANIS, E. (1966), Activation of some organophosphorus insecticides by liver microsomes from phenobarbital-treated mice. *Biochem. Pharmacol.*, 15, 749.

WADA, O., YANO, Y., URATA, G. and NAKAO, K. (1968), Behaviour of hepatic microsomal cytochromes after treatment of mice with drugs known to disturb porphyrin metabolism in liver. *Biochem. Pharmacol.*, 17, 595.

WADDELL, W. J. (1962), The metabolic conversion of secobarbital to 5-allyl-5-(3-hydroxy-1- methylbutyl)barbituric acid. *Fed. Proc.*, 21, 182.

WADDELL, W. J. (1963), The metabolic conversion of secobarbital to 5-(1-methylbutyl)barbituric acid and to 5-(2,3-dihydroxypropyl)-5-(1-methylbutyl) barbituric acid. *Fed. Proc.*, 22, 480.

WADDELL, W. J. (1965), The metabolic fate of 5 allyl-5-(1-methylbutyl)barbituric acid (Secobarbital). *J. Pharmacol. exp. Ther.*, 149, 23.

WEISBURGER, J. H., SCHMEHL, E. A. and PAI, S. R. (1965), Liver damage by the carcinogen N-hydroxy-N-2-fluorenylacetamide, pentobarbital sleeping time and morphology. *Toxicol. appl. Pharmacol.*, 7, 579.

WELCH, R. M., ROSENBERG, P. and COON, J. M. (1959), Inhibition of hexobarbital metabolism by chlorothion (p-nitro-m-chlorophenyl dimethyl thionophosphate). *Pharmacologist*, 1, 64.

WELLES, J. S., McMAHON, R. E. and DORAN, W. J. (1963), The metabolism and excretion of methohexital in the rat and dog. *J. Pharmacol. exp. Ther.*, 139, 166.

WIBERG, G. S., COLDWELL, B. B. and TRENHOLM, H. L. (1969), Toxicity of ethanol-barbiturate mixtures. *J. Pharm. Pharmacol.*, 21, 232.

WILLIAMS, R. T. (1959), *Detoxication Mechanisms*, 2nd ed., 593. Chapman and Hall, London.
WILLIAMS, R. T. and PARKE, D. V. (1964), The metabolic fate of drugs. *Ann. Rev. Pharmacol.*, 4, 85.
WINTERS, W. W., SPECTOR, E., WALLACH, D. P. and SHIDEMAN, F. E. (1955), Metabolism of thiopental-S^{35} and thiopental-2-C^{14} by a rat-liver mince and identification of pentobarbital as a major metabolite. *J. Pharmacol. exp. Ther.*, 114, 343.
WOOLES, W. R. and BORZELLECA, J. F. (1966), Prolongation of barbiturate sleeping time in mice by stimulation of the reticulo-endothelial system (RES). *J. reticuloendoth. Soc.*, 3, 41.
YAFFE, S. J., LEVY, G., MATSUZAWA, T. and BALIAH, T. (1966), Enhancement of glucuronide conjugating capacity in a hyperbilirubinemic infant due to apparent enzyme induction by phenobarbital. *New Engl. J. Med.*, 275, 1461.
YEARY, R. A., BENISH, R. A. and FINKELSTEIN, M. (1966), Acute toxicity of drugs in newborn animals. *J. Pediat.*, 69, 663.
ZEIDENBERG, P., ORRENIUS, S. and ERNSTER, L. (1967), Enhancement of glucuronylating enzymes and mitochondrial oxidative enzymes in livers of rats treated with phenobarbital. *Trans. N. Y. Acad. Sci.*, 29, 310.
ZINS, G. R. (1965), The *in vivo* production of a potent long-acting hypotensive metabolite from diallylmelamine. *J. Pharmacol. exp. Ther.*, 150, 109.

3. methods of chemical analysis for the barbiturates

This chapter deals with methods of analysis for the sedative-hypnotic barbiturates, which are applicable to patients suffering from the effects of acute barbiturate poisoning. Thus, methodology is considered in relation to measurement of the plasma barbiturate concentrations, to identification of the drugs and their metabolic products in the urine, and to measurement of barbiturate concentrations in the dialysate fluid from overdose patients. Special attention is given to plasma barbiturate levels, since they provide an index to the pharmacological status of the patient as well as to the physiological availability of the drug or drugs in the body, and this information may be of value in the treatment of the poisoned patient.

The absorption, distribution, and excretion of the individual barbiturate follows from its simple physico-chemical properties. Thus, the slightly water-soluble quinalbarbitone, which has a relatively low dissociation constant, is rapidly absorbed and taken up into the tissues, but lipid solubility confers comparatively rapid metabolism, which in turn controls plasma drug levels, with the result that the drug is short-acting, its metabolites being rapidly excreted in the urine. In comparison, barbitone, with a comparatively high water-solubility and dissociation constant, is less rapidly absorbed and taken up into the tissues, and since its rate of metabolism is very slow, plasma levels remain high. Barbitone is long-acting and is excreted unchanged via the kidneys. The different concentrations of the various barbiturates in the different biological situations therefore necessitate the availability of versatile methods of assay. The spectrophotometry, spectrophotofluorimetry, diagnostic chromatographic methods, and gas chromatography for those drugs are discussed in this chapter.

Coverage is limited to those barbiturates responsible for human poisonings (Fig. 1). In Britain, the four barbiturates most commonly taken in overdose are amylo-, pento-, quinal- and phenobarbitone; the first three of them being the agents for more than 60% of our cases. Some cases of barbitone and butobarbitone poisoning have however been reported. This chapter has been written with the overall biochemical-pharmacological considerations in view, and aims at exemplifying salient principles in the several subject areas rather than at completeness.

Chemical names	Structural formulae	Trivial names
5-Ethyl-5-(3′-methylbutyl) barbituric acid m.p. 156–158°C	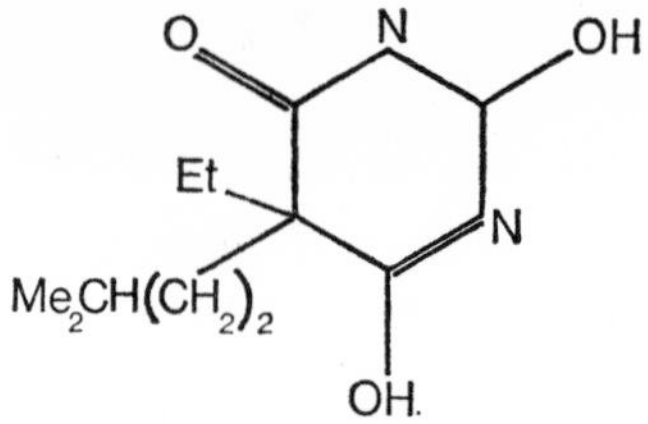	Amylobarbitone. (Amobarbital), 'Amytal', etc.
5-Ethyl-5-(1′-methylbutyl) barbituric acid m.p. 126–130°C	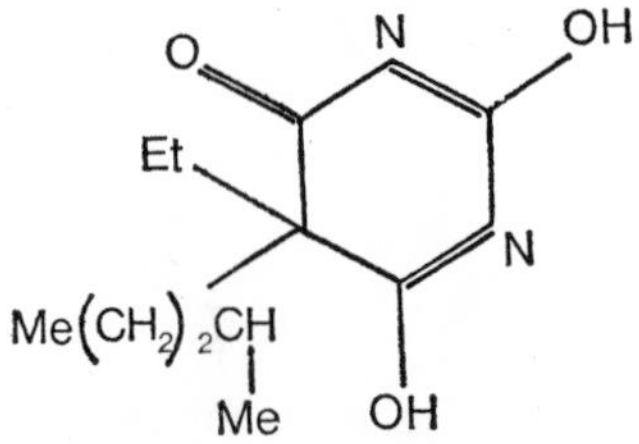	Pentobarbitone. (Pentobarbital), 'Nembutal' etc.
5-Allyl-5-(1′-methylbutyl) barbituric acid m.p. 100°C	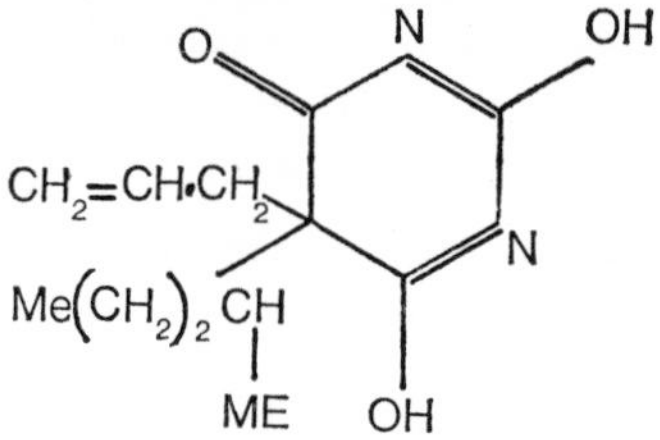	Quinalbarbitone. (Secobarbital), 'Seconal', etc.
5-Butyl-5-ethylbarbituric acid m.p. 122–125°C	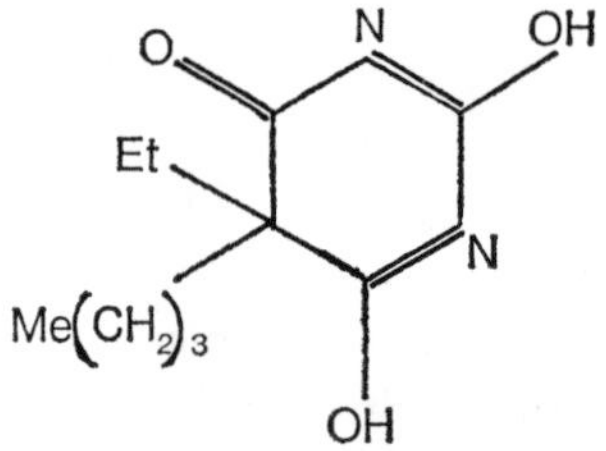	Butobarbitone. (Butethal), 'Soneryl', etc.
5-Ethyl-5-phenylbarbituric acid m.p. 174–178°C (174°C)	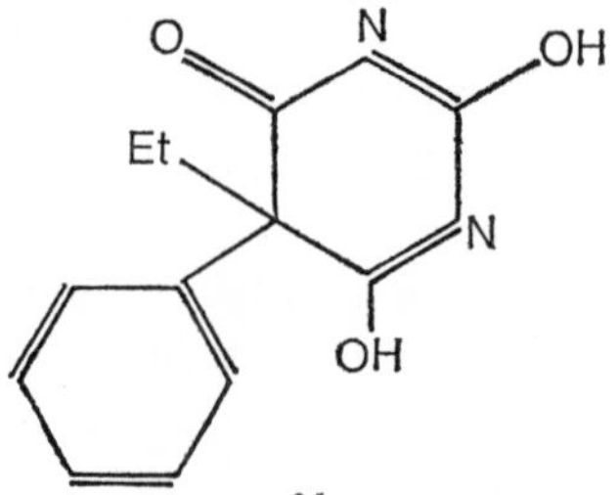	Phenobarbitone. (Phenobarbital), 'Luminal', 'Gardenal', etc.
5,5-Diethylbarbituric acid m.p. 188–192°C (191°C)	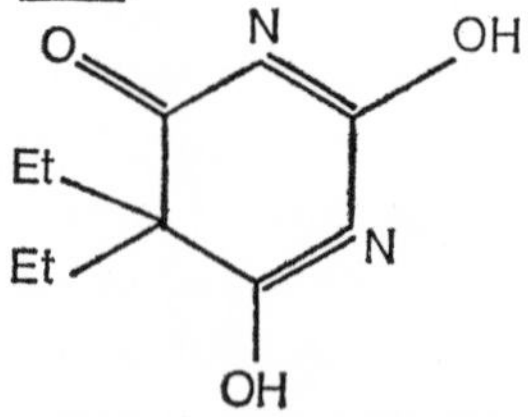	Barbitone. (Barbital), 'Veronal', etc.

Fig. 1. The common barbiturates. Melting-point data throughout from Butler and Mathers (1967, p. 109 *et seq.*), but values in parentheses from Heilbron and Bunbury (1943).

PHYSICO-CHEMICAL PROPERTIES

The action of barbiturates in the body is conditioned by their physico-chemical properties. On account of the comparatively high concentrations of the drugs and their metabolites occurring in the body fluids after moderate doses, and especially in the case of overdoses, a range of modern methods of biochemical analysis is applicable to their detection, separation, and measurement. The physico-chemical properties of the barbiturates and barbiturate metabolites also determine the conditions for their extraction from body fluids. Hence, brief discussion of the physico-chemical properties of the commonly used barbiturates is relevant.

Barbiturates have a small but significant solubility in water, ranging from approximately 0.50–6.25 mg/ml (Table 1), and, because of their weakly acidic properties and capacity for complex formation with proteins, the plasma solubilities would be expected to be considerably greater than those for water.

TABLE 1

Solubilities of common barbiturates (solubility data assembled from values, cited by Clarke, 1969, pp. 195, 231, 486 and 207 respectively).

Compounds	Solubility of undissociated form in water (μg/ml)
Quinalbarbitone	slightly sol.
Pentobarbitone	slightly sol.
Amylobarbitone	667
Butobarbitone	4000
Phenobarbitone	1000
Barbitone	6250

The acidity of barbituric acid, $k_{25}° = 1.0 \times 10^{-4}$; pKa, 4.98 (Morton, 1946, p. 988), which is stronger than the carboxylic acidity of acetic acid or benzoic acid, is diminished by substitution of the methylene group. Thus, barbitone ($k_{25}° = 3.7 \times 10^{-8}$; pKa, 7.14) (Morton, 1946, p. 488) shows weak acidity, and quinal-, pento- and amylobarbitones, which are also 5,5-dialkylbarbituric acids, are even weaker acids (pKa, 7.74, 7.88 and 7.72) (Waddell, 1965), but phenobarbitone (pKa, 7.23) (Butler, 1956) is almost as acidic as barbitone. There is a strong supposition that the metabolism of these compounds is mainly dependent on factors such as pKa (Wiberg, 1955), lipid solubility, and plasma protein binding.

Polarity increases from quinalbarbitone, which is a 'short-acting' barbiturate, through the 'intermediate-acting' barbiturates, pento-, amylo- and butobarbitones, to phenobarbitone and barbitone, which are 'long-acting' (Table 2). In general, the higher the solvent-aqueous partition coefficient of the barbiturate (Table 3) the higher its potency (or the lower its plasma concentration for a given anaesthetic condition). If a barbiturate-containing solvent extract of blood is extracted with two portions of

TABLE 2

Order of polarity and of potency of the barbiturates

Order of polarity	Compounds	Order of potency
	Quinalbarbitone	
	Pentobarbitone	
	Amylobarbitone	
	Butobarbitone	
	Phenobarbitone	
	Barbitone	

TABLE 3

Partition coefficients for barbiturates between chloroform and buffer pH 7.4 (Data reported by Dybing, 1955).

Compounds	Partition coefficients	% barbiturate in the solvent phase after shaking 3 ml buffer and 25 ml chloroform
Amylobarbitone	12.40	99
Pentobarbitone	5.44	97
Phenobarbitone	0.89	88
Barbitone	0.41	77

borax buffer and then with N-NaOH, most of the barbiturate of lowest potency, including phenobarbitone, will be in the first borax extract, some in the second borax extract, and very little in the NaOH; whereas most of the barbiturate of highest potency, including amylo-, pento-, and quinalbarbitones, will be present in the NaOH.

Barbiturates have been extracted from plasma, urine, or other biological material at a pH of 7.4 or lower with chloroform (Butler and Mathers, 1967, p. 107), ethylene dichloride (Butler and Mathers, 1967), dibutyl ether (Stevenson, 1961), or light petroleum containing isoamyl alcohol (Brodie *et al.*, 1953). Dibutyl ether is the solvent of choice (Stevenson, 1961), but chloroform is most commonly used. In one procedure, barbiturates are extracted directly from blood with chloroform in the presence of 0.5M pH 6.5 phosphate buffer (Podmore, 1962). Alternatively, barbiturate-containing blood, pH 7.4 buffer, and chloroform are shaken together, solid anhydrous Na_2SO_4 is added until the aqueous phase is adsorbed, and the chloroform phase is removed and combined with a second solvent extract of the blood-sodium sulphate cake (Broughton, 1956). From a consideration of the partition coefficients (Dybing, 1955; Stevenson, 1961), it follows that blood or plasma containing the commonly used barbiturates should be extracted with 20 volumes of chloroform to obtain 95% theoretical extraction for all the barbiturates. In practice, it is wise to make two such extractions.

MEASUREMENT OF PLASMA BARBITURATE CONCENTRATIONS BY ULTRAVIOLET SPECTROPHOTOMETRY

Barbiturates are extracted from the plasma and other body fluids at pH 7.4 or less with chloroform, and are re-extracted from the organic phase with strong alkali. The absorption spectra of these drugs in strong alkali are characteristic of one ionization species (A^{2-}), and those in the alkaline solution buffered to pH10.0 are characteristic of another ionization species (HA^-). A difference in absorbance between strong alkali and the buffer pH10.0 is characteristic of all barbiturates, with the exception of N-methyl and thio-derivatives. Quantitation is based on maximal absorbance difference at 260 mμ (Broughton, 1956; Butler and Mathers, 1967).

Thus, by means of the first method for extracting barbiturate-containing blood with chloroform (Podmore, 1962):

mg total barbiturates/100 ml blood = $10.8 \times (E_{pH13} - E_{pH10})$ at 260 mμ.

And with the second method for extraction, in which the aqueous phase was adsorbed on to Na_2SO_4 and the blood – Na_2SO_4 cake re-extracted with solvent (Broughton, 1956):

mg total barbiturates/100 ml blood = $16 \times (E_{pH13} - E_{pH10})$ at 260 mμ. The method of absorbance differences can also be applied to the buffered alkaline solution, pH10.0 and to the acid solution of the unionized species (H_2A) at pH 2.0 (Stevenson, 1961).
Thus:

mg total barbiturates/100 ml blood = $5.94 \times (E_{pH10} - E_{pH2})$ at 240 mμ (Podmore, 1962), and

mg total barbiturates/100 ml blood = $8.8 \times (E_{pH10} - E_{pH2})$ at 240 mμ (Broughton, 1956).

In the various equations, the empirical factors take into consideration: (1) the efficiency of extraction, and hence the partition distribution for that unit operation, (2) the proportion of the solvent phase recovered and (3) the relationship between the rate of change of concentration and that for the absorbance difference at two values of pH.

These empirical factors are a compromise for the various common barbiturates, and for a particular case the exact extinction factor ought to be used (Broughton, 1956; Stevenson, 1961).

Finally, the spectrum should be recorded between 220 and 420 mμ. A barbiturate is indicated only where a maximum positive difference in absorbance occurs at 260mμ, decreasing through zero at approximately 250 mμ (1st isobestic point) to a maximum negative difference in absorbance at approximately 240 mμ, and increasing through zero at about 227 mμ (2nd isobestic point) to positive absorbance differences at lower wavelengths (Broughton, 1956; Goldbaum, 1952; Butler and Mathers, 1967, p. 108).

It may be of interest that Wright and Johns (1953) and others had previously used ultraviolet spectrophotometric methods in which the light extinction was measured at 240 mμ at pH10 and in acid solution. Barbiturate was detected by the finding of an absorption maximum at that wavelength at pH10, and its concentration was proportional to the difference, $E_{pH10} - E_{pH2}$. However, salicylic acid and sulphonamides also absorb in that region of the spectrum and may therefore interfere with the detection and measurement of barbiturate by those means. Further, recovery of barbiturate from spiked blood was low (55–79%), and a correction had to be made for this (Wright and Johns, 1953). In comparison, recoveries of the various barbiturates, for example by the method of Broughton (1956), were 88–105%, and the washing of the barbiturate-rich solvent extract with phosphate buffer, which removed salicylic acid and a high proportion of sulphonamides and their metabolic products, did not result in substantial barbiturate loss. In the procedure described in this chapter, distortion of the barbiturate spectrum in the 240–260 mμ region by sulphonamides absorbing at 250–260 mμ in caustic alkali and borate buffer, indicates the presence of interfering drugs and, as previously stated, great importance is attached to the recording of the spectrum between 220 and 420 mμ.

If the foregoing extraction methods are rigorously pursued, interference by other drugs in the spectrophotometric estimation of plasma-barbiturate concentrations from overdose cases will be minimal; much greater interference would in fact be expected at lower plasma concentrations. A number of other drugs can however be extracted in varying proportion from chloroform under neutral or slightly acid conditions. The drugs, which might be expected to accompany the barbiturates in the subsequent alkaline extraction of the solvent, include salicylamide and phenylbutazone, as well as very small proportions of the non-barbiturate hypnotics, meprobamate (Equanil, Miltown), methyprylone (Noludar) and glutethimide (Doriden), and possibly of the tranquillizers, chlordiazepoxide (Librium), diazepam (Valium) and oxazepam (Serenid-D). Spectrophotometric distortion from such complication is predictably not very significant.

Some doubt has been expressed about the validity of blood barbiturate measurements, because the presence of pharmacologically inactive metabolites might lead to misleading results (Geall, 1966; Matthew and Lawson, 1966). If drug metabolites with an intact pyrimidine ring were extracted under the conditions that have been described, then the concentrations for the active, unchanged drugs, measured by spectrophotometry would be high. In this connection, p-hydroxyphenobarbitone has in fact been measured in urine by the method of differential absorption (Butler, 1956). This problem could not be resolved before the utilization of gas chromatography with its improved resolutions and highly sensitive detector systems. Reasonably good agreement has now been established between values for total barbiturate concentrations in plasma by ultraviolet spectrophotometry and by gas chromatography, but spectrophotometric assays tend to be high. (Reference is made to comparative measurement by the two techniques in the section dealing with gas chromatography.)

Leach and Toseland (1968) found that 3'-hydroxyamylobarbitone has different retention times from amylobarbitone on various columns, and the hydroxy-derivatives of other common barbiturates would also be expected to behave on the gas chromatograph differently from the unchanged drugs. Such metabolites have not however been found in extracts used for spectrophotometry. 3'-Hydroxyamylobarbitone has been studied, and its solubility and partition distributions prevent its recovery from blood or aqueous solution by chloroform extraction (Maynert, 1952). Although 3′-hydroxypentobarbitone can be extracted from urine saturated with salt by diethyl ether, it is not extracted with chloroform (Maynert, 1965; Maynert and Dawson, 1952). Similarly, although 3′-hydroxyquinalbarbitone can be separated from urine or water with ethyl acetate (Waddell, 1965), and p-hydroxyphenobarbitone from plasma, urine or water with diethyl ether (Butler, 1956), these substances are too polar to be extracted into chlorinated solvents. Accordingly there is but slight tendency for spectrophotometric measurement of the common barbiturates to be increased by substantial proportions of their hydroxylated metabolic products, provided that selective conditions are employed for the extraction of the unchanged drugs, but it might be emphasized that selectivity in measurement is imposed by the choice of solvent used for extraction.

However, spectrophotometric measurements of plasma barbiturate levels include small quantities of a barbiturate with the chromatographic properties of barbitone, which appears in the blood after administration of the 5-ethylbarbitones (Leach and Toseland, 1968). This might either be a minor metabolic product or an impurity of one of the intermediates used for the Grimaux (barbiturate) synthesis.

Information on plasma barbiturate levels must be assessed in the context of their application, i.e., the treatment of the unconscious patient, poisoned with barbiturates. (Measurement in relation to therapy is accordingly considered in this section of the chapter, because by tradition barbiturates have been measured by ultraviolet spectrophotometry.) The clinical state of the sick patient is fundamentally important, and plasma drug concentrations are valuable inasmuch as they indicate the approximate duration of coma. The physician has to decide, first, what supportive therapy is necessary for relatively short periods of unconsciousness or for more extended periods of barbiturate-induced hypnosis and, second, the possible application of such extra-renal procedures for accelerated body unloading of barbiturates as haemodialysis, peritoneal dialysis, or osmotic diuresis in those states where renal failure may arise or where deterioration of the clinical condition may occur under prolonged unconsciousness. Assessment of the severity of poisoning is best done on clinical/chemical grounds, but plasma blood concentration may be of value both in assessment of severity and in determining certain lines of management. In severely poisoned patients knowledge of the particular barbiturate or mixture of barbiturates responsible is desirable (Table 4), since there is a considerable difference in the clinical effects consequent upon the ingestion of a short-acting barbiturate compared with one which has a much longer action. Individual drugs cannot however be identified by a method which measures total barbiturate levels in the plasma and does not distinguish between the components. Additional information about partition distributions, which could be obtained at the same time, is indecisive (Stevenson, 1961). More specific information derives from measurements of total barbiturate concentrations in conjunction with chromatographic identifications of the individual drugs and their metabolites in the urine.

TABLE 4

*A page from a casebook of barbiturate poisonings**

Personal details			Clinical examination			Treatment		Hypnotic effect
Age (years)	Sex	Drug habits[1]	Depth of coma[2]	Blood level[3] (µg/ml)	Identification of drug	Hypotension[4]	Respiratory[5] depression	Duration[6] of coma (in hours)
17	♀		2	7	Seconal	b		12
50	♀	H	0	12	Seconal			0
24	♀		1–2	28	Amytal			39
27	♀	H	0	0	Amytal			0
26	♀	H	2	19	Tuinal	b		31
21	♀	H	2–3	31	Tuinal			20
24	♀		3	18	Tuinal			8
46	♀	A	4	11	Tuinal		IT	8
20	♀		2	19	Amytal			10
43	♀	H	0	8	Tuinal			0
24	♂		3	35	Amytal	b	IT	27.5
21	♀		2	23	Amytal			6
59	♀	H	3	23	Nembutal	a	V	20.5
55	♂	H	0	14	Tuinal[7]			0
31	♂	A	4	22	Tuinal		V	15
31	♂	A	4	13	Tuinal	a	V	17
62	♂	H	4	43	Tuinal	a	V	25
49	♀	H	3	11	Tuinal	b		6
20	♀	H	0	9	Amytal			0
71	♀	H	0		Tuinal			0
26	♀		0	18	Soneryl			0
24	♀		4	86	Soneryl		V	72
56	♀		1		Soneryl			0
52	♀	H	2	56	Phenobarbitone			7
72	♀	H	0	56	Phenobarbitone			0
39	♀	E	0–1	54	Phenobarbitone			0
29	♀		1	16	Phenobarbitone	b		0

* These data have been made available through the courtesy of Dr. S. S. Brown of the Department of Clinical Chemistry and Dr. A. T. Proudfoot of the Regional Poisoning Treatment Centre, the Royal Infirmary, Edinburgh.

[1] Addicted (A), epileptic (E), habituated (H).
[2] Empirical grading of coma : 0, least degree of confusion ; 4, no response to maximum painful stimulus.
[3] Blood level on admission to hospital.
[4] Treatment with Aramine (metaraminol) (a), patient on blocks (b).
[5] Intubated (IT), respiratory ventilation (V).
[6] Time after ingestion.
[7] Tuinal refers to a binary mixture of amylo- and quinalbarbitones.

Alternatively, plasma concentrations of the individual barbiturates can now be measured directly by gas chromatography, and this is discussed in the last section of this chapter.

Blood barbiturate levels of say 35µg/ml for short- to intermediate-acting drugs and of, say, 80 µg/ml for the long-acting ones, which are commonly encountered, are considered by Maher and Schreiner (1965) as 'potentially fatal'. At best, however, such statements can be regarded as relative generalizations only, and it must be stressed that the vast majority of patients poisoned by barbiturates can be confidently managed by intensive supportive therapy alone (Clemmesen and Nilsson, 1961; Matthew and Lawson, 1966). A further complication arises from the fact that the effects of barbiturates are potentiated by simultaneous ingestion of alcohol and/or tranquillizers. The data in Table 4 refer to cases which were managed by supportive therapy without accelerated body unloading of barbiturates. High blood levels were sometimes indicative of prolonged coma but not so invariably. Treatment for hypotension and respiratory depression was governed by the patient's condition, and did not necessarily follow the blood concentration and type of causative agent. Although moderate diuresis was tested in the case of the 24-year-old woman, severely poisoned with Soneryl (butobarbitone), only a small quantity of unchanged drug was rapidly removed, and diuresis was discontinued (Raeburn et al., 1969) (See below).

It has been suggested by Linton et al. (1964) that the application of osmotic diuresis may obviate the need for haemodialysis, but those workers recommend haemodialysis if the blood barbiturate level exceeds 40 µg/ml for short- to intermediate-acting barbiturates or 150 µg/ml for the long-acting ones, and also if the blood levels continue to rise or the clinical condition deteriorates during forced diuresis. Such suggestions, and those recommending dialysis if the patient has ingested certain quantities of barbiturates (Schreiner, 1958), should be interpreted with caution. If active measures to accelerate elimination are contemplated, then it is imperative that the barbiturate be first identified, since the efficacy of accelerated body-unloading depends on the extent to which unchanged drug can be removed, and individual drugs have different metabolic rates. Thus, short- and medium-acting barbiturates are inactivated in the liver at a rate equivalent to 13% of the body burden of active drug/hr (Mark, 1963), whereas long-acting barbiturates are mainly excreted unchanged. Assuming satisfactory renal function, forced alkaline diuresis should be carried out as a first measure in patients severely poisoned with a long-acting barbiturate. By those means, Raeburn et al. (1969) have reported the successful treatment of a 63-year-old woman with the highest recorded blood level of barbitone, 685 µg/ml[1], whereas Balme et al. (1962) have reported the treatment of barbitone poisoning by haemodialysis in a patient whose blood level was 600 µg/ml. On the other hand, forced diuresis (Linton et al., 1967; Mawer and Lee, 1968; Myschetzky and Lassen, 1963) and haemodialysis (Linton et al., 1964; Lee and Ames, 1965) can only remove small quantities of short- or intermediate-acting barbiturates (see Bloomer, 1965; Raeburn et al., 1969), and in practice, would be implemented only if the clinical condition were deteriorating and the blood barbiturate level were very high. In this connection, only a small quantity of unchanged drug was removed by moderate diuresis of a butobarbitone-poisoned patient, 86µg/ml of plasma (Raeburn et al., 1969), and Bloomer (1965) has presented evidence of the limited efficacy of forced diuresis and peritoneal dialysis in the case of pentobarbitone poisoning. Bloomer (1965) emphasizes that other workers have not distinguished between unchanged active barbiturate and unactive metabolic products, and that the drug clearance by those means has been exaggerated. This is readily understandable, if the drug had been extracted under non-specific conditions, and total barbiturate measured spectrophotometrically. Each overdose case ought therefore to be considered on its merits in conjunction with the relevant chemical information, but clinical judgement should prevail. Data on 'total barbiturate' concentrations in plasma can contribute to the assessment of a poisoned patient, but a knowledge of the identity of the component barbiturates is also essential, if the data are to be of real value.

MEASUREMENT OF DIALYSATE BARBITURATE CONCENTRATIONS BY SPECTROPHOTOFLUORIMETRY

Pesez (1938) first described the fluorimetric assay of barbiturates, and Udenfriend *et al.* (1957) later outlined extraction procedures for pentobarbitone, which are applicable to fluorimetric measurements. Maximum excitation and fluorescent wavelengths for the common barbiturates were reported by Udenfriend (1962). In a method for the spectrophotofluorimetric determination of amylobarbitone in plasma, Swagzdis and Flanagan (1964) wash the dibutyl ether extract with phosphate buffer, pH 8.0, and re-extract the drug into N–NaOH. With an excitation wavelength of 265 mμ, the fluorescence is measured at 410 mμ. These workers found that amylobarbitone concentration is proportional to fluorescence intensity in the range 0–3.0 μg/ml. Hence, spectrophotofluorimetry can be applied to measurement of low concentrations of barbiturates in large volumes of dialysate from haemodialysed patients, but the data obtained by these means again provide no information about the identity of individual drugs.

DIAGNOSTIC CHROMATOGRAPHIC METHODS

Better resolutions of barbiturates are obtained by paper chromatography than by thin-layer chromatography. The best separation of the commonly used barbiturates is effected in 17 minutes by high-temperature reverse-phase paper chromatography with tributyrin as the stationary phase and phosphate buffer pH 7.4 (M/15) as mobile phase, by the ascending method (Street and McMartin, 1963). However, even under the most favourable conditions (Jackson, 1969), amylo-, pento- and quinalbarbitones run close together, and amylo- and pentobarbitones overlap. Among many investigators using thin-layer chromatography, Frahm *et al.* (1961) with piperidine-light petroleum and Eberhardt *et al.* (1962) with isopropanol-ammonia-chloroform as the mobile phases have reported the successful separation of several barbiturates, but from a practical viewpoint, only the separation of intermediate-acting from long-acting bar-biturates has been accomplished (Gänshirt, 1962).

In those methods, barbiturates were detected ($< 10\,\mu g$) as dark absorbing areas under ultraviolet light and in the presence of ammonia. Those drugs, such as quinal-barbitone, with an unsaturated group attached to the pyrimidine ring, could be located as yellow spots by means of aqueous 0.1 % permanganate. If present in about $5\mu g$ quantity, all the commonly used barbiturates give a red colour with Co^{2+} (Dille-Koppanyi reagent) (Koppanyi et al., 1934), and the chloroform solubility of the resulting red complexes distinguishes between barbiturates and such other drugs as the hydantoins, the sulphonamides, methyprylone (Noludar), persedoin, etc., which also give that reaction. In the presence of ammonia, bluish-violet complexes result. Mercuric sulphate-diphenylcarbazone is also commonly used for barbiturates (e.g., Jackson, 1969), which give bluish-violet spots.

Amylo-, pento- and quinalbarbitones in blood and urine have however been identi-fied on thin-layer chromatograms by employing the sulphuric acid-catalysed 5-dealky-lation reaction (Petzold et al., 1963). The spotted chromatograms were treated at 125° with $4N-H_2SO_4$ and developed with acetone-butan-l-ol-ammonia (9:9:2, by vol.) by the ascending method. Dealkylation products of pento- and quinalbarbitones and unchanged amylobarbitone were located as purple-blue spots by spraying with silver acetate followed by diphenylcarbazone (Petzold et al., 1963).

Those chromatographic methods are diagnostic for individual barbiturates in the plasma and urine of poisoned patients. If diethyl ether or ethyl acetate is used for extracting the body fluid, then the presence of authenticated metabolites on the chromatograms can be used for confirmation of identity.
3'-Hydroxyamylobarbitone, (+), (—)-3'-hydroxyquinalbarbitone,
5-(2',3'-dihydroxypropyl)-5-(1'-methylbutyl)-barbituric acid,
(+), (—)-3'-hydroxypentobarbitone and p-hydroxyphenobarbitone are useful refer-ence compounds. The identification of the individual barbiturates is important in the treatment of severely poisoned patients.

IDENTIFICATION AND MEASUREMENT OF THE INDIVIDUAL BARBITURATES BY GAS CHROMATOGRAPHY

The necessity for the identification and measurement of the individual barbiturates in the plasma of poisoned patients has prompted the investigation of gas chromato-graphy for those purposes (Brochmann-Hanssen and Svendsen, 1962; Braddock and Marec, 1965; Cieplinski, 1963; Jain et al., 1964; McMartin and Street, 1966; Martin and Driscoll, 1966; Parker and Kirk, 1961; Parker et al., 1963a; 1963b). A fundamental requirement of both objectives is the clean separation of all relevant barbiturates on a single column, which should be easy to prepare, and which should give dependable service.

The most extensive separations were described by Brochmann-Hanssen and Svendsen, (1962), Parker et al. (1963b) and Parker and Kirk (1961). Brochmann-Hanssen and Svendsen (1962) used various individually prepared and selected columns, which had a low loading of stationary phases with different characteristics, and which afforded a high degree of resolution of the separate barbiturates. In that way, a range of barbiturates, including amylo-, pento- and quinalbarbitones appear to have been cleanly separated on (1.4%) Apiezon L, on (1.4%) phenyl silicone polymer SE-52, and probably, on (1.2%) methyl silicone polymer SE-30. Unfortunately, it has been difficult to reproduce the results obtained by using the columns prepared by Brochmann-Hanssen and Svendsen (1962). If good results are to be obtained, it is accordingly advisable to prepare a number of batches of coated support and columns, and to select only those with the optimum performance.

Underlying difficulties are further exemplified by the studies of the following workers, who also employed columns which had a low loading of the stationary phase. Thus, columns were packed with 60- to 80-mesh Chromsorb W, acid-washed and coated with 3.8% SE-30 silicone gum rubber (Braddock and Marec, 1965); with 100- to 120-mesh firebrick, acid-washed and coated with 5% of SE-30 (Parker and Kirk, 1961); with 100- to 120-mesh firebrick, acid-washed and coated with 1.5% SE-30 and 2% of the polar Carbowax 20M polyethylene glycols (Parker et al., 1963b; Jain et al., 1964); and with 100- to 120-mesh Chromsorb W, treated with a mixture of 2% SE-30 and 0.1% tristearin (McMartin and Street, 1966). In each study, the resolutions reported for the barbiturates, encountered in human poisonings, especially for amylo-, pento- and quinalbarbitones, were conspicuously poorer than those obtained by Brochmann-Hanssen and Svendsen (1962).

In an attempt to resolve the fundamental problem of peak tailing, Cieplinski (1963) added very small quantities of the more polar dimer (a C_{36} dibasic acid and trimer (a C_{54} tribasic acid) acids to SE-30 and neopentylglycol adipate columns. Using a Chromsorb W packing, coated with 0.75% trimer acid and 3% neopentylglycol adipate, Cieplinski (1963) obtained substantial improvement and, for example, an excellent resolution of amylo- and pentobarbitones was recorded. On the other hand, Martin and Driscoll (1966) tackled the problem of peak tailing by prior methylation of the barbiturate drugs, but retained the 5% loaded SE-30 column for chromatography. Although o-methylation marginally reduces peak tailing, blockage of the functional groups, which contribute to the molecular chromatographic properties, impairs resolution. The separation of amylo-, pento- and quinalbarbitones was not improved.

Although most investigators have used flame-ionization detectors, an argon ionization detector (Brochmann-Hanssen and Svendsen, 1962) and an ionization β-ray (^{90}Sr) detector (Parker and Kirk, 1961) have also been employed, but there is little to choose between those systems. However, the greater sensitivity afforded by electron capture (Gudzinowicz and Clark, 1965) permits smaller samples (100–800 mμg/μl) to be used, and under certain circumstances this could be advantageous.

Despite the undoubted difficulties, Brochmann-Hanssen and Svendsen (1962) had given a lead about the choice of stationary phases for gas-liquid chromatography, and by an extension of those methods they separated phenobarbitone and its p-hydroxy metabolite (Svendsen and Brochmann-Hanssen, 1962). Good separation of all barbiturates except amylo- and pentobarbitones, which were partially resolved as easily recognizable twin peaks, was obtained in the present author's laboratory at Guy's Hospital on Chromsorb W, acid-washed, silanized and coated more heavily with 15% SE-30. Those separations were good enough for identification purposes, but were inadequate for the measurement of component drugs in mixtures of amylo-, pento- (and possibly quinal-) barbitones. Such experiments established that a more heavily-loaded column was advantageous for the separation of structurally related barbiturates. This supposition underlies the work of Leach and Toseland (1968), who have recently achieved excellent resolutions of all the barbiturates associated with human poisoning (Fig. 2) on columns, packed with 80- to 100-mesh Chromsorb W, acid-washed, silanized and coated with 10% Apiezon L; they used a ^{90}Sr β-ionization detector. The more heavily loaded columns are easily prepared, and can be used continuously for many years. Unequivocal separation of amylo-, pento- and quinalbarbitones was repeatedly effected. The possibility of using lower loaded columns and running them under temperature-programmed conditions did not afford consistent retention data, and for that reason, the longer retention times on the more heavily loaded columns were not considered as limiting, especially when the good separations were taken into account. Gas chromatography is comparatively rapid, and yields much more exact information than other methods of assay.

If 0.5 to 5.0 µg of barbiturate are chromatographed, the instrument can be run well below its maximum sensitivity, but much smaller amounts than these can be identified (Gudzinowicz and Clark, 1965; McMartin and Street, 1966). The larger quantities are preferable, because they allow the interference, which may arise from the production of multiple, often unidentifiable, peaks, to be reduced, and also because smaller quantities of barbiturates would prolong the retention times. Liquid and solid-sample injection can be utilized.

The peaks obtained by Leach and Toseland (1968) for the barbiturates approximate to Gaussian curves, and their symmetry vindicates their usefulness for quantitative purposes. A solution of a standard barbiturate, say barbitone, is run immediately before or after the test sample, which has been chromatographed, and the relative retention time is calculated. From such data, the barbiturate (or barbiturates) is (are) identified. After such provisional identification, aliquots of a standard barbiturate solution are injected into the gas chromatograph, until two consecutive peak heights are the same. The peak areas of the standard and test are then calculated (Scott and Grant, 1964). A base line is constructed from the base of one peak to the beginning of the next one, and the peak area is then calculated as the product of the peak height and peak width at half-peak height. Identity can then be validated by the relation of the peak to that of the standard. The use of, say, barbitone or phenobarbitone as

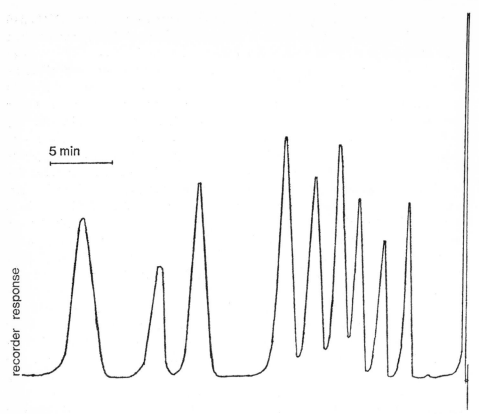

Fig. 2. Representative chromatogram of the more common barbiturates. The order of emergence from right to left is solvent, barbitone, diallylbarbitone, butobarbitone, amylobarbitone, pentobarbitone, quinalbarbitone, hexobarbitone, methylphenobarbitone and phenobarbitone.

Chromatography conditions: column packed with 10% Apiezon L on Chromosorb W; temperature 205°; flow rates, N_2, 11 lb/in², H_2, 60 ml/min and air, 400 ml/min; detector, flame ionization.

standard is sufficiently accurate for most calculations, but greater accuracy is obtainable by using another barbiturate with a retention time similar to that of the barbiturate(s), which is (are) being determined. Thus, pentobarbitone can be used for short retention-time barbiturates, unless pentobarbitone is one of the drugs being investigated, when amylobarbitone can be used. Cyclobarbitone may be used as standard for phenobarbitone measurements. This procedure gives peaks of almost identical geometry, which facilitates calculation of peak areas, and also affords more convincing proof of identity. Comparison of blood barbiturate concentrations by spectrophotometry and gas chromatography is relevant (Table 5); spectrophotometric values are corrected for the molar absorbance of the individual barbiturates (Stevenson, 1961). Integrators can profitably be employed for peak-area calculations. The results are promising, but some difficulties may be encountered in the case of mixtures of barbiturates with peaks close together. Hence, the column is run at a temperature, which

TABLE 5

Comparison of blood levels of barbiturates by gas chromatography (GC) and spectrophotometry (UV)

Barbiturate	GC (μg/ml)	UV (μg/ml)
Amytal	8	11
	26	23
	34	37
	19	20
	26	23
	14	16
	18	18
	30	33
	22	24
	28	25
Soneryl	31	29
	22	24
	13	15
	17	15
	19	23
	38	39
Nembutal	22	24
	28	27
	29	25
	30	34
	31	33
	19	17
	16	19
	7	10
	17	21
	26	23
	20	19
	27	30
Tuinal Amylo – (A)	20 (A)	29 (Total)
Quinal – (Q)	9 (Q)	
	15 (A)	26
	13 (Q)	
	8 (A)	17
	5 (Q)	
	14 (A)	22
	10 (Q)	
Phenobarbitone	80	84
	46	47
	51	53

gives optimum peak resolution, constant temperature control being superior to temperature-programmed conditions.

It should be restated that a knowledge of plasma barbiturate levels and of the identity of the particular barbiturate(s) responsible for poisoning can be important in the treatment of the severely poisoned patient. This has already been discussed in the section of this chapter dealing with spectrophotometric measurement of plasma barbiturate concentrations. It is only necessary to emphasize here that by means of gas chromatography the concentration of each individual barbiturate can be measured directly. Further, complications due to the presence of metabolites and contaminants with an intact pyrimidine ring do not arise, because they have entirely different retention times.

In the same way that gas chromatography has been applied to the measurement in plasma of both acetylsalicylic acid and its metabolite, salicylic acid (Rowland and Riegelman, 1967), and of both 5,5-diphenylhydantoin ('Epanutin') and its metabolite, 5-(p-hydroxyphenyl)-5-phenylhydantoin (Grimmer et al., 1969), so it can also be used for the measurement of both individual barbiturates and their metabolites. Study of 3'-hydroxyamylobarbitone on the 10% Apiezon L column showed that this metabolite and its 0-acetoxy derivative have retention times which are different from that of the parent drug (Leach and Toseland, 1968). Solvents of suitable polarity are required for extracting barbiturate metabolites. By means of gas chromatography on a 5% DC-200 silicone column, 5-(1'-methylbutyl) barbituric acid and a metabolite of unknown structure have been identified in the liver of a quinalbarbitone-suicide case (Niyogi, Cordova and Rieders, 1965). 1.4% Apiezon L was used to separate phenobarbitone and p-hydroxyphenobarbitone from the urine of treated patients, and also to follow the oxidative N-demethylation of N-methyl substituted barbiturates (Svendsen and Brochmann-Hanssen, 1962).

Hence, gas chromatography not only provides a means for the identification and measurement in plasma of the individual barbiturates but, by also providing information about their metabolic products, affords confirmatory evidence for those identifications.

CONCLUSIONS

The scope and limitations of the various methods that have been described in this chapter for the measurement of plasma concentrations, and for the recognition of the individual barbiturates that are commonly involved in acute poisonings, have been clearly defined. It is accordingly concluded that the most exact measurements of the concentrations of each individual barbiturate in the body fluids can be made by proper use of gas chromatography, but that the choice of stationary liquid phase and of the proportion which should be incorporated on the support is critical. Much has also been said about the quantitative extraction of barbiturates into suitable solvents, and the separation therefrom of drugs with some similar chemical properties. However, measurements of unchanged barbiturates by gas chromatography are unaffected by the presence of barbiturate metabolites and/or contaminants with an intact pyrimidine ring, because they have entirely different retention times from the parent drugs. Gas chromatography has therefore advantages both of specificity and of accuracy, compared with spectrophotometric measurement, and is much quicker to operate than the somewhat clumsy combination of spectrophotometric and chromatographic methods which is otherwise necessary to supply the same sort of information. Whilst spectrophotofluorimetry provides much more sensitive measurement of barbiturate than spectrophotometry does, it suffers from the same defect as the latter in not being diagnostic for the individual drugs. The powerful technique of gas chromatography can thus be used to provide all the chemical information required by the clinician for help in the management of an unconscious poisoned patient, and in the minimum of time. In this connection, attention is drawn to sequential measurements of plasma barbiturate concentrations, by means of which predictive information about the possible time of arousal can be supplied.

REFERENCES

BALME, R. H., LLOYD-THOMAS, H. G. and SHEAD, G. V. (1962), Severe barbitone poisoning treated by haemodialysis. *Brit. med. J.*, 1, 231.

BLOOMER, H. A. (1965), Limited usefulness of alkaline diuresis and peritoneal dialysis in pentobarbital intoxication. *New Engl. J. Med.*, 272, 1309.

BRADDOCK, L. I. and MAREC, N. (1965), The gas chromatographic analysis of sub-microgram quantities of barbiturates using a flame ionization detector. *J. Gas Chromat.*, 3, 274.

BROCHMANN-HANSSEN, E. and SVENDSEN, A. B. (1962), Separation and identification of barbiturates and some related compounds by means of gas-liquid chromatography. *J. pharm. Sci.*, 51, 318.

BRODIE, B. B., BURNS, J. J., MARK, L. C., LIEF, P. A., BERNSTEIN, E. and PAPPER, E. M. (1953), The fate of pentobarbital in man and dog and a method for its estimation in biological material. *J. Pharmacol. exp. Ther.*, 109, 26.

BROUGHTON, P. M. G. (1956), A rapid ultraviolet spectrophotometric method for the detection, estimation and identification of barbiturates in biological material. *Biochem. J.*, 63, 207.

BUTLER, T. C. (1956), The metabolic hydroxylation of phenobarbital. *J. Pharmacol. exp. Ther.*, 116, 326.

BUTLER, W. P. and MATHERS, A. P. (1967), *Methods of analysis for alkaloids, opiates, marihuana, barbiturates and miscellaneous drugs*. IRS, Washington, D.C., public. No. 341.

CIEPLINSKI, E. W. (1963), Prevention of peak tailing in the direct gas chromatographic analysis of barbiturates. *Analyt. Chem.*, 35, 256.

CLARKE, E. G. C. (1969), *Isolation and Identification of Drugs*. Pharmaceutical Press, London.

CLEMMESEN, C. and NILSSON, E. (1961), Therapeutic trends in the treatment of barbiturate poisoning: the Scandinavian method. *Clin. Pharmacol. Ther.*, 2, 220.

DYBING, F. (1955), Estimation of barbiturates in clinical chemistry. *Scand. J. clin. Lab. Invest.*, 7, Suppl. 20, 114.

EBERHARDT, H., FREUNDT, K. J. and LANGBEIM, J. W. (1962), Nachweis von Schlafmitteln als Reinsubstanzen und nach Körperpassage. *Arzneimittel-Forsch.*, 12, 1087.

FRAHM, V. M., GOTTESLEBEN, A. and SOEHRING, K. (1961), Erfahrungen mit der Dünnschichtchromatographie beim Nachweis von Arzneimitteln. *Arzneimittel-Forsch.*, 11, 1008.

GÄNSHIRT, H. (1962), Arzneimittel. In: E. Stahl (Ed), *Dünnschicht-chromatographie; Ein Laboratoriumshandbuch*, 315. Springer, Berlin.

GEALL, M. (1966), Management of barbiturate intoxication. *Hosp. Med.*, 1, 51.

GOLDBAUM, L. R. (1952), Determination of barbiturates. Ultraviolet spectrophotometric method with differentiation of several barbiturates. *Analyt. Chem.*, 24, 1604.

GRIMMER, G., JACOB, J. and SCHÄFER, H. (1969), Die gaschromatographische Bestimmung von 5,5-Diphenylhydantoin und 5-(p-Hydroxyphenyl)-5-phenylhydantoin im Blut. *Arzneimittel-Forsch.*, 19, 1287.

GUDZINOWICZ, B. J. and CLARK, S. J. (1965), The gas chromatographic analysis of low concentrations of barbiturates using an electron affinity detector. *J. Gas Chromat.*, 3, 147.

HEILBRON, I. M. and BUNBURY, H. M. (1943), *Dictionary of Organic Compounds*, rev. ed. Eyre and Spottiswoode, London.

JACKSON, J. V. (1969), The barbiturates. In: I. Smith (Ed), *Chromatographic and Electrophoretic Techniques*, 3rd ed., vol. I, *Chromatography*, 494. Heinemann, London.

JAIN, N. C., FONTAN, C. R. and KIRK, P. L. (1964), Rapid extraction method for barbiturates from blood for gas-liquid chromatographic analysis. *Microchem. J.*, 8, 28.

KOPPANYI, T., DILLE, J. S., MURPHY, W. S. and KROP, S. (1934), Studies on barbiturates, part 2, contributions to methods of barbital research. *J. Amer. pharm. Ass. (Sci. ed.)*, 23, 1074.

LEACH, H. and TOSELAND, P. A. (1968), The determination of barbiturates and some related drugs by gas chromatography. *Clin. chim. Acta*, 20, 195.

LEE, H. A. and AMES, A. C. (1965), Haemodialysis in severe barbiturate poisoning. *Brit. med. J.*, 1, 1217.

LINTON, A. L., LUKE, R. G. and BRIGGS, J. D. (1967), Methods of forced diuresis and its application in barbiturate poisoning. *Lancet*, II, 377.

LINTON, A. L., LUKE, R. G., SPEIRS, I. and KENNEDY, A. C. (1964), Forced diuresis and haemodialysis in severe barbiturate intoxication. *Lancet*, I, 1008.

McMARTIN, C. and STREET, H. V. (1966), Gas-liquid chromatography of submicrogram amounts of drugs. II. Analysis of barbiturates and related drugs in biological media. *J. Gas Chromat.*, 23, 232.

MAHER, J. F. and SCHREINER, G. E. (1965), Editorial review. The clinical dialysis of poisons. *Trans. Amer. Soc. artif. intern. Org.*, 11, 349.

MARK, L. C. (1963), Metabolism of barbiturates in man. *Clin. Pharmacol. Ther.*, 4, 504.

MARTIN, H. F. and DRISCOLL, J. L. (1966), Gas chromatographic identification and determination of barbiturates. *Analyt. Chem.*, 38, 345.

MATTHEW, H. and LAWSON, A. A. H. (1966), Acute barbiturate poisoning: a review of two years' experience. *Quart. J. Med.*, 35, 539.

MAWER, G. E. and LEE, H. A. (1968), Value of forced diuresis in acute barbiturate poisoning. *Brit. med. J.*, 2, 790.

MAYNERT, E. W. (1952), Ethyl(3'-hydroxyisoamyl) barbituric acid as the principal metabolite of Amytal. *J. biol. Chem.*, 195, 397.

MAYNERT, E. W. (1965), The alcoholic metabolites of Pentobarbital and Amobarbital in man. *J. Pharmacol. exp. Ther.*, 150, 118.

MAYNERT, E. W. and DAWSON, J. M. (1952), Ethyl(3'-hydroxy-1'-methylbutyl) barbituric acid as metabolite of Pentobarbital. *J. biol. Chem.*, 195, 389.

MORTON, A. A. (1946), *The Chemistry of Heterocyclic Compounds*. McGraw-Hill, New York.

MYSCHETZKY, A. and LASSEN, N. A. (1963), Urea induced osmotic diuresis and alkalization of urine in acute barbiturate intoxication. *J. Amer. med. Ass.*, 185, 936.

NIYOGI, S. K., CORDOVA, V. F. and RIEDERS, F. (1965), Detection of a secobarbital metabolite in human liver by gas chromatography. *Nature (Lond.)*, 206, 716.

PARKER, K. D. and KIRK, P. L. (1961), Separation and identification of barbiturates by gas chromatography. *Analyt. Chem.*, 33, 1378.

PARKER, K. D., FONTAN, C. R. and KIRK, P. L. (1963a), Rapid gas chromatographic method for screening of toxicological extracts for alkaloids, barbiturates, sympathomimetic amines, and tranquilizers. *Analyt. Chem.*, 35, 356.

PARKER, K. D., FONTAN, C. R. and KIRK, P. L. (1963b), Improved gas chromatographic column for barbiturates. *Analyt. Chem.*, 35, 418.

PESEZ, M. (1938), Sur quelques nouvelles réactions colorées des dérivées barbituriques. *J. Pharm. Chim. (Paris)*, 27, 247.

PETZOLD, J. A., CAMP, W. J. R. and KIRCH, E. R. (1963), Identification of some barbiturates in blood by use of thin-layer chromatography. *J. pharm. Sci.* 52, 1106.

PODMORE, D. A. (1962), Rapid paper chromatography of barbiturates. *Clin. chim. Acta*, 7, 176.

RAEBURN, J. A., MATTHEW, H. and CAMERON, J. C. (1969), Severe barbiturate poisoning: contrasts in management. *Clin. Toxicol.*, 2, 133.

ROWLAND, M. and RIEGELMAN, S. (1967), Determination of acetylsalicylic acid and salicylic acid in plasma. *J. pharm. Sci.*, 56, 717.

SCHREINER, G. E. (1958), The role of hemodialysis (artificial kidney) in acute poisoning. *Arch. intern. Med.*, 102, 896.

SCOTT, R. P. W. and GRANT, D. W. (1964), Measurement of elution peaks in gas-liquid chromatography. *Analyst*, 89, 179.

STEVENSON, G. W. (1961), Spectrophotometric determination of blood barbiturate. *Analyt. Chem.* 33, 1374.

STREET, H. V. and McMARTIN, C. (1963), Quantitative estimation and identification of barbiturates in blood in emergency cases. *Nature (Lond.)*, 199, 456.

SVENDSEN, A. B. and BROCHMANN-HANSSEN, E. (1962), Gas chromatography of barbiturates. II. Application to the study of their metabolism and excretion in humans. *J. pharm. Sci.*, 51, 494.

SWAGZDIS, J. E. and FLANAGAN, T. L. (1964), Spectrophotofluorimetric determination of low concentrations of Amobarbital in plasma. *Analyt. Biochem.*, 7, 147.

UDENFRIEND, S. (1962), *Fluorescence Assay in Biology and Medicine*. Academic Press, New York.

UDENFRIEND, S., DUGGAN, D. E., VASTA, B. M. and BRODIE, B. B. (1957), A spectrophotofluorometric study of organic compounds of pharmacological interest. *J. Pharmacol. exp. Ther.*, 120, 26.

WADDELL, W. J. (1965), The metabolic fate of 5-allyl-5-(1'-methylbutyl)barbituric acid (Secobarbital). *J. Pharmacol. exp. Ther.*, 149, 23.

WIBERG, K. B. (1955), The deuterium isotope effect. *Chem. Rev.*, 55, 713.

WRIGHT, J. T. and JOHNS, R. G. S. (1953), A study of barbiturate intoxication by an ultra-violet spectrophotometric technique. *J. clin. Path.*, 6, 78.

BIBLIOGRAPHY OF TECHNIQUES

BERLMAN, I. B. (1965), *Handbook of Fluorescence Spectra of Aromatic Molecules*. Academic Press, New York.

SZYMANSKI, H. A. (1964), *Biomedical Applications of Gas Chromatography*, vol. 1. Plenum Press, New York; also vol. 2 (1968).

UDENFRIEND, S. (1962), *Fluorescence Assay in Biology and Medicine*. Academic Press, New York.

4. pharmacokinetics of barbiturates

Lester C. Mark

The barbiturates are ubiquitous in our civilization and in our patients. After ingestion, they appear in all organs, tissues, and fluids throughout the body (Table 1) (Brodie et al., 1950; 1953). In this chapter, the factors involved in accomplishing this distribution will be considered, starting with the pertinent physicochemical properties (extent of ionization, lipid solubility, and protein binding), continuing with the pharmacokinetic sequence, which they dominate, of absorption, distribution to tissues (including sites of action in the brain and storage sites elsewhere), biotransformation, and excretion (Brodie and Hogben, 1957; Brodie et al., 1960), and concluding with their therapeutic implications in barbiturate poisoning.

PHYSICOCHEMICAL CHARACTERISTICS

DISSOCIATION CONSTANT (pK$_a$)*

The barbiturates are weak acids, most of which range in pK$_a$ from about 7.8 to 8.1; an important exception is phenobarbital, whose pK$_a$ is 7.2 (Waddell and Butler, 1957). All of these drugs exist largely as undissociated molecules in the physiologic range of pH. It is in this unionized form that they pass through lipoid membranes such as the blood-brain and other blood-tissue barriers, the rate of transfer depending upon the lipid solubility (see below) of the undissociated molecule (Brodie et al., 1960; Mark, 1963a).

LIPID SOLUBILITY

When the oil-to-water partition ratios of various barbiturates were determined by distributing 4 mg of each drug between peanut oil (5 ml) and pH 7.4 phosphate buffer

---

* The pK$_a$ of a drug is defined as that pH at which 50% of the drug is ionized and 50% is not.

TABLE 1

Barbiturates in tissues (dog). Data from Brodie et al. (1950; 1953). The studies were made 2½ hr (dog A), 3 hr (dog C) and 3½ hr (dog B) after intravenous administration of barbiturate.

	Thiopental		Pentobarbital
Dog	*A*	*B*	*C*
Weight	8.4 kg	14.0 kg	10.7 kg
Dose	0.65 g	0.7 g	0.43 g
Tissue	Concentration		Concentration
	mg/l	*mg/l*	*mg/l*
Plasma	14.7	19.0	34.4
Plasma water	3.4	4.8	18.7
Cerebrospinal fluid	2.9	—	18.2
	mg/kg	*mg/kg*	*mg/kg*
Red blood cells	—	—	36.0
Liver	27.8	—	64.4
Brain	23.9	—	42.3
Heart	18.4	—	38.4
Lung	13.6	—	20.8
Kidney	17.6	—	45.8
Spleen	13.0	—	41.4
Muscle	22.1	—	27.5
Lumbodorsal fat	—	119	37.3
Omental fat	—	192	—
Perirenal fat	—	222	—

(20 ml) (Mark *et al.*, 1958), the drugs ranged in sequence from barbital, which is more water- than lipid-soluble, through phenobarbital, equally soluble in both media, and pentobarbital, more soluble in the lipid phase, to the highly lipid-soluble anesthetic barbiturate, thiopental (Table 2). These values are, of course, only relative, varying with the experimental conditions (solvent, pH, temperature) chosen by the investigator, but the rank-order of each drug remains essentially unchanged.

The anesthetic barbiturates, whose undissociated molecules are so highly lipid-soluble, pass readily through the blood-brain and other blood-tissue barriers. Less lipid-soluble barbiturates, which penetrate the brain more slowly, are useful as seda-

TABLE 2

Oil-to-water partition ratios of barbiturates (Mark et al., 1958)

Barbital	0.26	Thiobarbital	2.3
Phenobarbital	1.0	Thiophenobarbital	11.0
Pentobarbital	5.8	Thiopental	63.0

tive-hypnotic agents. For example, dogs do not fall asleep until 30 to 40 minutes after therapeutic doses of barbital intravenously, or 20 to 30 minutes after phenobarbital, these being the times required for passage across the blood-brain barrier (Mark *et al.*, 1958). This is explained by the low lipid solubility of these drugs. The other barbiturates in Table 2, being more lipid-soluble, enter the brain sooner, with more prompt onset of sleep.

PROTEIN BINDING

The clinically useful barbiturates are all bound to varying degrees to plasma protein, presumably plasma albumin. Thus, Goldbaum and Smith (1954), who measured binding of a series of barbiturates to bovine serum albumin *in vitro*, found them to range from barbital (5% bound) through phenobarbital (20%) and pentobarbital (37%) to thiopental (65% bound), the same rank-order previously observed with lipid solubility as the criterion.

Binding of barbiturates to plasma protein is an unstable type of bonding, readily reversible with changes in concentration. It may be considered a means of barbiturate transport in the bloodstream, somewhat analogous to oxygen transport by hemoglobin (except that oxyhemoglobin is a chemical compound, while albumin and the barbiturate form a loose structural complex held together by forces of physical attraction acting at their surfaces) (Mark *et al.*, 1969). Tissue proteins also bind barbiturates, to about the same extent as the binding onto plasma proteins (Goldbaum and Smith, 1954). This probably contributes to the accumulation of barbiturates in tissues throughout the body.

From the preceding, it should now be apparent that two key factors in barbiturate pharmacokinetics are the lipid solubility of the drug in question and the concentration of unbound, undissociated molecules at whatever site is being examined.

ABSORPTION

The barbiturates are readily absorbed from the gastrointestinal tract. Being weak acids, they exist largely as undissociated molecules in the highly acid gastric juice. Their rate of passage across the gastric mucosa, which acts as a lipoid barrier between the lumen and the plasma (Brodie and Hogben, 1957; Schanker, 1960), is proportional to their solubility in lipids. As might be expected from its low lipid-solubility, barbital is absorbed most slowly of all. When the barbiturate molecules leave the gastric juice, at whose pH of 1 they are largely unionized, they cross the gastric mucosa to enter the bloodstream. Here the usual pH (7.35 to 7.4) is closer to the pK_a of the barbiturate, resulting in its increased ionization. Thus, for pentobarbital, whose pK_a is 7.9, about 80 per cent of the drug in plasma remains unionized, while for phenobarbital, whose pK_a is 7.2, about 40% remains unionized in the plasma. For both drugs, a concentration gradient exists between the unionized drug in the stomach and the unionized drug in the bloodstream, facilitating absorption of the barbiturate.

In the small intestine and colon, the environmental pH is less acid (about 6.5), but still sufficiently far removed from the barbiturate range of pK_a values for the drug to remain largely unionized. As in the stomach, the concentration gradient across the mucosa continues to facilitate drug absorption (Schanker *et al.*, 1958; Schanker, 1959).

Comparable studies of rectal absorption of barbiturates are not available. Clinical usage has, however, demonstrated rapid absorption of thiopental administered rectally for preanesthetic hypnosis (Mark *et al.*, 1949) and of suppository preparations of other barbiturates, especially in children.

Parenteral administration of barbiturates is also effective. Although, here again, quantitative data are lacking, the accepted usage of intramuscular or even subcutaneous injection of barbiturates for preoperative medication attests to the efficacy of these routes of administration.

The process of absorption may of course be completely bypassed by direct intravascular injection. This procedure, which is tantamount to instantaneous absorption, is useful when a prompt response is essential, as in clinical anesthesia and in the control of convulsions or delirium.

DISTRIBUTION INTO TISSUES

Lipid solubility is the dominant factor in tissue distribution of the barbiturates. It controls both the rate of absorption into the bloodstream and the rate of departure from the bloodstream across various blood-tissue barriers, including the blood-brain barrier (Brodie *et al.*, 1960).

With intravenously administered anesthetic barbiturates (*e.g.*, thiopental), whose high lipid-solubility enables their rapid transit across the blood-brain and other blood-tissue barriers, the rate of drug uptake by each tissue depends primarily upon the rate of blood flow to the tissue. The sequence of events is as follows: from the moment of intravascular administration, thiopental begins to pass into its locus of action (*i.e.*, into the brain) (Mark and Brand, 1964) and into pharmacologically inert tissues in the three body compartments (vital organs, lean body mass, adipose tissue). These events occur simultaneously but at different rates, depending primarily upon the circulation to the component structures within each compartment. Maximal concentrations appear in the brain practically instantaneously (*i.e.*, within one to two circulation times), with prompt onset of sleep (Mark *et al.*, 1957). Yet perfusion of the brain, although rich, is far from uniform, as demonstrated autoradiographically in animals by Landau *et al.* (1955), using as the indicator substance trifluoriodomethane-[131]I. In the conscious state, the highest rates of blood flow were found in the visual, auditory and somatosensory areas of the cerebral cortex, the geniculate bodies and the inferior colliculus. Correspondingly, Roth and Barlow (1961) observed high radiodensity (indicating high concentrations of drug) in the same areas examined similarly one minute after the intravenous injection of thiopental-^{14}C; at 30 minutes, distribution was uniform. It is interesting to note that, during light thiopental anesthesia, significant reductions in blood flow were observed in all of the above-named structures, especially the three sensory areas of the cortex (Landau et al., 1955).

Other organ tissues comprising the remainder of the richly perfused visceral compartment also receive thiopental rapidly. Thus, maximal drug concentrations were observed in the liver immediately following administration (Brodie et al., 1952). Although similar measurements have not been attempted with other vital organs, analogous findings may be presumed: thiopental concentrations in this highly vascular compartment quickly equilibrate with those in plasma.

Concurrently from the beginning, thiopental is also being distributed to the poorly perfused tissue components of the lean body mass (i.e., muscle, connective tissue, bone, etc.) and of the depot fats, with a corresponding fall in drug levels in blood, brain and other viscera. Drug concentrations in muscle reach a peak about 20 to 30 minutes after the end of injection in the dog (Brodie et al., 1952) and in man (Price et al., 1960), thereafter declining parallel to concentrations in plasma and viscera. Meanwhile, the drug is also entering adipose tissues, whose rate of blood flow is essentially the same as that to resting muscle (Perl et al., 1960). Unlike muscle, however, fatty tissues exhibit continued uptake by fat beyond the point at which muscle ceases to acquire thiopental. Thus, Mark and Brand (1964) could account for 50% of an administered dose in adipose tissues within 90 minutes after the end of administration, analogous to the findings of Shideman et al. (1953) of near maximal localization in human subcutaneous fat within 30 to 90 minutes.

According to Mountcastle (1968), skeletal muscle accounts for 42% of the total body weight of a normal man, while fat contributes 18%. Together they provide a substantial reservoir for the redistribution of thiopental from the viscera, including brain, thus contributing importantly to early awakening after a small dose of the drug. Because of its slow rate (9 to 15% per hour) (Mark, 1963a), biotransformation of thiopental is unimportant in these early events. After larger dosage, with delayed awakening, beyond 30 minutes thiopental is leaving both viscera and lean tissues, but up to about 90 minutes continues to enter fat at a considerable rate. Awakening during this period is mediated primarily by the distribution of the drug into adipose tissue depots. After still larger dosage, awakening is of course greatly delayed; beyond 90 minutes, fat continues to accumulate thiopental too slowly to be helpful. The further decline in plasma concentration and disappearance of thiopental from the body now depend solely upon the slow process of drug metabolism, and postanesthetic depression is apt to be greatly prolonged.

The preceding description of the pharmacokinetics of the highly lipid-soluble anesthetic barbiturates can be applied to the other commonly used barbiturates, with two important differences. Being less lipid-soluble, their rate of passage across the blood-brain barrier is slower, rendering them less useful as anesthetic agents (Mark *et al.*, 1958); and their accumulation is little or no more extensive in adipose tissues than in other tissues of the body (Table 1, C). Clinically, the hypnotic effect, once achieved, remains stable for a few hours, rather than the few minutes noted with the anesthetic barbiturates. Exhaustive documentation of these pharmacokinetic conclusions is lacking, but they have been confirmed in the case of pentobarbital in rats (Goldstein and Aronow, 1960).

BIOTRANSFORMATION

The chemical pathways of inactivation of barbiturates by drug-metabolizing enzymes residing in liver microsomes were discussed in Chapter 2. Suffice to note here that the barbiturates can be arranged into two groups according to their rates of metabolism, one group ranging from 10 to 70% per *day* (the so-called long- and medium-acting barbiturates), the other from 0.5 to 20% per *hour* (the anesthetic and so-called short-acting barbiturates) (Mark, 1963a). None of these is truly rapid: the barbiturates as a class are relatively stable *in vivo*.

EXCRETION

Since the glomerular filtrate is equivalent to protein-free plasma water (Chinard, 1952), that portion of any barbiturate in the bloodstream not bound to plasma proteins passes freely across the glomerulus. As noted above, the more lipid-soluble barbiturates are also more extensively bound to plasma proteins, with consequent reduction in concentration of free, filterable barbiturate in both plasma water and glomerular filtrate. Increased lipid solubility also facilitates reabsorption across the wall of the kidney tubule, which behaves like a lipoid barrier (Brodie, 1964), with resultant decrease in drug excretion in the urine. For example, following administration of the relatively lipid-soluble barbiturate pentobarbital in doses of 2.5 g to several human subjects, less than 1% of the original dose appeared in the urine over a 48-hour period (Brodie *et al.*, 1953). Conversely, the kidney does normally dispose of considerable fractions of some barbiturates, including barbital, allobarbital (Dial), aprobarbital (Alurate), phenobarbital and phenmethylbarbital (Rutonal) (Mark, 1963a), all of which are relatively poorly soluble in lipids.

It should be emphasized here that barbiturate metabolites resulting from drug oxidation in the liver have lost their pharmacologic activity (Mark, 1963a). Renal excretion of these inactive molecules and of other pharmacologically inert debris, such as might result from hydrolytic cleavage of the barbituric acid ring, contributes in no way to a further lessening of barbiturate effects.

THERAPEUTIC IMPLICATIONS

Pharmacokinetic considerations both suggest and impose limitations on potentially useful manipulations in the treatment of barbiturate poisoning. For example, as noted above, drugs with low lipid solubility, such as barbital and phenobarbital, are reabsorbed to a relatively small extent across the renal tubule, resulting in their substantial excretion in the urine. In addition, elimination of these barbiturates can be greatly enhanced by osmotic diuresis (Myschetzky and Lassen, 1963). On the other hand, more lipid-soluble barbiturates, such as secobarbital and pentobarbital, are readily reabsorbed from the renal tubule; as noted above, less than one per cent of the original dose appears unchanged in the urine. A two-, five-, or even ten-fold increase in renal clearance, readily demonstrable with increasing rates of urine flow (Cirksena et al., 1964), results at best in an unimportant increase in the urinary excretion of these barbiturates (Bloomer, 1966; Mark and Papper, 1967). Again, therapeutic manipulation of urinary pH was suggested by Waddell and Butler (1957), who first noted the unique pK_a, 7.2, of phenobarbital. Remember that a shift in pH towards the alkaline side of the pK_a increases ionization of the acid barbiturate. At a urinary pH of 8, readily achievable therapeutically, 86% of the poorly lipid-soluble phenobarbital is ionized and only a small fraction (14%) is present in the undissociated, reabsorbable form (Albert, 1960). This explains why renal excretion of phenobarbital (but not of barbiturates with higher pK_a values) is greatly enhanced by urinary alkalinization (Bloomer, 1966; Mark and Papper, 1967).

Pharmacokinetic considerations also influence the course of peritoneal dialysis, which utilizes the living peritoneum and mesentery as dialyzing membranes separating the patient from appropriate lavage solutions introduced into the peritoneal cavity (Maxwell et al., 1959; Boen, 1961). In acute barbiturate intoxication, a concentration gradient exists initially between the high barbiturate levels in the blood and the barbiturate-free dialysis fluid. However, commercially available solutions for peritoneal dialysis all range in pH from 5.1 to 6.2, a range in which barbiturates are largely undissociated. Since the concentration of unionized barbiturate in the peritoneal dialysate is considerably higher than that in the plasma, non-ionic back-diffusion into the bloodstream occurs, with disappointing yield of barbiturate in the dialysate (Gosselin and Smith, 1966). Barbiturate retrieval can be considerably augmented by adding human serum albumin or tromethamine (THAM) to the dialysis fluid (Berman and Vogelsang, 1964; Knochel et al., 1964; Nahas et al., 1965). The albumin provides an abundance of binding sites for the barbiturate, reducing the amount of unbound barbiturate within the dialysate and thereby maintaining a downhill concentration gradient from the bloodstream into the peritoneal cavity. The THAM provides an intraperitoneal pH of 9.8 to 8.5, well on the alkaline side of both the pH of the plasma and the pK_a of the barbiturate, so that less than 5% of the phenobarbital is present in the undissociated, reabsorbable form. Both mechanisms result in excellent yield of barbiturate in the dialysate. Unfortunately, the quantity of albumin required for an adequate course of peritoneal dialysis is prohibitively expensive, while THAM is not yet clinically available for this purpose.

For a more complete discussion of the application of these therapeutic measures in the clinical management of acute barbiturate poisoning, the reader is referred to the appropriate chapters of this book.

REFERENCES

ALBERT, A. (1960), *Selective Toxicity*, 209. Methuen, London.
BERMAN, L. B. and VOGELSANG, P. (1964), Removal rates for barbiturates using two types of peritoneal dialysis. *New Engl. J. Med.*, 270, 77.
BLOOMER, H. A. (1966), A critical evaluation of diuresis in the treatment of barbiturate intoxication. *J. Lab. clin. Med.*, 67, 898.
BOEN, S. T. (1961), Kinetics of peritoneal dialysis in comparison with the artificial kidney. *Medicine (Baltimore)*, 40, 243.
BRODIE, B. B. (1964), Distribution and fate of drugs: therapeutic implications. In: T. B. Binns (Ed) *Absorption and Distribution of Drugs*, 199. Livingstone, Edinburgh.
BRODIE, B. B. and HOGBEN, C. A. M. (1957), Some physico-chemical factors in drug action. *J. Pharm. Pharmacol.*, 9, 345.
BRODIE, B. B., MARK, L. C., PAPPER, E. M., LIEF, P. A., BERNSTEIN, E. and ROVENSTINE, E. A. (1950), The fate of thiopental in man and a method for its estimation in biological material. *J. Pharmacol. exp. Ther.*, 98, 85.
BRODIE, B. B., BERNSTEIN, E. and MARK, L. C. (1952), The role of body fat in limiting the duration of action of thiopental. *J. Pharmacol. exp. Ther.*, 105, 421.
BRODIE, B. B., BURNS, J. J., MARK, L. C., BERNSTEIN, E. and PAPPER, E. M. (1953),The fate of pentobarbital in man and dog and a method for its estimation in biological material. *J. Pharmacol. exp. Ther.*, 109, 26.
BRODIE, B. B., KURZ, H. and SCHANKER, L. S. (1960), The importance of dissociation constant and lipid-solubility in influencing the passage of drugs into the cerebrospinal fluid. *J. Pharmacol. exp. Ther.*, 130, 20.
CHINARD, F. P. (1952), Derivation of an expression for the rate of formation of glomerular fluid (GFR). Applicability of certain physical and physico-chemical concepts. *Amer. J. Physiol.*, 171, 578.
CIRKSENA, W. M., BASTIAN, R. C., MALLOY, J. T. and BARRY, K. G. (1964), Use of mannitol in exogenous and endogenous intoxications. *New Eng. J. Med.*, 270, 161.
GOLDBAUM, L. R. and SMITH, P. K. (1954), The interaction of barbiturates with serum albumin and its possible relation to their disposition and pharmacological actions. *J.Pharmacol. exp.Ther.*, 111, 197.
GOLDSTEIN, A. and ARONOW, L. (1960), The durations of action of thiopental and pentobarbital. *J. Pharmacol. exp. Ther.*, 128, 1.
GOSSELIN, R. E. and SMITH, R. P. (1966), Trends in the therapy of acute poisoning. *Clin. Pharmacol. Ther.*, 7, 279.
KNOCHEL, J. P., CLAYTON, L. E., SMITH, W. L. and BARRY, K. G. (1964), Intraperitoneal THAM: An effective method to enhance phenobarbital removal during peritoneal dialysis. *J. Lab. clin. Med.*, 64, 257.
LANDAU, W. M., FREYGANG,W. H., ROWLAND, L. P., SOKOLOFF, L. and KETY, S. S. (1955), Local circulation of the living brain; values in the unanesthetized and anesthetized cat. *Trans. Amer. neurol. Ass.*, 80, 125.
MARK, L. C. (1963a), Metabolism of barbiturates in man. *Clin. Pharmacol. Ther.*, 4, 504.
MARK, L. C. (1963b), Factors modulating barbiturate action. *Far East. J. Anesth.*, 4(2), 1.
MARK, L. C. and BRAND, L. (1964), Where does the Pentothal go? *Bull. N. Y. Acad. Med.*, 40, 476.
MARK, L. C. and PAPPER, E. M. (1967), Changing therapeutic goals in barbiturate poisoning. *Pharmacol. for Physicians*, 1(3), 1.

MARK, L. C., FOX, J. L., and BURSTEIN, C. L. (1949), Preanesthetic hypnosis with rectal Pentothal in children. *Anesthesiology*, 10, 401.

MARK, L. C., BURNS, J. J., CAMPOMANES, C. I., NGAI, S. H., TROUSOF, N., PAPPER, E. M. and BRODIE, B. B. (1957), The passage of thiopental into brain. *J. Pharmacol. exp. Ther.*, 119, 35.

MARK, L. C., BURNS, J. J., BRAND, L. CAMPOMANES, C. I., TROUSOF, N., PAPPER, E. M., and BRODIE, B. B. (1958), The passage of thiobarbiturates and their oxygen analogs into brain. *J. Pharmacol. exp. Ther.*, 123, 70.

MARK, L. C., PEREL, J. M., BRAND, L., and DAYTON, P. G. (1969), Distribution and metabolism of thiohexital (Letter to the Editor). *Anesthesiology*, 31, 384.

MAXWELL, M. H., ROCKNEY, R. E., KLEEMAN, G. R. and TWISS, M. R. (1959), Peritoneal dialysis; technique and applications. *J. Amer. med. Ass.*, 170, 917.

MOUNTCASTLE, B. B. (1968), *Medical Physiology*, 12th ed., Vol. 1, 289. Mosby, St. Louis.

MYSCHETZKY, A. and LASSEN, N. A. (1963), Urea-induced, osmotic diuresis and alkalinization of urine in acute barbiturate intoxication. *J. Amer. med. Ass.*, 185, 936.

NAHAS, G. G., GJESSING, J., GIROUX, J. J., VEROSKY, M. and MARK, L. C. (1965), The passage of THAM across the peritoneum during dialysis. *Clin. Pharmacol. Ther.*, 6, 560.

PERL, W., Lesser, G. T. and STEELE, J. M. (1960), The kinetics of distribution of the fat-soluble inert gas cyclopropane in the body. *Biophys. J.* 1, 111.

PRICE, H. L., KOVNAT, P. J., SAFER, J. M., CONNER, E. H. and PRICE, M. L. (1960), The uptake of thiopental by body tissues and its relation to the duration of narcosis. *Clin. Pharmacol. Ther.*, 1, 16.

ROTH, L. J. and BARLOW, C. F. (1961), Drugs in the brain. *Science*, 134, 22.

SCHANKER, L. S. (1959), Absorption of drugs from the rat colon. *J. Pharmacol. exp. Ther.*, 126, 283.

SCHANKER, L. S. (1960), On the mechanism of absorption of drugs from the gastrointestinal tract. *J. med. pharm. Chem.*, 2, 343.

SCHANKER, L. S., TOCCO, T. J., BRODIE, B. B. and HOGBEN, C. A. M. (1958), Absorption of drugs from the rat small intestine. *J. Pharmacol. exp. Ther.* 123, 81.

SHIDEMAN, F. E., GOULD, T. C., WINTERS, W. D., PETERSON, R. C. and WILNER, W. K. (1953), The distribution and *in vivo* rate of metabolism of thiopental. *J. Pharmacol. exp. Ther.*, 107, 368.

WADDELL, W. J. and BUTLER, T. C. (1957), The distribution and excretion of phenobarbital. *J. clin. Invest.*, 36, 1217.

5. *mode of action and acute toxic effects of barbiturates*

Lester C. Mark

Most drugs, including the barbiturates, are cellular poisons. To be therapeutically useful, the 'poisoning' must be *selective* for the specific target cell in the living body, without injury to other cells with which they are associated (Albert, 1960). Unless the target cells are invading organisms or cancer cells, the 'poisoning' must also be *reversible,* so that the effect produced can wear off when it is no longer needed.

In the case of the barbiturates, the spectrum of drug effects may be depicted as follows (Mark, 1969): sedation ⟷ hypnosis ⟷ anesthesia ⟷ poisoning → death.

Any of these effects can be achieved deliberately or accidentally by any barbiturate given in appropriate dosage. Yet the precise mechanism by which they are produced at the cellular or molecular level is unknown. While the question remains unanswered, therapy for overdosage can only be symptomatic.

Many years ago, Quastel and Wheatley (1932) noted that low concentrations of barbiturates inhibited the oxidation of glucose, lactate and pyruvate but not of succinate by a suspension of brain cells *in vitro.* This early observation suggested to Soskin and Taubenhaus (1943) that the administration of sodium succinate might furnish a substitute for the inhibited substrates, hence providing a useful antidote for barbiturate poisoning. Despite a brief flurry of enthusiasm (Barrett, 1949), the failure of others (*e.g.,* Giarman *et al.,* 1954) to confirm the postulated antagonistic effects of succinate finally led to its abandonment in therapy. Subsequently, Brody (1955) demonstrated that barbiturates depress the formation by brain slices *in vitro* of high energy phosphates, such as adenosine triphosphate (ATP) and phosphocreatine, which are essential to cellular function. This finding, however, is contrary to studies *in vivo* by McIlwain (1953), who found increased concentrations of phosphocreatine in the brains of anesthetized animals. Greig (1958) sought to reconcile these differences by suggesting that during anesthesia, when function is depressed, there is no demand for high energy phosphates, so they are not hydrolyzed, thus accounting for their accumulation *in vivo.* Her concept was based on the premise that decreased oxidative metabolism is the result and not the cause of psychodepression produced by barbiturates and other anesthetic agents.

The conflict between cause and effect was fueled but not settled by the studies of Landau *et al.* (1955), who measured blood flow to various brain areas in the cat. During consciousness, the highest rates of blood flow were found in the visual, auditory and somatosensory areas of the cerebral cortex, the geniculate bodies and the inferior colliculus; during light thiopental anesthesia, the blood flow to these structures was reduced 30 to 50%, with the greatest reductions in the three cortical areas subserving important sensory functions. These alterations in perfusion reflect comparable depression in metabolic rate and functional activity without defining the mechanism of its production.

Despite the lack of precise information concerning the molecular basis of barbiturate action, sites of action on a higher organizational and functional level have been defined by French *et al.* (1953) in the ascending reticular activating system. Located in the central core of the brain stem, this multisynaptic system extends from the spinal cord to the corpus striatum, with extensive but diffuse projections to the cerebral cortex. The importance of the system to the state of wakefulness was first demonstrated by Moruzzi and Magoun (1949), who produced electroencephalographic and clinical arousal in sleeping or lightly sedated cats by electric stimulation of the reticular formation in the brain stem. Conversely, selective ablation of the area resulted in irreversible unconsciousness. Potentials evoked in the ascending reticular system by electric stimulation of the sciatic nerve were suppressed by the administration of pentobarbital. Although other impulses in more laterally situated pathways reached the sensory cortex with unimpaired or even augmented intensity at first, later these, too, were altered. Inferring from the evidence that the multisynaptic interneuronal systems in the reticular formation and the cortex are more susceptible to the anesthetic agents employed (ether or pentobarbital), they concluded that drug-induced depression of these two areas contributed importantly to the anesthetic state (French *et al.*, 1953).

Increasing depressant effects on the brain would be expected with increasing dosage of barbiturate. Such is indeed the case, as noted by Kiersey *et al.* (1951). These authors described 5 different levels of barbiturate anesthesia, each with its distinctive electroencephalographic (EEG) pattern, as follows: Level I, corresponding to light anesthesia, during which the resting EEG pattern is suddenly replaced by a continuous succession of low voltage (10 to 25 μv) fast activity (10 to 25 cps), as shown in Fig. 1. Level II, moderate anesthesia, is marked by the appearance of high voltage (50 to 200 μv) slow waves (2 to 6 cps). Deep anesthesia, level III, is marked by the appearance of periods of electric silence or burst suppression of up to 3 seconds in duration. Levels IV and V in the danger zone are characterized by silent periods lasting up to and longer than 10 seconds respectively.

It would seem reasonable to expect a continuing correlation between EEG patterns and concentrations of drug in the plasma (which, of course, are in equilibrium with and hence reflect drug concentrations in the brain) with increasing depth of anesthesia. Such a correlation has been established with inhaled anesthetics, *e.g.*, ether

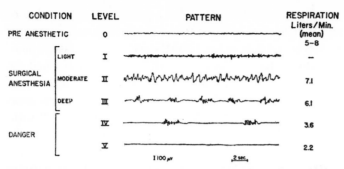

Fig. 1. Electroencephalographic patterns during thiopenal anesthesia. (From Kiersey *et al.*, 1951, with kind permission of the authors and *The British Journal of Anaesthesia.*)

(Faulconer, 1952) and cyclopropane (Possati *et al.*, 1953), but not with the intravenous anesthetic barbiturate, thiopental (Brand *et al.*, 1961). Thus, plasma thiopental concentrations ranged from 6 to 36 mg/l with EEG pattern I, 7 to 48 with pattern II, 10 to 50 with pattern III and 28 to 42 mg/l with pattern IV. Doubtless indicative of individual variations in susceptibility to the barbiturate, the wide and overlapping ranges of plasma drug levels obtained with each EEG pattern made it impossible to prognosticate accurately either the EEG pattern or the clinical status for any isolated plasma level of thiopental. A further observation was made that, with prolonged maintenance of a constant EEG pattern and clinical depth of anesthesia, plasma thiopental concentrations tended to rise successively higher, especially after the first hour. This probably represents a form of acute tolerance to the drug, a phenomenon previously demonstrated after large initial doses of thiopental (Brodie *et al.*, 1951). In the latter study, after receiving a large dose of thiopental, subjects awoke at plasma levels of drug considerably in excess of levels which adequately maintained a deep state of anesthesia after a smaller dose. The mechanism of this phenomenon remains obscure, although it is possible that a true tissue adaptation is involved: in a manner as yet undetermined, the central nervous system develops partial resistance to the depressant effect of a large dose of thiopental.

PHARMACOLOGIC AND ACUTE TOXIC EFFECTS OF BARBITURATES

The barbiturates as a class are sedative-hypnotic drugs, some of which are useful adjuncts to clinical anesthesia. The spectrum of barbiturate effects noted at the beginning of this chapter is, in essence, a dose-response curve of drug action, ranging from mild pharmacologic to maximal toxic effect. With the exception of certain methylated derivatives possessing convulsant properties, the barbiturates are all central nervous system depressants. In ordinary sleep doses they produce a gentle sleep without depression of reflex activity or muscle tone, while other organ systems exhibit only slight or no functional impairment, as in natural sleep. Parenthetically, it should be emphasized that barbiturate-induced sleep differs from physiologic sleep, with its recurring periods of rapid eye movement (REM); following barbiturate administration, the REM phase is almost completely suppressed (Oswald *et al.*, 1963).

In acute barbiturate intoxication, all degrees of depression of the central nervous system may be observed, from mild incoordination to profound coma. The patients may be classified as conscious (but intellectually impaired), stuporous (but rousable by painful stimulus), or comatose (unconscious and unrousable) (Locket and Angus, 1952), with obvious prognostic and therapeutic implications. Overdosage may be a pharmacologic accident, especially in the elderly, due to 'automatism' (Richards, 1934), in which the prescribed tablet or capsule produces not sleep, but an amnesic state. Aware of the need for medication but forgetful that it has been taken, the patient continues to repeat the dose at intervals until the supply has been exhausted (but see Chapter 17 on Barbiturate Automatism, p. 263).

CENTRAL NERVOUS SYSTEM

As noted above, the degree of depression may vary from mild incoordination, with slurred speech and disorientation, to profound coma, with absence of deep tendon, pupillary, pharyngeal, laryngeal and even cranial reflexes, and with positive Babinski sign. Periods of burst suppression may occur in the EEG (Fig. 1).

RESPIRATORY SYSTEM

The anatomic localization of the several elements of the respiratory center(s) within the reticular formation of the pons and medulla would seem to render these structures peculiarly liable to depression during surgical anesthesia. On the other hand, the wakeful state maintained by the reticular activating system may itself contribute to the regulation of breathing. Fink (1961) found rhythmic respiration persisting in conscious human subjects whose chemical (carbon dioxide) drive was eliminated by hyperventilation. It is thus difficult to determine whether respiratory depression during barbiturate anesthesia or barbiturate poisoning is due to the action of the drug on the reticular activating system as a whole, the respiratory center in particular, or both (Ngai, 1963). During experimentally excessive barbiturate depression, using thiopental, pentobarbital or enibomal (Narkotal), Gordh and Åström (1955) found the respiratory response to hypoxia (mediated by chemoreceptors in the carotid body and aortic arch) almost unimpaired although, at the same time, response of the respiratory center to carbon dioxide excess was greatly reduced or even abolished. These findings have therapeutic significance: attempted stimulation of respiration by inhalation of carbon dioxide has no place in the treatment of barbiturate poisoning. In addition, although the fears of some clinicians may be justified that oxygen inhalation, by removing the hypoxic stimulus, might further impair the already depressed respiratory function, the latter should be treated by appropriate support, including mechanical ventilation if necessary, rather than by withholding oxygen therapy.

CARDIOVASCULAR SYSTEM

Large doses of barbiturates can depress the cardiac and vasomotor centers in the brain stem, with resultant diminution in cardiac output, hypotension, and peripheral vasodilatation (Price, 1960). Although sufficiently high concentrations of barbiturates do exert a direct depressant action on isolated heart or heart-lung preparations *in vitro*, the doses utilized are usually far in excess of those compatible with life in man (Hardman *et al.*, 1959). Shubin and Weil (1965) attributed hypotension in barbiturate poisoning either to an absolute reduction in plasma volume or to a relative hypovolemia in relation to an expanded vascular bed, with cardiac output initially reduced and peripheral vascular resistance normal or increased. They obtained prompt increase in cardiac output, blood pressure, and urinary flow by the administration of large amounts of fluid (5 to 6 liters in 12 hours); vasopressor agents were generally detrimental to these effects.

GASTROINTESTINAL SYSTEM

Reduction in gastrointestinal tone and motility following barbiturate administration again reflect the central depression. Thus, Rosenblum and Cummins (1954) found comparable reduction in motor activity of the sigmoid colon in man during sleep and following a hypnotic dose of barbiturate. As a corollary, the clinician should remember that restoration of gastrointestinal function during recovery from acute barbiturate intoxication, with resumption of peristalsis and absorption of retained drug residue, may result in relapse of symptoms.

GENITOURINARY SYSTEM

Renal function is unimpaired during sedation, hypnosis, or light anesthesia with barbiturates. In deep anesthesia and barbiturate poisoning, urinary output may be markedly diminished, because of decreased renal blood flow secondary to systemic hypotension and to the increased secretion of antidiuretic hormone (ADH). The latter may itself reflect the altered hemodynamics, since reduction in the circulating blood volume appears to stimulate the secretion of ADH (Share, 1962). This information provides yet another indication for increased hydration of the poisoned patient.

HYPOTHERMIA

Hypothermia, a not uncommon concomitant of acute barbiturate poisoning, results from depression of the temperature-regulating center in the pons. The effect may be aggravated by prolonged exposure of the victim prior to his discovery.

LIVER

The barbiturates seem to exert no appreciable influence on liver function, except in the area of drug metabolism. Abundant evidence in animals, as well as some in man, has shown that barbiturates are potent stimulators of drug-metabolizing enzymes residing in liver microsomes (Conney, 1967). Both the amount of enzyme protein and the activity of the enzymes are greatly increased, resulting in more rapid metabolism of the drugs studied. To this should be appended the interesting observation that drugs such as the barbiturates can stimulate their own metabolism. The inducing effect is not instantaneous, requiring about three days of pretreatment with barbiturates in experimental animals. The fascinating possibility arises that prolonged barbiturate coma may also result in enzyme induction, providing an incidental contribution to therapy. Indirect support for this view comes from the finding of Remmer (1962) that the metabolism of the analgesic drug dipyrone was enhanced in patients with barbiturate poisoning.

OTHER TOXICOLOGIC CONSIDERATIONS

In cases of barbiturate poisoning, appreciable concentrations of the offending drug will be found in all body tissues and fluids (see Chapter 4). Potentially fatal blood concentrations have been designated as 3 mg% (*i.e.*, 30 mg/l) for the so-called short-acting, more lipid-soluble barbiturates, such as pentobarbital, secobarbital and amobarbital, and 10 mg% (100 mg/l) for the so-called long-acting, less lipid-soluble barbiturates, such as phenobarbital and barbital (Schreiner, 1958). Nevertheless, because of the wide variations in individual response to barbiturate, these figures must not be taken literally. Patients do die following massive overdosage of barbiturates, the mechanism of death undoubtedly consisting of a combination of asphyxia and cardiovascular collapse. However, the patient who reaches the hospital alive has, in a sense, conducted a therapeutic trial on himself: having withstood the primary onslaught, he is no longer in imminent danger of death from the ingested drug *per se*, whatever the blood level. Indeed, with proper supportive care to maintain respiration, circulation and excretion, all but 1 or 2% should survive (Brand and Mark, 1967). In the exceptions, death is usually attributable to irreversible cardiac, neurologic or renal damage from the combined effects of anoxia, shock, and exposure sustained prior to therapy.

REFERENCES

ALBERT, A. (1960), *Selective Toxicity*, 3. Methuen, London.
BARRETT, R. H. (1949), Sodium succinate – analeptic for barbiturate poisoning in man. *Ann. intern. Med.*, 31, 739.
BRAND, L. and MARK, L. C. (1967), Barbiturate dependence and intoxication. In: P. G. H. Wolber (Ed), *Tice's Practice of Medicine*, Vol. IX, chap. 23. Harper and Row, New York.

BRAND, L., MAZZIA, B. D., VAN POZNAK, A., BURNS, J. J. and MARK, L. C. (1961), Lack of correlation between electroenphalographic effects and plasma concentrations of thiopentone. *Brit. J. Anaesth.*, 33, 92.

BRODIE, B. B., MARK, L. C., LIEF, P. A., BERNSTEIN, E. and PAPPER, E. M. (1951), Acute tolerance to thiopental. *J. Pharmacol. exp. Ther.*, 102, 215.

BRODY, G. M. (1955), Uncoupling of oxidative phosphorylation in the mechanism of drug action. *Pharmacol. Rev.*, 7, 335.

CONNEY, A. H. (1967), Pharmacological implications of microsomal enzyme induction. *Pharmacol. Rev.*, 19, 317.

FAULCONER, A., JR. (1952), Correlation of concentrations of ether in arterial blood with electroencephalographic patterns occurring during ether-oxygen and during nitrous oxide, oxygen and ether anesthesia of human surgical patients. *Anesthesiology*, 13, 316.

FINK, B. R. (1961), Influence of cerebral activity in wakefulness on the regulation of breathing. *J. Appl. Physiol.*, 16, 15.

FRENCH, J. D., VERZEANO, M. and MAGOUN, H. W. (1953), A neural basis of the anesthetic state. *Arch. Neurol. Psychiat. (Chic.)*, 69, 519.

GIARMAN, N. J., ROWE, R. P. and YOUNG, J. (1954), The effect of sodium succinate and some of its derivatives on thiopental anesthesia. *Anesthesiology*, 15, 122.

GORDH, T. and ÅSTRÖM, A. (1955), Respiratory effects of oxygen deficiency and carbon dioxide excess during ether and barbiturate anesthesia in the dog. *Anesthesiology*, 16, 245.

GREIG, M. E. (1958), Theories of Anesthesia. In: V. A. Drill (Ed), *Pharmacology in Medicine*, chap. 3. McGraw-Hill, New York.

HARDMAN, H. F., MOORE, I. J. and LUM, B. K. B. (1959), A method for analyzing the effect of pH and of the ionization of drugs upon cardiac tissue with special reference to pentobarbital. *J. Pharmacol. exp. Ther.*, 126, 136.

KIERSEY, D. K., BICKFORD, R. G. and FAULCONER, A., JR. (1951), Electroencephalographic patterns produced by thiopentone sodium during surgical operations: description and classification. *Brit. J. Anaesth.*, 23, 141.

LANDAU, W. N., FREYGANG, W. H., ROWLAND, L. P., SOKOLOFF, L. and KETY, S. S. (1955), The local circulation of the living brain: values in the unanesthetized and anesthetized cat. *Trans. Amer. neurol. Ass.*, 80, 125.

LOCKET, S. and ANGUS, J. (1952), Poisoning by barbiturates: success of conservative treatment. *Lancet*, 1, 580.

McILWAIN, H. (1953), The effect of depressants on the metabolism of stimulated cerebral tissues. *Biochem. J.*, 53, 403.

MARK, L. C. (1969), Archaic classification of barbiturates. *Clin. Pharmacol. Ther.*, 10, 287.

MORUZZI, G. and MAGOUN, W. H. (1949), Brain stem reticular formation and activation of the E.E.G. *Electroenceph. clin. Neurophysiol.*, 1, 455.

NGAI, S. H. (1963), General anesthetics. Effects upon physiological systems. In: W. S. Root and F. G. Hofmann (Ed), *Physiological Pharmacology*, Vol. I, chap. A2. Academic Press, New York.

OSWALD, I., BERGER, R. J., JARAMILLO, R. A., KEDDIE, K. M. G., OLLEY, P. C. and PLUNKETT, G. B. (1963), Melancholia and barbiturates: a controlled EEG, body and eye movements study of sleep. *Brit. J. Psychiat.*, 109, 66.

POSSATI, S., FAULCONER, A. JR., BICKFORD, R. G. and HUNTER, R. C. (1953), Electroencephalographic patterns during anesthesia with cyclopropane: correlation with concentration of cyclopropane in arterial blood. *Curr. Res. Anesth.*, 32, 130.

PRICE, H. L. (1960), General anesthesia and circulatory homeostasis. *Physiol. Rev.*, 40, 187.

QUASTEL, J. H. and WHEATLEY, A. H. M. (1932), Narcosis and oxidations of brain. *Proc. roy. Soc. Med.*, 112, 60.

REMMER, H. (1962), Drugs as activators of drug enzymes. In: B. B. Brodie and E. G. Erdös (Ed), *Metabolic Factors Controlling Duration of Drug Action*. Proc. 1st Int. Pharmacol. Meeting, Stockholm, Vol. VI, 235. MacMillan, New York.

RICHARDS, R. (1934), A symptom of poisoning by hypnotics of the barbituric acid group. *Brit. med. J.*, 1, 331.

ROSENBLUM, M. J. and CUMMINS, A. J. (1954), The effect of sleep and amytal on the motor activity of the human sigmoid colon. *Gastroenterology*, 27, 445.

SCHREINER, G. E. (1958), The role of hemodialysis (artificial kidney) in acute poisoning. *Arch. intern. Med.*, 102, 896.

SHARE, L. (1962), Vascular volume and blood level of antidiuretic hormone. *Amer. J. Physiol.*, 212, 791.

SHUBIN, H. and WEIL, M. H. (1965), The mechanism of shock following suicidal doses of barbiturates, narcotics and tranquillizer drugs, with observations on the effects of treatment. *Amer. J. Med.*, 38, 853.

SOSKIN, S. and TAUBENHAUS, M. (1943), Sodium succinate as antidote for barbiturate poisoning and in control of duration of barbiturate anesthesia. *J. Pharmacol. exp. Ther.*, 78, 49.

6. formulation and presentation of the barbiturates

C. McArdle

THE NATIONAL PHARMACOPOEIAS

Since the original synthesis of malonylurea in 1863 (Baeyer, 1863), the medicinal potential of barbituric acid was dormant until the synthesis of diethylmalonylurea at the turn of the twentieth century (Fischer and Von Mering, 1903). This product was found to possess excellent hypnotic qualities. A further decade passed before the appearance of phenobarbitone, but a rapid expansion in the barbiturate field certainly occurred between the first and second World Wars until, at the present day, many appear to hold a permanent place in the pharmocopoeias of the world. The perusal of one particular U.K. index of ethical preparations, the *Monthly Index of Medical Specialities*, shows that no less than 169 proprietary formulations containing barbiturates are listed, the majority of which are in tablet and/or capsule form, with a minority as powders, elixirs, syrups, injections and suppositories.

The administration of drugs in the form of capsules and compressed tablets is now generally accepted as an ideal form of presentation and has largely replaced the powder, pill and mixture. The factors leading to this change are fairly self-evident: convenience to the patient, increased qualities of storage and stability, and more accurate dosage. The barbiturate group of drugs is no exception. A conservative estimate of usage of barbiturates in the United Kingdom (excluding hospital usage) is that in 1968 some 90,000 kg were prescribed, of which tablets and capsules accounted for 97.5% and injections some 2% (Lainton, 1969).

It is profitable to examine more closely the problems of formulation of tablets in particular. Since very few substances can be compressed without prior granulation, the first stage to be aimed at is the preparation of good granules. Most medicinal substances require the addition of one or more substances to assist in the preparation of granules and the compression of tablets. Such excipients must play their part in ensuring that the active principle is made readily available for absorption after the tablet has been swallowed. Each excipient must be scrutinized for chemical and pharmacological incompatibilities. The physical form of the drug itself is important and such factors as particle size may have an important bearing on the physiological availability after disintegration. The excipients used may be divided into:

(a) Diluents. For instance, where the drug dose is measured in milligrams, a diluent is used to give the tablet sufficient bulk for ease of handling. Examples of such diluents are methylcellulose, lactose, sucrose and mannitol.

(b) Adhesives. A prime requisite of the compression process is the binding together of powdered ingredients in order to produce free-flowing granules. Adhesives serve this purpose. Sodium alginate, sodium carboxymethylcellulose, gelatin solution, freshly prepared mucilage of starch, acacia and tragacanth gums find wide use today in this respect.

(c) Disintegrants. In order to ensure, after a tablet or tablets have been swallowed, that they break down into small particles within a reasonable time, a disintegrant is added and examples of such disintegrants are the starch grains of potato, maize and tapioca.

(d) Wetting agent. It may well be that one or more of the ingredients in a formulation is water-repellant and to overcome this a suitable non-toxic wetting agent is introduced.

(e) Lubricants are used to reduce friction between the tablet and the wall of the die during the compression and ejection cycle. They also prevent the adherence of tablet matter to the dies and punches. Examples are polyethylene glycol 6000, stearic acid, and its magnesium and calcium salts.

Tablets may have to be coated for a number of reasons such as an unpleasant taste, odour or appearance. Certain drugs may need protection from moisture, light, or carbon dioxide. The traditional process is that of sugar coating – a tedious operation requiring much skill and experience. To some extent this has been replaced by film coating, first introduced commercially in 1953 (Gross and Endicott, 1960). The materials used for film coating should be odourless, tasteless, and white or colourless and should be pharmaceutically inert and soluble in, or permeable to, gastro-intestinal secretions. Cellulose derivatives are usually the substances of choice in film coating, and many patents exist for the use of polymeric materials. Film coating, however, does not protect from oxygen, water vapour or carbon dioxide, and sugar coatings represent the only satisfactory alternative if such protection is required. Those tablets which have an emetic side effect or are sensitive to acid need to be enteric coated to prevent disintegration in the stomach.

With regard to tablets and capsules, certain controls are now standard requirements in most pharmacopoeias and these involve such factors as uniformity of tablet weight, active agent content and rate of disintegration.

Research into further problems, such as dissolution rate (in order to better control physiological availability) and microbial contamination of drugs not applied or administered as sterile products, is being actively pursued by workers in many countries (Hersant, 1969).

Thus it will be seen that the art of tablet making demands the knowledge and expertise of a number of related disciplines. The pharmacist, the organic chemist, the physical chemist, all have their part to play.

Dealing next with the division of the barbiturates into groups, it is conventional to use the groupings 'very short-acting', 'short-acting', 'intermediate-acting', and 'long-acting'. Table 1 shows which of the barbiturates are official in the various pharmacopoeias of the world, and given here are the detailed characteristics of the individual 'official' barbiturates, together with information on dosage and presentation.

VERY SHORT-ACTING

HEXOBARBITONE SODIUM (Mono-sodium derivative of 5-cyclohex-1'-enyl-1:5-dimethylbarbituric acid)

Characteristics: A white, crystalline, odourless, very hygroscopic powder with a bitter taste. An aqueous solution is strongly alkaline and slowly decomposes.
Dosage: 200 mg to 1 g, by intravenous injection. Also given by rectal injection with a maximum dose of 2 g.
Presentation: As a sterile dry powder for injection in strengths of 500 mg and 1 g.

NARCOBARBITAL (5-(2-bromoallyl)-5-isopropyl-1-methylbarbituric acid)

Characteristics: A white powder, with a bitter taste.
Dosage: Up to 1 g, by intravenous injection as a 10% sterile solution of the sodium derivative.
Presentation: As an injection.

TABLE 1

Barbiturates official in the pharmacopoeias of the world

Pharmacopoeia

Barbiturate	U.S.P.	Swiss. P.	Span. P.	Russ. P.	Roum. P.	Port. P.	Pol. P.	Nord. P.	Neth. P.	Mex. P.	Jug. P.	Jap. P.	Ind. P.	I.P.	Hung. P.	Ger. P.	Fr. P.	Cz. P.	Chin. P.	Chil. P.	Braz. P.	Belg. P.	B.P.	Aust. P.
Very short-acting																								
Buthalitone sodium																								
Hexobarbitone sodium	x				x		x	x	x		x	x			x		x			x	x	x	x	x
Methohexitone sodium		x		x			x																x	
Narcobarbital																		x						
Sodium thiamylal																								x
Thialbarbitone sodium																								x
Thiopentone sodium	x	x		x					x	x	x	x	x	x	x		x	x		x	x	x	x	x
Short-acting																								
Cyclobarbitone					x		x		x		x	x	x		x		x	x						x
Cyclobarbitone calc.		x			x		x	x	x			x	x	x	x	x							x	x
Heptabarbitone								x				x												
Hexobarbitone		x					x	x	x			x	x	x	x	x		x		x	x			x
Pentobarbitone calc.												x												
Pentobarbitone sod.	x	x		x						x		x	x	x				x			x		x	x
ditto free acid			x					x									x							
Quinalbarbitone	x													x			x							
Quinalbarbitone sodium	x	x	x	x										x			x							x

Intermediate-acting																								
Allobarbitone	x						x			x			x			x		x					x	
Allylbarbituric acid																								
Amylobarbitone		x					x			x	x		x				x							x
Amylobarbitone sodium		x						x			x		x							x	x			x
Aprobarbitone																x	x							
Aprobarbitone sodium																								
Butallylonal									x															
Butobarbitone		x						x		x						x								
Ibomal									x															
Nealbarbitone		x																						
Probarbital sodium																								
Secbutobarbitone sodium																								
Talbutal																								
Vinbarbitone																								
Vinbarbitone sodium																								
Long-acting																								
Barbitone	x		x	x	x	x	x		x	x		x	x	x	x	x	x	x	x	x	x	x	x	
Barbitone sodium	x	x		x			x		x		x	x	x	x		x		x		x	x	x	x	
Metharbitone																								
Methylphenobarbitone	x		x		x				x			x		x		x	x	x					x	
Phenobarbitone	x	x	x	x	x	x	x	x	x	x	x	x	x	x	x	x	x	x	x	x	x	x	x	x
Phenobarbitone sodium	x	x	x	x	x	x	x		x	x	x	x	x	x	x	x	x	x		x		x	x	x
Phenylmethyl barbituric acid																x								

METHOHEXITONE SODIUM (Sodium a-dl-1-methyl-5-allyl-5-(1-methyl-2-pentynyl) barbituric acid)

Characteristics: A white crystalline substance. Aqueous solutions are alkaline pH 11.1 to 11.4.

Dosage: 30 mg to 120 mg, by slow intravenous injection. The injection is a sterile solution of a mixture of 100 parts by weight of methohexitone sodium and 6 parts by weight of anhydrous sodium carbonate.

Presentation: As a sterile dry powder for injection in strengths of 500 mg, 2.5 g, and 5 g.

THIALBARBITONE SODIUM (Mono-sodium derivative of 5-allyl-5-cyclohex-2'-enyl-2-thiobarbituric acid)

Characteristics: A pale yellow, hygroscopic powder with an alliaceous odour. A 2.5% w/v in (carbon dioxide free) water has a pH of about 10.5.

Dosage: 0.2 to 1 g, by intravenous injection, usually as a 10% solution, prepared immediately before use.

Presentation: As a sterile powder in vials of 1 g and 2 g.

THIOPENTONE SODIUM (Mono-sodium derivative of 5-ethyl-5-(1-methylbutyl)-2-thiobarbituric acid)

Characteristics: A yellowish-white, hygroscopic powder with a characteristic alliaceous odour and a bitter taste. Solutions in water are alkaline to litmus. Decomposition occurs on standing, and precipitation occurs on boiling.

Dosage: 100 mg to 500 mg, by intravenous injection. 40 mg per kg body-weight by rectal injection with a maximum of 2 g. (B.P.)

45 mg per kg body-weight by rectal injection in a 5 to 10% solution to a total of 3 g. (U.S.P.)

Presentation: For injection as a sterile dry powder containing 6 parts of anhydrous sodium carbonate and 100 parts of thiopentone sodium, in strengths of 500 mg, 1 g, 2.5 g, and 5 g.

Suppositories in strengths of 125 mg, 250 mg, and 500 mg, and also as a rectal suspension in a buffered emulsion of light liquid paraffin.

SHORT-ACTING

CYCLOBARBITONE (5-cyclohex-1'-enyl-5-ethylbarbituric acid)

Characteristics: A white, crystalline powder, odourless, with a slightly bitter taste. Aqueous solutions are acid to litmus.

Dosage: 200 mg to 400 mg.

Presentation: As tablets.

CYCLOBARBITONE CALCIUM (Calcium derivative of 5-cyclohex-1'enyl-5-ethyl barbituric acid)

Characteristics: An almost white, almost odourless powder with a persistent bitter taste. A saturated solution in water is alkaline to litmus.

Dosage: 200 mg to 400 mg (usual).

(Ger. P. states 400 mg single dose and 1.2 g daily dose.)

Presentation: As tablets.

HEXOBARBITONE (5-cyclohex-1′enyl-1:5-dimethylbarbituric acid)

Characteristics: Colourless, odourless, tasteless, prismatic crystals. A saturated solution in water is neutral to methyl red.

Dosage: 250 mg to 500 mg (usual).

(Ger. P. states single dose 750 mg and daily dose 1.5 g.)

Presentation: As tablets in a strength of 250 mg.

PENTOBARBITONE CALCIUM (Calcium derivative of 5-ethyl-5-(1-methylbutyl) barbituric acid)

Characteristics: A fine, white, odourless, crystalline powder with a bitter taste. A saturated solution in water is alkaline to litmus.

Dosage: 100 mg to 200 mg (usual).

(Jap. P. states maximum single dose 500 mg and maximum daily dose 1 g.)

Presentation: As tablets.

PENTOBARBITONE SODIUM (Mono-sodium derivative of 5-ethyl-5-(1-methylbutyl) barbituric acid)

Characteristics: A white, odourless, crystalline powder or granules with a slightly bitter taste. A solution in water is alkaline to litmus and to phenolphthalein, and slowly decomposes.

Dosage: 100 mg to 200 mg. (B.P.)

Oral range 15 mg to 300 mg. I/V range 100 mg to 200 mg. (U.S.P.)

Maximum single dose 500 mg and maximum daily dose 1 g. (Jap. P .and Rus. P.)

Presentation: As tablets of 100 mg, as capsules in strengths of 30 mg, 50 mg, and 100 mg, and as ampoules 5 % in 2 ml, 5 ml, 20 ml, and 50 ml (adjusted to pH 10 to 10.5). Elixir 0.4%. (U.S.P.)

Note: Four pharmacopoeias, namely Fr., Neth., Nord., and Span., specify the free acid.

QUINALBARBITONE (5-allyl-5-(1-methylbutyl) barbituric acid)

Characteristics: A white, amorphous, odourless powder having a slightly bitter taste. A saturated solution is acid to litmus.

Dosage: 50 mg to 200 mg.

Presentation: As an elixir containing 440 mg per cent in a flavoured vehicle.

QUINALBARBITONE SODIUM (Mono-sodium derivative of 5-allyl-5-(1-methylbutyl) barbituric acid)

Characteristics: A white, odourless powder with a bitter taste. Hygroscopic.

Solutions in water are alkaline to litmus and to phenolphthalein. Solutions decompose on standing.

Dosage: 50 mg to 200 mg.

Presentation: As capsules, usually available in strengths of 30 mg, 50 mg, and 100 mg. As tablets in strengths of 50 mg, and 100 mg. As a sterile powder for parenteral use, usually available in a strength of 250 mg.

INTERMEDIATE-ACTING

ALLOBARBITONE (5,5-diallylbarbituric acid)

Characteristics: A white, crystalline, odourless powder with a slightly bitter taste. A saturated solution in water is acid to litmus.

Dosage: 30 mg to 200 mg.

Presentation: As tablets.

AMYLOBARBITONE (5-ethyl-5-isopentylbarbituric acid)

Characteristics: A white, odourless, crystalline powder with a bitter taste. Its solutions are acid to litmus.

Dosage: There is a wide variation of dosage in the various pharmacopoeias. 100 mg to 200 mg as a hypnotic, with up to 600 mg daily as a sedative. (B.P.) Dose range 100 mg to 300 mg. (U.S.P.) Maximum single or daily dose 300 mg. (Nord. P.) Maximum single dose 500 mg and a maximum in 24 hours, 1 g. (Cz.P., Fr.P., Hung. P. and Jap.P.)

Presentation: As tablets and capsules in a variety of strengths; elixirs, and also as a sterile powder for parenteral use.

AMYLOBARBITONE SODIUM (Mono-sodium derivative of 5-ethyl-5-isopentylbarbituric acid)

Characteristics: A white, odourless, granular powder with a bitter taste. Hygroscopic.

Dosage: 100 mg to 200 mg, as a hypnotic; up to 600 mg daily as a sedative.

Presentation: As tablets and capsules in strengths of 60 mg and 200 mg. As a sterile powder, usually available in strengths of 60 mg, 125 mg, 250 mg, 500 mg, and 1 g. Suppositories, containing 200 mg, have also been used.

APROBARBITONE (5-allyl-5-isopropylbarbituric acid)

Characteristics: A fine, white, odourless, crystalline powder with a slightly bitter taste. Stable in air. A saturated solution in water is acid to litmus.

Dosage: Usual dose 60 mg, but Nord.P. has a maximum single or daily dose of 300 mg, and Neth.P. has a maximum daily dose of 600 mg.

Presentation: As tablets.

BUTALLYLONAL (5-(2'-brom-allyl)-5-(1''-methyl-propyl) barbituric acid)

Characteristics: A fine, white, crystalline powder with a slightly bitter taste.

Dosage: 600 mg daily.

Presentation: As tablets.

BUTOBARBITONE (5-butyl-5-ethylbarbituric acid)

Characteristics: A fine, white, crystalline powder with a very slight odour and a slightly bitter taste. A saturated solution is acid to litmus.
Dosage: Usual dose 100 mg to 200 mg, but Fr.P. states a maximum daily dose of 600 mg.
Presentation: As tablets in a strength of 100 mg. Suppositories in strengths of 200 mg and 300 mg have also been used.

IBOMAL (5-(2'-brom-allyl)-5-isopropyl barbituric acid)

Characteristics: A white, crystalline powder with a slightly bitter taste.
Dosage: Ger.P. states single dose 400 mg and daily dose 800 mg.
Presentation: As tablets.

NEALBARBITONE (5-allyl-5-neopentylbarbituric acid)

Characteristics: A white, or slightly cream coloured powder with a very slight odour and a bitter taste.
Dosage: As a hypnotic, up to 200 mg. As a sedative, 60 mg to 180 mg daily in divided doses.
Presentation: As tablets.

LONG-ACTING

BARBITONE (5,5-diethylbarbituric acid)

Characteristics: A white, odourless, crystalline powder with a faintly bitter taste. A saturated solution is acid to litmus.
Dosage: Usual dose 300 mg to 600 mg, but Ger.P. states a maximum daily dose of 1 g.
Presentation: As tablets in strengths of 300 mg and 500 mg.

BARBITONE SODIUM (Mono-sodium derivative of 5,5-diethylbarbituric acid)

Characteristics: A white, crystalline, odourless powder with a bitter taste. A solution in water is alkaline to litmus.
Dosage: As a hypnotic, 300 mg to 600 mg. As a sedative, up to 900 mg daily in divided doses is usual, but Ger.P. states a maximum daily dose of 1 g.
Presentation: As tablets in strengths of 300 mg and 500 mg, as a 10% solution for parenteral use, and as a 5% solution for rectal administration.
Note: This substance is incompatible with ammonium salts, salts of heavy metals and acids, and with chloral hydrate, and is therefore best given without admixture.

METHYLPHENOBARBITONE (5-ethyl-1-methyl-5-phenylbarbituric acid)

Characteristics: A white, odourless, tasteless, crystalline powder. A saturated solution in water is acid to litmus.
Dosage: Usual dose 60 mg to 200 mg, but Ger.P. states single dose 400 mg and maximum daily dose 800 mg.
Presentation: As tablets in strengths of 30 mg, 60 mg, and 200 mg.

PHENOBARBITONE (5-ethyl-5-phenylbarbituric acid)

Characteristics: A white, crystalline, odourless powder with a slightly bitter taste. A saturated solution in water is acid to litmus.

Dosage: Usual dose, up to 350 mg daily in divided doses but U.S.P. states 15 mg to 100 mg, and Ger.P. states maximum single dose 400 mg, with a maximum daily dose of 800 mg.

Presentation: As tablets, usually available in strengths of 15 mg, 30 mg, 60 mg, and 100 mg. Elixir 0.4% w/v. (U.S.P.). Powder 1 in 10 w/w in starch or lactose. (Jap.P.)

PHENOBARBITONE SODIUM (Mono-sodium derivative of 5-ethyl-5-phenyl barbituric acid)

Characteristics: A white, odourless, hygroscopic powder with a bitter taste. A solution in water is alkaline to litmus and to phenolphthalein.

Dosage: Usual dose up to 350 mg daily in divided doses. By intravenous, intramuscular, or subcutaneous injection 50 mg to 200 mg, but U.S.P. states 15 mg to 300 mg, and parenteral 100 mg. Ger.P. states maximum single dose 400 mg, and maximum daily dose 1 g. Fr.P. states intramuscular single dose of 300 mg, with a maximum daily dose of 600 mg. Chil.P. and Swiss P. state a maximum single dose of 200 mg.

Presentation: Available as tablets in strengths of 30 mg and 100 mg, as injections, and as mixtures.

PHENYLMETHYLBARBITURIC ACID (5-methyl-5-phenylbarbituric acid)

Characteristics: A white, crystalline powder with a slightly bitter taste. A saturated solution in water is acid to litmus.
Dosage: Single dose 200 mg, with a maximum daily dose of 1 g.
Presentation: As tablets.

Other 'non-official' barbiturates in use are those listed below.

VERY SHORT-ACTING

BUTHALITONE SODIUM (Mono-sodium derivative of 5-allyl-5-isobutyl-2-thiobarbituric acid)

Characteristics: A pale yellow, hygroscopic powder with a very slight odour.
Dosage: Up to 1 g.
Presentation: For intravenous injection as a sterile dry powder containing 6 parts of anhydrous sodium carbonate and 100 parts of buthalitone sodium.

SODIUM THIAMYLAL (Mono-sodium derivative of 5-allyl-5-(1-methyl-butyl)-2-thiobarbituric acid)

Characteristics: A white powder with a disagreeable odour.
Dosage: 3 to 6 mls of a 2.5% solution intravenously.
Presentation: As a sterile mixture of sodium thiamylal with anhydrous sodium carbonate as a buffer, available in ampoules of 500 mg, 1 g, 5 g and 10 g.

SHORT-ACTING

HEPTABARBITONE (5-cyclohept-1-enyl-5-ethylbarbituric acid)

Characteristics: A white, crystalline powder with a slightly bitter taste.
Dosage: As a hypnotic, 200 mg to 400 mg. As a sedative, 50 mg to 100 mg.
Presentation: As tablets in a strength of 200 mg.

INTERMEDIATE-ACTING

ALLYLBARBITURIC ACID (5-allyl-5-isobutylbarbituric acid)

Characteristics: A white, crystalline powder with a slightly bitter taste.
Dosage: 200 mg to 400 mg daily.
Presentation: As tablets in a strength of 200 mg.

APROBARBITONE SODIUM (Mono-sodium derivative of 5-allyl-5-isopropylbarbituric acid)

Characteristics: A white, hygroscopic, odourless powder with a slightly bitter taste. Solutions in water are alkaline to litmus.
Dosage: Usual dose 20 mg to 80 mg, with a maximum daily dose of 300 mg.
Presentation: As a solution for oral or rectal administration.

Probarbital sodium (Mono-sodium derivative of 5-ethyl-5-isopropyl barbituric acid)

Characteristics: A white, hygroscopic powder with a bitter taste.
Dosage: 250 mg.
Presentation: As tablets.

Secbutobarbitone sodium (Mono-sodium derivative of 5-ethyl-5-sec-butylbarbituric acid)

Characteristics: A white powder with a bitter taste.
Dosage: As a sedative 30 mg, and as a hypnotic 100 mg.
Presentation: As tablets in strengths of 15 mg, 30 mg, 50 mg and 100 mg, and as capsules in a strength of 100 mg. Also as an elixir 6 mg/ml.

Talbutal (5-allyl-5-sec-butylbarbituric acid)

Characteristics: A white, crystalline powder with a slightly bitter taste. A saturated solution in water is acid to litmus.
Dosage: As a hypnotic 120 mg. As a sedative 30 mg to 50 mg.
Presentation: As tablets in strengths of 30 mg, 50 mg and 120 mg.

Vinbarbitone (5-ethyl-5-(1-methylbut-1-enyl) barbituric acid)

Characteristics: A white powder with a characteristic odour and a bitter taste.
Dosage: 60 mg.
Presentation: As capsules in strengths of 30 mg, 100 mg and 200 mg.

VINBARBITONE SODIUM (Mono-sodium derivative of 5-ethyl-5-(1-methylbut-1-enyl) barbituric acid)

Characteristics: A white, hygroscopic powder with a bitter taste. An aqueous solution is alkaline to phenolphthalein.
Dosage: As a sedative, 60 mg, and as a hypnotic, 100 mg to 200 mg.
Presentation: As a sterile solution for injection in a strength of 60 mg/ml, and as an elixir, 8.3 mg/ml.

LONG-ACTING

METHARBITONE (5,5-diethyl-1-methylbarbituric acid)

Characteristics: A white, crystalline powder with a faint aromatic odour.
Dosage: 100 mg, up to three times daily.
Presentation: As tablets in a strength of 100 mg.

PROBLEMS OF IDENTIFICATION

In addition to the official and semi-official tablets and capsules, many 'unofficial' or proprietary products with a barbiturate content are available throughout the world also in tablet and/or capsule form. Methods for the rapid identification of such solid dosage forms have been published by Hefferren (1962), Collier (1962), and McArdle and Skew (1961). Each of these is based on the physical characteristics of the tablet/capsule and, in the latter method, such characteristics are recorded on a punched card (see Fig. 1). Further useful information, such as taste, weight, diameter, thickness,

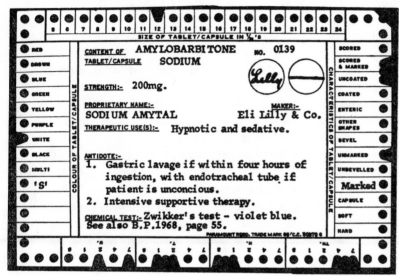

Fig. 1.

colour of inner core of tablets, type and colour of powder or granules in the case of capsules, therapeutic incompatibilities, and spectrophotometric and chromatographic information where such is thought to be desirable, is recorded on the reverse of the card. The method of operating this scheme is as follows:

A card is initially prepared for all authentic specimens of tablets and capsules as received from the manufacturer, punchings being made in accordance with the physical characteristics observed (see Fig. 1). Manufacturers samples are then stored in small plastic containers, each sample bearing a number corresponding to that of the appropriate card.

To identify an unknown tablet:

1. Measure the diameter of the tablet with a micrometer.
2. Refer the micrometer measurement to the appropriate size in 1/32nds of an inch as per card.
3. Insert a needle through the appropriate size hole, thus enabling all cards punched

at that particular size to drop. Discard any cards remaining on the needle. (This step is unnecessary if cards are filed in size order.)

4. Insert the needle through the appropriate colour hole, again rejecting all cards remaining on the needle.

5. Similarly, insert the needle through the holes on the right-hand side of card appropriate to the physical characteristics of the unknown tablet.

This, if not having positively identified the unknown, will have considerably narrowed the field of possibilities; examination of the colour of the inner core of the unknown tablet, along with its taste, weight, diameter and thickness, followed by comparison with the detail on the reverse of the remaining cards, will further assist positive identification.

To identify an unknown capsule, a procedure similar to that for tablets is adopted, thus:

1. The diameter of a capsule is taken at the widest point of the shortest axis and again referred to a size in 1/32nds of an inch.

2. With capsules, two needles must be inserted for colour, one for the colour of each half, but in the case of a single-colour capsule, the needles would be inserted through the actual colour and also at 'S' ('S' standing for single).

3. Needles are then inserted on the right-hand side of the card through: Capsule; Hard or Soft (as appropriate); Marked, if appropriate; and where a capsule has a band round the centre, then this is classified as a scoring and a needle should be inserted through the hole marked 'Scored'. To select any particular numbered card, the system used is '7, 4, 2, 1,' for each of thousands, hundreds, tens and units (marked on the bottom of the card). Two needles must be used for each digit required, each digit being made up as follows:

1 = 1 and S	6 = 2 and 4
2 = 2 and S	7 = 7 and S
3 = 1 and 2	8 = 1 and 7
4 = 4 and S	9 = 2 and 7
5 = 1 and 4	0 = 4 and 7

For instance, a card numbered 0139 would have needles inserted as follows: at 4 and 7; 1 and S; 1 and 20; 2 and 7.

Final confirmation of the tablet/capsule content can then be made by means of official pharmacopoeial tests or by the use of instant thin-layer chromatography.

DETECTION AND IDENTIFICATION OF BARBITURATES USING THIN-LAYER CHROMATOGRAPHY

This is a rapid and simple method of qualitative analysis, particularly when only minute portions of material for test are available.

The stages involved are:

(a) Preparation of standards: usually to a strength of 10 mg/ml, in chloroform or, if the barbiturate is present in the tablet or capsule as the sodium salt, in 17% glacial acetic acid in methanol.

(b) Extraction of the drug by organic solvents.

(c) The separation of the barbiturate or barbiturates involved, using instant thin-layer chromatoplates.

(d) The identification of the spots on the chromatoplates after spraying with reagents.

The solvent system used is very frequently a personal choice of the operator and a great deal of published work is available on such systems (Bogan *et al.*, 1964; Curry and Fox, 1968; Sunshine *et al.*, 1963). The method preferred by the author is that of D. R. Calavan, the procedure being:

Medium: I.T.L.C. – S.G. (glass microfibre sheets impregnated with silica gel adsorbent) activated at 110°C for 30 minutes.

Solvent: Iso-octane – glacial acetic acid 100:7.

Quantity applied: 5 µl.

Migration distance: 12 cm.

Differential spot reactions: The sprays used are:

(a) Mercuric sulphate reagent. (Suspend 5 g mercuric oxide in 100 ml distilled water. Add 20 ml conc. H_2SO_4 while stirring. Cool and dilute with water to 250 ml.)

(b) Overspray with diphenylcarbazone reagent (5 mg diphenylcarbazone in 50 ml chloroform).

(c) Potassium permanganate reagent (0.1% aqueous solution).

(d) Fluorescence. Fluorescein reagent 10 mg 27-dichlorofluorescein in 100 ml distilled water, plus 5 ml of 5N NaOH. Viewed under shortwave UV light (254 mµ) barbiturates give a purple spot against a yellow-green background.

Some examples of the colours given are as follows:

Compound	Mercuric sulphate reagent	Diphenylcarbazone reagent	Potassium permanganate reagent
Amylobarbitone	White	Violet	—
Aprobarbitone	None	Blue	Yellow
Cyclobarbitone	White	Blue	Yellow
Pentobarbitone	White	Violet	—
Phenobarbitone	White	Violet	—
Quinalbarbitone	White	Blue	Yellow
Secbutobarbitone	White	Violet	—
Thiopentone	White	—	Yellow

These colour reactions, in conjunction with the relevant R_f values for the solvent system used should be sufficient to establish positive identification.

Melting Points

Extraction of the powdered tablet with a suitable solvent (for solubilities see Table 2), evaporation of same and, after drying, the determination of the melting point of the substance, can also be an important aid to identification (see Table 3).

TABLE 2

Solubilities

Barbiturate	Water	Ethanol	Chloroform	Ether
Long-acting				
Barbitone	160	15	75	40
Barbitone sodium	5	600	0	0
Metharbitone	830	23		40
Methylphenobarbitone	Slight	240	40	200
Phenobarbitone	1,000	10	40	15
Phenobarbitone sodium	3	25	0	0
Phenylmethylbarbituric acid	0	60		
Intermediate-acting				
Allobarbitone	800	20		30
Allylbarbituric acid	Slight			
Amylobarbitone	1,500	5	20	6
Amylobarbitone sodium	Very	2	0	0
Aprobarbitone	350	2½	40	5
Aprobarbitone sodium	Very	Slight		0
Butallylonal	Slight	Freely	Soluble	Freely
Butobarbitone	250	1	3	10
Ibomal	V. Slight	Soluble		Slight
Nealbarbitone	5,000	4	80	5
Probarbital sodium	Very	Slight	0	0
Secbutobarbitone sodium	2	7	0	0
Talbutal	0	Soluble	Soluble	Soluble
Vinbarbitone	Slight	Soluble		0
Vinbarbitone sodium	Soluble	Soluble	Slight	Slight
Short-acting				
Cyclobarbitone	800	4	20	15
Cyclobarbitone calcium	100	0	0	0
Heptabarbitone	Sparingly	30	75	Soluble
Hexobarbitone	3,000	45	4	20
Pentobarbitone calcium	Slight	Slight		0
Pentobarbitone sodium	Very	Very		0
Quinalbarbitone	Slight	Very	0	0
Quinalbarbitone sodium	3	5		0
Very short-acting				
Buthalitone sodium	Freely			
Hexobarbitone sodium	Very	Very	Slight	Slight
Methohexitone sodium	Soluble			
Narcobarbital	Slight	20	Soluble	Soluble
Sodium thiamylal	Freely			
Thialbarbitone sodium	Very	Very	Slight	0
Thiopentone sodium	1.5	Soluble		

Very soluble	= Less than 1	Sparingly soluble	= 30–100
Freely soluble	= 1–10	Slightly soluble	= 100–1,000
Soluble	= 10–30	Very slightly soluble	= 1,000–10,000

TABLE 3

Melting points

Melting point range	Barbiturate
100	Quinalbarbitone
108–110	Talbutal
115	Narcobarbital
122–125	Butobarbitone
129	Pentobarbitone sodium (free acid)
130–133	Butallylonal
132–133	Sodium thiamylal (free acid)
138–139	Allylbarbituric acid
141–143	Aprobarbitone
145	Hexobarbitone
147	Buthalitone sodium (free acid)
151–155	Metharbitone
155–157	Nealbarbitone
155–158	Amylobarbitone
160–163	Vinbarbitone
165–168	Secbutobarbitone sodium (free acid)
171–174	Cyclobarbitone
172	Heptabarbitone
172–174	Allobarbitone
174–177	Phenobarbitone
178–181	Methylphenobarbitone
179–182	Ibomal
189–192	Barbitone
226	Phenylmethylbarbituric acid

REFERENCES

BOGAN, J., RENTOUL, E. and SMITH, H. (1964), Detection of barbiturates and related drugs by thin-layer chromatograph. *J. forens. Sci. Soc.*, 4, 147.
CALAVAN, D. R. (1969), *Clinical Toxicology Manual* (unpublished work).
CLARKE, E. G. C., and BERLE, J. (1969), *Isolation and Identification of Drugs*. Pharmaceutical Press, London.
COLLIER, W. A. L. (1962), Index of imprints used on tablets and other solid dosage forms. *Lancet*, I, 473.
CURRY, A. S. and FOX, R. H. (1968), Thin layer chromatography of the common barbiturates. *Analyst*, 93, 834.
FISCHER, E. and VON MERING, J. (1903), Therapie der Gegenwart (Cit. *Merck Index*, 1968).
GROSS, H. M. and ENDICOTT, C. J. (1960), *Drug and Cosmetic Industry*, 86 (2), 170–171, 264, 288, 291.
HEFFERREN, J. J. (1962), Identification guide for solid dosage forms. *J. Amer. med. Ass.*, 182, 1146.
HERSANT, E. F. (1969), Drug standards for the future. *Pharm. J.* ,vol. 203, 5523, 239.
LAINTON, K. F., (1969), Personal communication.
MCARDLE, C. and SKEW, E. A. (1961), A scheme for rapid tablet identification. *Lancet*, II, 924.
M.I.M.S. (1969), *Monthly Index of Medical Specialities*. Haymarket Press, London.
SUNSHINE, I. ROSE, E. and LEBAU, J. (1963), *Clin. Chem.*, 9, 312.
VON BAEYER, A. (1863), Wiebergs Annalen der Chemie, 127, 199 (Cit. *Merck Index*, 1968, p. 119, Merck, Rahway, N. J.).

7. clinical features of acute barbiturate poisoning

S. Moeschlin

OCCURRENCE

Acute poisoning by intentional ingestion of an overdose of barbiturates or similar hypnotics is steadily increasing in all so-called developed countries. Barbiturate poisoning can be treated very effectively today; thus the shift of suicides to this group has reduced the number of fatalities from other poisons such as corrosives, and also from other methods such as shooting, hanging and throat-cutting.

Accidental poisoning from barbiturates in children is less frequent than from other drugs. Homicidal poisonings are rare. Occasionally hypnotics are misused in order to stimulate illnesses and to obtain benefits (Laubenthal, 1951). A special criminal form to provoke narcosis for the purpose of robbery, etc., is the deliberate administration of barbiturates or other hypnotics dissolved in a pint or bottle of beer (Peters, 1969). Due to the well-known potentiating effect of alcohol this usually provokes deep sleep after a few minutes.

The number of patients suffering from acute barbiturate poisoning admitted to Swiss hospitals each year amounts to approximately 0.25% of the total admissions or to 0.3 per thousand of the population.

Chronic poisoning by daily misuse in addicts is rising in an alarming way in most developed countries, but this aspect will not be discussed in this chapter and the reader is referred to other papers (Moeschlin, 1964).

FATAL DOSE IN UNTREATED CASES

Fortunately most short-acting barbiturates developed in recent years are rapidly metabolized and eliminated. It is nevertheless wrong to assume that these short-acting preparations can be prescribed unhesitatingly, as relatively harmless drugs, to patients who may have suicidal ideas. The toxicity of these weaker and more rapidly metabolized drugs is still a question of the dose. Fatalities in such cases, discovered too late, still occur, for example from 20 g of heptabarbital (i.e., 80 tablets) or 10–20 g glutethimide (Doriden)). Although not a barbiturate, the danger of glutethimide in high doses must be particularly emphasized, as respiratory arrest is not uncommon in this now frequent form of poisoning. Poisoning due to this drug in Switzerland and Germany has in the last few years become more common than barbiturate poisoning (Ibe *et al.*, 1961; Reutter, 1961). The most dangerous preparations are still barbital and the other long-acting barbiturates, as their therapeutic index is extremely small. Little metabolism occurs in the liver, as they are largely excreted unchanged by the kidneys.

Phenobarbital is the preparation which takes the longest time for excretion. It can still be detected in the urine after as long as nine days (Staub, 1956). Table 1 gives the approximate lethal doses of some of these drugs in untreated cases. Combinations with tranquillizers or alcohol are much more dangerous. Fortunately, if treatment is begun at an early stage, before shock or severe respiratory depression develops, even severe poisoning is rarely fatal.

TABLE 1

Lethal doses of some hypnotics in untreated adults

Hypnotic	Lethal dose (without treatment)
Slowly eliminated, dangerous substances	
Barbital (Veronal) and Aprobarbital (Somnifen)	6 to 8 g
Allobarbital (Dial)	6 to 8 g
Phenobarbital (Luminal)	4 to 6 g
Glutethimide (Doriden) (eliminated in 3 days)	approx. 10 to 20 g (Ibe specifies 7 to 10 g but this dose is probably too low); depression of respiratory centre.
Rapidly eliminated, comparatively less dangerous substances (in descending order of toxicity) and analogous derivatives	
Chloral hydrate	approx. 5 g
Secobarbital (Seconal)	approx. 5 to 10 g
Cyclobarbital (Phanadorm)	approx. 20 g (80 tablets)
Heptobarbital (Medimin)	approx. 20 g (80 tablets)
Apronalide (Sedormid)	approx. 40 to 45 g
Hexobarbital (Evipan)	
Other mild hypnotics (Persedon; methyl prylonum – Noludar; etc.)	

Blood levels of different barbiturates may be of great help in the initial assessment of the severity of poisoning and in the evaluation of therapeutic measures. However, as stressed below, the clinical state of the patient is paramount. Setter *et al.* (1966) found that serum phenobarbital levels in 150 patients ranged from 1.9 to 29 mg/100 ml. A grade 1 or 2 coma, based on the criteria of Reed *et al.* (1952), was recorded in all but one patient with a serum level below 7 mg/100 ml, and a grade 3 or 4 coma in all but one patient with levels above 11 mg/100 ml. The duration of coma shows a linear relationship to the blood barbiturate level. Amylobarbitone intoxications were usually not severe unless the blood level exceeded 5.0 mg/100 ml, when deep coma was always present. The same was true for butobarbital. Coma was always grade 3–4 with serum secobarbital or pentobarbital levels above 3.0 mg/100 ml. Matthew and Lawson (1970), however, pointed out the lack of correlation between serum barbiturate level and the degree of unconsciousness. Higher blood levels of any specific barbiturate can be well tolerated by those who habitually take the drug. This is especially true of addicts and psychiatric patients. Some epileptics may still be awake at serum phenobarbital levels above 7.0 mg/100 ml. This last point shows clearly that the essential criteria in judging the severity of barbiturate poisoning are the clinical features.

On the other hand many patients now frequently take a combination of barbiturates and tranquillizers or other sedatives. These patients are more deeply intoxicated than one would predict from the blood level and they often improve slowly. However, if alcohol has also been involved, they may recover more rapidly than anticipated. Thus the blood levels are useful only in conjunction with clinical data. Serial blood levels, however, can give a quantitative guide to the response to therapy.

The mortality from barbiturate poisoning in hospital has shown a steady decrease over the last two decades. This is not so much due to the development of less toxic and more rapidly metabolized short-acting barbiturates, but more to the enormous progress in therapeutic measures, initiated by the Scandinavian school (Clemmesen and Nilsson, 1961), and later developed by many others. In an excellent and critical clinical study of 776 patients by Matthew and Lawson (1966) the mortality was only 0.8%. This figure may vary between 0.5 and 2.5% in different hospitals depending on the age distribution, combination with other sedative drugs, feasibility of rapid transportation, and adequate therapeutic measures.

In a way, we doctors can welcome the fact that attempts at suicide, which we shall never be able to prevent, have shifted more and more to poisoning by hypnotics, as this is probably the most 'agreeable' and at the same time the most 'uncertain' method of taking one's life, and as prolonged sleep will often help the patient to overcome his psychological problems.

CLINICAL FEATURES

From the practical point of view three or four grades of severity of poisoning are usually distinguished. The poisoning may begin as mild poisoning gradually changing into a more severe stage. Reed et al. (1952), modifying previous classifications of European authors, distinguished the following groups, basing their classification of severity of poisoning primarily on the degree of depression of the central nervous system:

Grade 0: Asleep but can be roused to speak.
Grade 1: Patient comatose, but responds to painful stimuli, has all tendon reflexes, and vital signs are stable.
Grade 2: Patient does not respond to painful stimuli but all deep tendon reflexes are present and vital signs are stable.
Grade 3: No response to painful stimuli and tendon reflexes are absent or almost totally absent, but vital signs are stable.
Grade 4: No response to painful stimuli, all deep tendon reflexes are absent, and supportive measures for maintenance of blood pressure and respiration are required.

Matthew and Lawson (1966) grade the patients according to their conscious level in the following way:
Grade 1: Drowsy but response to verbal commands.
Grade 2: Response to mild painful stimulation.
Grade 3: Minimal response to maximum painful stimulation.
Grade 4: No response to maximum painful stimulation.

They used rubbing of the patient's sternum with the knuckles as standard painful stimulus. This classification is of greater practical value, because the tendon reflexes and those of the cornea and pupils are too variable to be useful indices of the severity of poisoning. In this we agree from our experience with Matthew and Lawson (1966).

MILD POISONING

In mild cases, grade 1 of Reed, grade 1 and 2 of Matthew, the patient reveals the features of light anaesthesia. The deep tendon reflexes are present, the corneal reflexes are usually still active, and the patient responds to painful stimulation. The pupillary light reflex is present. Respiration and blood pressure are unchanged. These groups generally recover uneventfully. However, mild poisoning may slowly progress into a more severe form.

MODERATE POISONING

In moderate poisoning, grade 2–3 of Reed and grade 3 of Matthew, the deep tendon reflexes may still be partially present. Corneal reflexes are often already absent; however the pupillary reflexes are still present. The most essential sign is that the patient shows minimal response to painful stimulation. Respiration may be decreased but still adequate. Blood pressure remains normal.

SEVERE POISONING

In severe poisoning the patient is deeply comatose and does not respond to maximum painful stimulation. In the initial state the face is often reddened, then ashy-pale and finally cyanotic. Breathing becomes shallow, often slow at first and at a later stage usually rapid. Also the pulse rate tends to increase and, as the circulation begins to fail, becomes more rapid and of lower volume until finally it is barely palpable. The behaviour of the pupils varies. Usually they are constricted but, contrary to morphine poisoning, they still show a slight reaction to light. Often they are unequal and occasionally they are extremely dilated, these being, on the whole, unfavourable signs. In severe barbiturate poisoning the tendon reflexes gradually disappear. In most cases the corneal reflex is lost before the deep tendon reflexes, but there is no constant pattern. In serious poisoning the laryngeal and tracheal reflexes also vanish, leading to an accumulation of mucus in the bronchial tree which, if not treated, may precipitate respiratory failure.

Shock

Shock due to a direct toxic effect can develop at an early stage if a very large dose has been taken. More often, however, shock develops at a later stage secondary to peripheral vascular or respiratory or, rarely, cardiac failure. Typical of severe barbiturate poisoning, especially from barbital, is the development of a hypovolaemic shock: the haematocrit value increases and the total protein of the blood falls. Early detection of hypovolaemic shock is essential because of the importance of treatment with large amounts of plasma in addition to other measures. In all forms of shock the fall of blood pressure may lead to the impairment or cessation of renal function.

Other complications

As a result of capillary damage by the reduced blood flow and perhaps also by a toxic action, blisters of the skin and bedsores may develop, not only in the usual areas but also below the shoulder blades and over the spinal column (Holten, 1952; Beveridge and Lawson, 1965). The gluteal region is particularly endangered in late detected cases who have lain for a long time in the same position. They are rare in early discovered and adequately treated cases.

In rare cases, even in young people, extensive ischaemic muscular necrosis of large areas and whole extremities may occur. In all these cases, the combined effects of arterial compression by the immobility of the body together with the reduced general circulation and pronounced hypothermia contribute to the eventual necrosis.

We observed the case of a 22-year-old Italian who was found in deep phenobarbital coma after having lain for 36 hours in an unheated lavatory, squeezed between the wall and the w.c., during a very cold winter. On admission to hospital he was in severe hypovolaemic shock with anuria. After adequate treatment of the shock and peritoneal dialysis for several days, and despite severe hypostatic pneumonia, he recovered gradually. However, the left leg remained cold; the femoral and popliteal pulses were absent, and the patient died after three weeks. At autopsy the muscles of the whole of the left leg were yellow and necrotic and the left femoral artery was completely occluded by thrombosis below the inguinal region. The urine had contained myoglobin during the early part of his illness, resulting in renal damage, confirmed at autopsy. These ischaemic lesions are also very well known occurrences in severe carbon monoxide poisoning (Moeschlin, 1964) and they are particularly common in combined intoxications by barbiturate and carbon monoxide. Howse and Seddon (1966) have described four similar cases in carbon monoxide or barbiturate poisoning.

Pulmonary oedema

This is a relatively common complication of barbiturate poisoning. In some instances it may be due to overload of therapeutically administered fluid. Occasionally it may result from cardiac failure and also, especially in young people, from a toxic central origin as is sometimes seen in brain tumours. There is no doubt that barbiturates themselves in high doses can provoke pulmonary oedema, especially the barbiturates of the short-acting type (Setter *et al.*, 1966).

Pneumonia and pulmonary abscess

Both complications are possible in barbiturate poisoning. However, since the introduction of better care to prevent hypostasis and occlusion of bronchi, by repeated bronchial aspiration and change of body position, they are much less common. Some patients may have aspirated vomitus prior to hospital admission and they will usually develop aspiration pneumonia. Gastric lavage in the early phase, if performed carefully and in the typical position and in comatose patients with previous intubation, has never produced aspiration in our cases.

Blood changes

The white blood-cell count often reveals a leukocytosis, even in the absence of infection, of as much as 15,000–30,000/cu.mm with a distinct shift to the left. The probable cause is a relative acidosis as seen in other poisonings and the neutrophils show an absence of coarse toxic granulations. If distinct toxic granulations appear it is always a clear sign of bacterial infection (usually respiratory) but it can be cysto-pyelonephritis, which so often follows bladder catheterization). Hence daily examination of the blood smear is of value in all severe cases. The checking of the blood gases is of great value in cyanotic patients if there is any doubt of diminished oxygen saturation. In occasional instances the blood sugar may be reduced (Colldahl, 1947). Rarely we found a positive Wassermann reaction which rapidly returned to negative. The electrolytes need to be carefully monitored.

Urine

As already mentioned, the urine may contain albumin and some tubular casts in the initial phase. Some preparations, such as large amounts of barbital, may provoke mild signs of reversible tubular necrosis but it is always difficult to exclude other causes of renal damage, such as shock. Myoglobinuria with renal damage may occur in some rare cases with ischaemic muscular necrosis (see above and see also Fahlgren, 1957). Excretion of the different hypnotics varies considerably according to their metabolism. It is remarkably slow with phenobarbital and barbital if no forced diuresis is applied. The careful studies of Staub (1950) reveal that phenobarbital can be detected in the urine until the ninth day after ingestion. For the other barbiturates he found an average excretion at the eighth day of 2–4% of the amount normally eliminated on the first day after ingestion.

Foetus

Abortion is rare after acute barbiturate poisoning if it has not been combined with other poisons and if no severe anoxaemia or shock has occurred. Martland (1950) was able to demonstrate that barbiturates accumulate up to double concentration in the foetus.

Electroencephalogram (EEG)

The EEG in the comatose phase shows typical signs of depression. As the absorption progresses Krump (1956) claimed 'irritation phenomena' become apparent after 10 to 24 hours, the slow theta and delta activity being superimposed and interrupted by bursts of high voltage and high-frequency waves (12–15 and 18–24 cycles per second). Unlike the effects of mild poisoning, the amplitudes are augmented and the frequency is reduced as the severity of poisoning increases (Swank and Foley, 1948). In very severely poisoned patients, the tracing is flat. The EEG is therefore able to offer valuable prognostic and differential diagnostic information.

Electrocardiogram (ECG)

The changes which can occur in barbiturate poisoning are chiefly the result of concomitant shock or anoxia and are seldom due to a direct toxic effect. This is not the case in combined poisonings with thymoleptics such as imipramine, which can produce evidence of myocardial change and arrhythmias. The ECG may therefore reveal pathological findings, such as changes in the Q and T waves with flattening of the T wave or negativity. Clearly some patients with previous coronary vascular disease may show changes corresponding to the ECG after exercise. Usually all changes disappear after recovery of the patient from the poisoning.

Cerebro-spinal fluid

As we have demonstrated previously (Moeschlin, 1942 and 1957), the lumbar puncture may be of prognostic value in severe cases admitted a considerable time after ingestion. Usually if no severe brain degeneration has occurred, only a slight parenchymatous curve may be found with no distinct increase in total protein. The finding of a high total protein after correction of dehydration is usually a bad sign, indicating severe brain damage of probably irreversible type. There is likely to be necrosis of ganglion cells, occasionally encephalomalacia in the pallidum and other cerebral parts, and lesions of cerebral vessels (Scheidegger, 1937). Clinically it must be assumed, if this elevation in the total protein in the spinal fluid corresponds with other neurological changes and a flat EEG tracing, that further treatment will be ineffective if these toxic-degenerative changes have developed beyond a certain point. In this unit we would recommend curtailment of treatment after careful estimation of the clinical situation in such prognostically highly unfavourable cases. If, despite these findings, such cases are treated with all the measures of intensive care available today, severe permanent organic brain sequelae, such as dementia, Parkinsonism, Korsakoff syndrome, stupor and decerebration, may result. These may necessitate permanent hospital or psychiatric care, which we encountered in two such tragic cases.

Toxic psychoses

Severe states of excitement or even true toxic psychoses resembling acute schizophrenia are occasionally observed as consciousness is regained. Sometimes despite tranquillizers such patients have to be transferred to a psychiatric clinic. In one patient of 23 years, who had taken 17 g of barbital with suicidal intention and been comatose for 132 hours, this state of excitement with hallucinations persisted for three weeks.

Psychiatric management

Every patient on recovery from acute barbiturate poisoning has to be treated carefully in convalescence by a psychiatrist, to avoid depressive relapses and to help the patient psychologically. Often the former depression improves by the provoked 'sleeping-cure'. Although suicide is frequently denied, interviews obtained on early awakening while the patients are semi-confused often reveal positive information, which may not be obtained later on (Kessel, 1965).

Polyneuritis

Isolated neuritis or polyneuritis can occasionally occur in the convalescent phase. We observed a patient with typical paralysis of the left ulnar nerve after recovery. He had been found comatose, having lain on his left side on the floor for about 48 hours in a cold room in winter. The combined influence of cold, mechanical pressure, and the toxic influence of the barbiturate are responsible for most cases of polyneuritis after barbiturate poisoning. Recovery is usually complete but may take several weeks.

Thrombophlebitis and pulmonary embolization

This complication occurred in 5–6% of our patients; Hadden et al. (1969) reported this event in 3 out of 50 patients suffering from severe barbiturate poisoning. Especially severe cases with prolonged treatment are exposed to this complication which can be prevented by anticoagulant therapy.

COMBINED POISONING

Simultaneous ingestion of other sedative drugs or tranquillizers, narcotics and especially alcohol, gives rise to dangerous potentiation of the toxic effects of the barbiturates. Opiates, owing to their depressant action on the respiratory centre, are particularly dangerous in this respect, as are alcohol (Fisher *et al.*, 1948) and carbon monoxide. Under these conditions, doses of hypnotics that are in themselves not dangerous may even today cause fatal poisoning. After consumption of large quantities of alcohol, *e.g.*, three-quarters of a bottle of whisky, death has occurred from a routine dose of only four barbiturate tablets in non-treated patients. Special diagnostic difficulties may arise in combined poisoning with barbiturate and alcohol or carbon monoxide. If there is any doubt, the appropriate laboratory tests have to be performed. It is frequently not appreciated that steroid preparations may have a potentiating effect in acute barbiturate poisoning. Dhunér and Nordqvist (1957) demonstrated that cortisone, if given on awakening, may cause the patient to relapse into deep sleep. Thus in barbiturate poisoning or even anaesthesia, no cortisone should be given before, during or shortly after awakening.

DURATION OF COMA

This depends largely on the nature of the preparation and its metabolism and excretion and today especially on the therapeutic measures. Thus patients severely poisoned by phenobarbital, who would have slept up to 130–140 hours, may awake after only 12–24 hours if given a forced diuresis. Setter *et al.* (1966) observed an average duration of coma of 42 hours in patients who were hospitalized within 18 hours after ingestion. Hadden *et al.* (1969) reported a mean duration of 36 hours in 50 patients. However, in poisoning by the medium- and shorter-acting barbiturates, methods attempting to shorten the period of unconsciousness are almost invariably unrewarding (Matthew and Lawson, 1970).

DIFFERENTIAL DIAGNOSIS

In doubtful cases, in which the history is unhelpful, the following other possibilities must be borne in mind. Barbiturate poisoning differs from morphine poisoning in that the skin colour in the beginning is rather red, in comparison to the pallor of morphine poisoning. The pupils are not maximally constricted and the reaction to light is initially not completely abolished in barbiturate intoxication. Respiratory depression is usually more pronounced in morphine poisoning. The differentiation may present considerable difficulties, but a therapeutic test with nalorphine may be helpful. Carbon monoxide poisoning can usually be excluded if the light-red colour is only limited to the skin of the face and not spread out 'bright red' over the whole body. Naturally, in doubtful cases the blood carboxyhaemoglobin level has to be checked.

Severe poisoning from alcohol, ether, or other liquid hydrocarbons, which presents a picture similar to that of poisoning from hypnotics, can often be diagnosed by the typical odour of the breath. Estimations of the expired air by the well-known 'Draeger gas detector' (Moeschlin, 1964) with different test tubes may give a rapid answer in questionable cases, especially in the combined form of alcohol and barbiturate poisoning. Diabetic coma and hyperosmolar coma are easily recognized by the deep acidotic respiration; in case of doubt, blood sugar estimation will give the answer. As mentioned before, the blood sugar in barbiturate poisoning is normal or often below normal. An odour of acetone in the breath and a slightly positive acetone test in the urine may also be found in poisoning from hypnotics and is due to starvation, but the urine is usually free of sugar.

Differentiation from apoplectic coma is perhaps the most difficult, particularly in elderly persons. Special problems arise if the pathology is in the silent zone or if there is total areflexia and anamnestic information is lacking. Occasionally, unilateral constriction of a pupil may indicate the diagnosis, or it may be indicated in other cases by the result of the lumbar puncture. In all these instances the circumstances in which the patient was found must be carefully established in order to obtain further information. Moreover, gastric washings, urine, and blood must be examined for the presence of barbiturates.

Krump (1956) particularly emphasized the significance of the EEG in the differentiation from carbon monoxide poisoning and endotoxic comas as seen in uraemia, diabetes, and hepatic failure. In endotoxic comas the reduction in frequency precedes loss of consciousness, whereas in barbiturate poisoning there is an unusual contrast between deep coma and the irritation phenomena in the EEG. These differences are obscured only in the preterminal stage.

PROGNOSIS

Prognosis in barbiturate poisoning is determined chiefly by the age of the patient, the dose, and the nature of the barbiturate swallowed; also by the interval elapsing between ingestion and discovery. If a patient who has taken a high dose of a dangerous preparation is found after three to four days, the prognosis is grave. Further factors which may give rise to an unfavourable course are severe hypothermia or pre-existing cardiac failure. However, as mentioned above, patients treated within 24 hours after the ingestion nearly always show a favourable outcome. Hyperthermia and a persistent rise in pulse rate to 140–160 in patients with clear respiratory passages are often deleterious signs. If coma persists over several days despite the anticipated fall in the blood barbiturate level, lumbar puncture should be performed. Severe changes in the spinal fluid indicate serious, mostly irreversible, central damage and thus a very unfavourable prognosis.

IDENTIFICATION

Barbiturates can be detected spectrographically in the urine early in the illness (Helldorf et al., 1949). Today, however, paper chromatography has also achieved great significance in the detection of the non-barbituric hypnotics, such as glutethimide (Doriden).

It is a puzzling and alarming feature of our hectic modern world that the number of sedatives on the one hand and stimulants on the other is increasing so rapidly and steadily.

REFERENCES

BEVERIDGE, G. W. and LAWSON, A. A. H. (1965), Occurrence of bullous lesions in acute barbiturate intoxication. Brit. med. J., 1, 835.

CLEMMESEN, C. and NILSSON, E. (1961), Therapeutic tendency in the treatment of barbiturate poisoning. The Scandinavian method. Clin. Pharmacol. Ther., 2, 220.

COLLDAHL, H. (1947), Acta med. scand., 120, 257.

DHUNÉR, K. G. and NORDQVIST, P. (1957), Sleep re-induced by cortisone and glucose in patients intoxicated with barbiturates and related drugs. Acta anaesth. scand., 1, 55.

FAHLGREN, H., HED, R., and LANDMARK, C. (1957), Myonecrosis and myoglobinuria in alcohol and barbiturate intoxication. Acta med. scand., 158, 405.

FISHER, R. S., WALKER, J. T., and PLUMMER, C. W. (1948), Quantitative estimation of barbiturates in blood by ultraviolet spectrophotometry. Amer. J. clin. Path., 18, 462.

HADDEN, J., JOHNSON, K., SMITH, S., PRICE, L., and GIARDINA, E. (1969), Acute barbiturate intoxication. J. Amer. med. Ass., 209, 893.

HELLDORF, J., IDESTRÖM, C. M., and REIS, G. VON (1949), Clinical study of barbiturates and their demonstration in blood in barbiturate intoxication. Nord. Med., 1795.

HOLTEN, C. (1952), Cutaneous phenomena in acute barbiturate poisoning. Acta dermato-venereol. (Stockh.), 32, 162.

HOWSE, A. J. G. and SEDDON, H. (1966), Ischaemic contracture of muscle associated with carbon monoxide and barbiturate poisoning. Brit. med. J., 1, 192.

IBE, K., NEUHAUS, G., and REMMER, H. (1961), Akute Doriden-Vergiftung. Internist (Berl.), 2, 247.

KESSEL, N. (1965), Self-poisoning, part I. Brit. med. J., 2, 1265.

KRUMP, J. E. (1956), Kongressband der Tagung der Dtsch. Ges. Innere Medizin, Weisbaden, 133. Springer, Berlin.

LAUBENTHAL, F. (1951), Schlafmittelmissbrauch. Dtsch. med. Wschr., 76, 976.

MARTLAND, H. S. (1950), Placental barrier in carbon monoxide, barbiturate, and radium poisoning; some barbiturate and radium poisoning. Amer. J. Surg., 80, 270.

MATTHEW, H. and LAWSON, A. A. H. (1966), Quart. J. Med., 35, 539.

MATTHEW, H. and LAWSON, A. A. H. (1970), Treatment of Common Acute Poisonings, 18. Livingstone, Edinburgh.

MOESCHLIN, S. (1942), Die Sedormid-Thrombozytopenie anhand von Sternalpunktaten, Belastungs- und Transfusionsversuchen. Schweiz. med. Wschr., 72, 119.

MOESCHLIN, S. (1957), Phenacetinsucht und Phenacetinschäden. Schweiz. med. Wschr., 87, 123.

MOESCHLIN, S. (1964), Poisoning. Diagnosis and Treatment, 410. Grune and Stratton, New York.

PETERS, J. (1969), Personal communication.

REED, C. E., DRIGGS, M. F. and FOOTE, C. C. (1952), Acute barbiturate intoxication: a study of 300 cases based on physiologic system of classification of severity of intoxication. Ann, intern. Med., 37, 290.

REUTTER, F. (1961), On acute hypnotic poisoning. Internist, (Berl.), 2, 240.

SCHEIDEGGER, S. (1937), Veränderungen des Zentralnervensystems bei Vergiftungen durch Schlafmittel (Barbitursäurevergiftung). Schweiz. Arch. Neurol. Psychiat., 39, 388.

SETTER, J. G., MAHER, J. F., and SCHREINER, G. E. (1966), Barbiturate intoxication. *Arch. intern. Med.*, 117, 223.

STAUB, H. (1950), *Schweiz. Arch. Neurol. Psychiat.*, 65, 330.

SWANK, R. L. and FOLEY, J. M. (1948), Respiratory, electroencephalographic and blood gas changes in progressive barbiturate necrosis in dogs. *J. Pharmacol. exp. Ther.*, 92, 381.

8. *the skin in acute barbiturate poisoning*

Cutaneous manifestations of hypersensitivity to barbiturates are extensively documented. However the occurrence of bullous lesions in acute barbiturate intoxication has received little recognition. One of the earliest reports of blisters and skin ulceration in barbiturate poisoning was published in 1932 by Villaret. There have been a number of brief reports of similar lesions since then (Anderson, 1941; Reed *et al.*, 1952), but it is only recently that more detailed clinical studies have indicated that characteristic bullous lesions occur in 4–7% of those suffering from acute barbiturate intoxication (Holten, 1952; Lowther, 1959; Beveridge and Lawson, 1965).

In the majority of cases the blisters appear within 24 hours of ingestion of the barbiturate, and in a series of 290 cases studied in detail there was no evidence that any particular type of barbiturate was involved (Beveridge and Lawson, 1965). All the patients who developed blisters had been unconscious, but the occurrence of blisters did not appear to be related to the depth of coma, the occurrence of complications such as hypotension or hypoxia, or the ultimate recovery of the patient. The lesions had developed on sites where there had been some pressure but were relatively infrequent in maximum pressure areas such as the greater trochanters, sacrum, and scapular area. The most typical sites were on the limbs, particularly on the fingers and toes where two skin surfaces had been in contact, or on the heels, knees, and malleoli where the legs had been in apposition. The appearance of frank bullae was preceded by a marginate patch of erythema which became slightly raised. This appearance may on occasion resolve without progressing to bulla formation. Typical blisters are tense and have only a slight margin of erythema around the edge. In some situations, particularly on the hands and feet, large blisters may develop (see Fig. 1). The bullae contain a pale yellow fibrinous fluid and examination of this fluid has on occasions shown a concentration of barbiturate above that of the plasma. The base of the bulla exhibits a raw exudative surface comparable to a superficial burn and in most cases this heals without scarring, but in a few instances, particularly if secondary infection occurs, the lesions may be very persistent and leave scarring with occasional keloid formation, as has been reported by Blau *et al.* (1962).

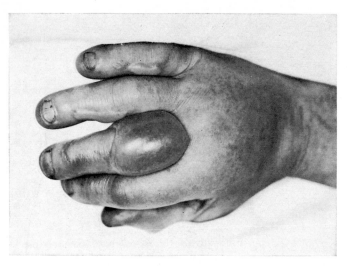

Fig. 1. A group of typical blisters. *(*Photograph by kind permission of the Editor, British Medical Journal).

There have been few reports on the histology of bullae occurring in barbiturate poisoning. Histological material from five patients was examined by Beveridge and Lawson (1965) and this showed a constant picture. In the roof of the blister the stratum corneum remained, but deep to this the epidermis showed marked signs of necrosis, the cytoplasm of the epidermal cells had become intensely eosinophilic, there was either loss of nuclear staining or occasional pyknotic nuclei, and in some areas all semblance of the epidermal cellular structure had disappeared. These changes extended through the full depth of the epidermis with almost complete loss of epidermal structure at the site of the bulla except for remnants of hair follicles and sweat ducts (see Fig. 2). The bulla fluid was acellular except for occasional nuclear fragments. In a very early blister it appears that the bulla has formed partly as a result of oedema occurring in the papillary layer of the dermis in addition to epidermal necrosis (see Fig. 3). In this material, which was all obtained from early lesions, there was no evidence of vascular damage or a marked inflammatory infiltrate in the dermis. Holten (1952), in addition to these changes, reported the presence of an inflammatory infiltrate around dermal vessels, but this was from post-mortem material, and may have been a secondary feature. Soltz-Szots and Sluga (1963), in a biopsy, noted fibrinoid degeneration in small vessels and extravasation of red cells, but this was not seen in any of the other histological material reported. More recently Leavell (1969), in sections from one case, has drawn attention to marked sweat gland necrosis and describes a section where, in relation to a sweat duct which has undergone necrosis, there is within the epidermis the formation of intra-epidermal and sub-epidermal vesicles, which may represent the earliest stage of bullous formation.

A number of different views have been expressed on the cause of these blisters.

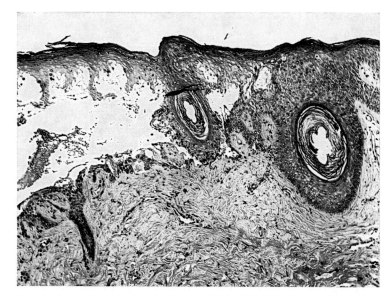

Fig. 2. A section from the margin of an intact bulla showing massive epidermal necrosis with remnants of a sweat duct and hair follicle (Haematoxylin and eosin x 80).

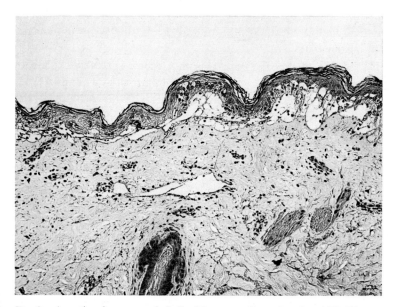

Fig. 3. A section from an early bulla (Haematoxylin and eosin x 100).(Photograph by kind permission of the Editor, British Medical Journal).

Some authorities such as Sorensen (1963) consider that they are solely the result of pressure; however, the rapid onset of the lesions and the fact that they do not necessarily occur over maximal pressure areas, and also do not clinically resemble decubitus ulcers, make it unlikely that this is the only factor. Lowther (1959) expressed the view that the lesions might in some way be related to depression of the central nervous system and therefore comparable to the skin lesions seen in association with other forms of severe brain damage (Robertson, 1953), and following leucotomy (Zeigler and Osgood, 1945; Mc Lardy, 1950). These lesions, however, develop more slowly and lead to massive and progressive necrosis of skin and subcutaneous tissues in the affected areas. The main histological feature in the lesions occurring in barbiturate intoxication, namely massive epidermal necrosis, is comparable to the changes noted in toxic epidermal necrolysis (Lyell, 1956). In Lyell's disease, which can be due to a number of aetiological factors, including drugs, Lyell (1967) considers that the damage to epidermal cells is probably the direct result of a toxin and not a manifestation of allergy. In the patients who had developed blisters, Beveridge and Lawson (1965) have shown, by means of patch tests and the administration of a challenging dose after their recovery, that there was no evidence of hypersensitivity to the barbiturates which they had ingested. In view of the histology it would seem likely that the skin changes are the direct result of the barbiturate, and an increased concentration in certain sites might result in the development of blisters. It could be that barbiturate interferes with the metabolism of the epidermal cells by inhibiting the pyruvic oxidase system. Recently Naylor (1970), in some interesting studies measuring the oxygen tension on the surface of the skin with a polarographic electrode, has shown that, after testing a number of drugs with a sedative effect, barbiturate was the most effective in reducing oxygen consumption of the skin.

The method of localization of the skin lesions has not been adequately explained, although pressure is probably an important factor. Soltz-Szots and Sluga (1963) suggest that both central depression of the vasomotor centre and the local loss of the ability to vasoconstrict peripherally, may lead to pooling of blood and a local increase in concentration of barbiturate. They quote animal studies in which piglets suffering from barbiturate poisoning readily developed blisters on the application of mechanical pressure which proceeded to necrosis within 48 hours of ingesting the barbiturate. In view of the recent observations of sweat gland necrosis in early lesions (Leavell, 1969), it is postulated that eccrine sweat glands, by excreting barbiturate, might increase the concentration of barbiturate, particularly if there are blockages of the ducts such as might occur when the fingers or two parts of the limbs were in contact. This is still hypothetical, and further investigations of the effect of barbiturates on the function of eccrine sweat glands will be required to determine their role from the point of view of excretion, and the effect that dysfunction may have on the temperature changes seen in barbiturate intoxication.

In most other forms of poisoning with sedative drugs, blisters have not been observed; however, recently in acute poisoning with tricyclic anti-depressants similar lesions have been reported in 4 % of the cases (Noble and Matthew, 1970). Blisters have occasionally been reported in carbon monoxide poisoning (Meigs and Hughes, 1952), but in our experience the lesions have developed later than the first 48 hours and have usually been characterized by wide areas of necrosis rather than discrete bullous formation. In conclusion, therefore, it is felt that, while the bullous lesions seen in acute barbiturate intoxication are not perhaps absolutely specific, they are sufficiently characteristic to strongly suggest this diagnosis.

ACKNOWLEDGEMENTS

Figures 1 and 3 are reproduced from Beveridge, G. W. and Lawson, A. A. H. (1965), Occurrence of bullous lesions in acute barbiturate intoxication. *Brit. med. J.*, i, 835, with the permission of the Editor, British Medical Journal.

REFERENCES

ANDERSON, J. P. (1941), The treatment of barbiturate intoxication with special reference to picrotoxin. A report of 20 cases. *Ann. intern. Med.*, 14, 2037.
BEVERIDGE, G. W. and LAWSON, A. A. H. (1965), Occurrence of bullous lesions in acute barbiturate intoxication. *Brit. med. J.*, I, 835.
BLAU, S., KANOF, N. B., and EIBER, H. B. (1962), Keloids in barbiturate coma. *Arch. Derm.*, 85, 747.
HOLTEN, C. (1952), Cutaneous phenomena in acute barbiturate poisoning. *Acta derm.-venereol. (Stockh.)*, 32, Supp. 29, p. 162.
LEAVELL, U. W. (1969), Sweat gland necrosis in barbiturate poisoning. *Arch. Derm.*, 100, 218.
LOWTHER, C. P. (1959), Barbiturate poisoning. *Scot. med. J.*, 4, 163.
LYELL, A. (1956), Toxic epidermal necrolysis: An eruption resembling scalding of the skin. *Brit. J. Derm.*, 68, 355.
LYELL, A. (1967), A review of toxic epidermal necrolysis in Britain. *Brit. J. Derm.*, 79, 662.
McLARDY, T. (1950), Uraemic and trophic deaths following leucotomy. Neuro-anatomical findings. *J. Neurol. Neurosurg. Psychiat.*, 13, 106.
MEIGS, J. W. and HUGHES, J. P. M. (1952), Acute carbon monoxide poisoning: Analysis of one hundred and five cases. *Arch. Industr. Hyg.*, 6, 344.
NAYLOR, P.D.F. and EVANS, N.T.S. (1970), The action of locally applied barbiturates on skin-oxygen tension and rate of oxygen utilization. *Brit. J. Derm.* 82, 600.
NOBLE, J. and MATTHEW, H. (1970), Acute poisoning by tricyclic antidepressants. *Clin. Toxicol.*, 2/4, 403
REED, C. E., DRIGGS, M. F., and FOOTE, C. C. (1952), Acute barbiturate intoxication. A study of 300 cases based on a physiologic system of classification of the severity of the intoxication. *Ann. intern. Med.* 37, 290.
ROBERTSON, E. E. (1953), Skin lesions in organic brain disease. *Brit. med. J.* I, 291.
SOLTZ-SZOTS, J. and SLUGA, W. (1963), Ungewöhnlicher Verlauf einer bartituratintoxikation. *Z. Haut.u. Geschl.-Kr.* 35, 299.
SORENSEN, B. F. (1963), Skin symptoms in acute narcotic intoxication. *Dan. med. Bull.*, 10, 130.
VILLARET, M., BITH, H., and DESOILLE, M. (1932), Ulcérations cutanées dues aux barbituriques. *Paris méd.*, 2, 340.
ZEIGLER, L. H. and OSGOOD, C. A. (1945), Oedema and trophic disturbances of the lower extremities complicating prefrontal leucotomy. *Arch. Neurol. Psychiat. (Chic.)*, 53, 262.

9. shock associated with barbiturate intoxication

H. Shubin and M. H. Weil

Shock which occurs as a complication of barbiturate poisoning is associated with profound coma and respiratory depression.

MECHANISM OF HYPOTENSION

The cardiac output is reduced. This is not due to heart failure, for central venous pressure is not elevated. Measurements of blood volume often reveal a reduction in the plasma component. When plasma volume is restored, both the blood pressure and cardiac output increase. Even when the blood volume initially is normal, augmentation of plasma volume results in an increase in blood pressure and cardiac output. These findings suggest that the hemodynamic defect is due to a deficit in effective blood volume, reflecting either an absolute decrease in plasma volume or an expansion of the capacity of the vascular bed accounting for relative hypovolemia (Shubin and Weil, 1965). The more frequent cause is a disproportion between blood volume and capacity of the vascular bed, and this hemodynamic defect accounts for the reduction in cardiac output and consequent fall in blood pressure.

PHYSICAL EXAMINATION

The patient characteristically is in a deep state of coma corresponding to the Grade 4 category of Matthew and Lawson (1966). Corneal and deep tendon reflexes are absent and pupillary response to light is minimal. Miosis, midriasis and normal size pupils are found with almost equal frequency. In a recent study (unpublished) of 33 patients in our Shock Research Unit, the rectal temperature was reduced to levels averaging only 35°C, and the skin was cool with the temperature over the great toes averaging only 26°C. Cyanosis of the earlobes, nose, or fingers is common. Spontaneous respiration, if present, tends to be shallow and rapid. A modest increase in heart rate is usually observed, but rates in excess of 130 per minute are uncommon. On clinical measurement, the blood pressure is typically reduced to levels of less than 80 mm Hg, systolic. However, the indirect pressure measurements which depend on detecting Karotkoff sounds are typically 10 to 20 mm Hg less than those obtained on direct measurement after insertion of a catheter into an artery. Moist rales are unusual; however, rhonchi and wheezes may be indicative of atelectasis or pneumonia, which is often due to aspiration of oral or gastric contents.

LABORATORY STUDIES

The serum levels of barbiturate do not necessarily reflect the severity of hypotension, respiratory depression, or coma. In our study of 33 patients, the mean level of short-acting barbiturate ranged from 2.2 to 11.2 (mean 3.8) mg% and long-acting barbiturate from 7.6 to 24.0 (mean 12.5) mg%. Serum levels above 3.5 mg% for short-acting barbiturates and above 10 mg% for long-acting barbiturates have been considered as potentially lethal levels (Berman et al., 1956).

The electrocardiogram often reveals non-specific ST-segment and T-wave changes. Serum oxalacetic transaminase and serum lactic dehydrogenase activity is elevated in the majority of patients. This reflects the more general tissue injury which is characteristic of circulatory deprivation and does not have specific significance with regard to the diagnosis of acute myocardial infarction (Shubin and Weil, 1963).

PATIENT MONITORING

Severe metabolic and respiratory acidosis frequently occurs in patients with shock and respiratory depression, thereby increasing the incidence of cardiac arrhythmias. Continuous electrocardiographic monitoring is warranted, therefore, in spite of the fact that the majority of patients are less than 40 years of age and without demonstrable ischemic heart disease. In some instances, the electrocardiogram may fail as an immediate indicator of 'cardiac arrest'. Electrocardiographic activity may continue for a minute or two after effective mechanical activity has ceased. Assessment of mechanical performance by a simple non-invasive technique is valuable. We have favored the finger plethsmograph for this purpose. Hemodynamic alterations are also reflected in a reduction in skin temperature of the large toes.The changes in skin temperature at this site often parallel changes in cardiac output (Joly and Weil, 1969).

Objective assessment of the hemodynamic and the respiratory status of a patient in shock and his response to therapy is facilitated by the use of arterial and central venous catheters (Weil and Shubin, 1967). The most important of these is a central venous catheter. A detailed description of the methods of its insertion and practical use, based on the experience in our center, has been published (Weil et al., 1965).

Repetitive measurements of central venous pressure (CVP) are especially valuable in assessing the patient's capacity to accept fluid loads. Although the central venous pressure *per se* may not necessarily reflect left ventricular and diastolic pressure, changes in central venous pressure in response to fluid challenge have served as a reliable indicator of the heart's competence to accept such fluid volumes when it is challenged.

A catheter inserted percutaneously for a distance of approximately 10 cm into the femoral or brachial artery is used to obtain measurements of arterial pressure. This catheter is also used for repetitive sampling of arterial blood in order to measure PO_2, PCO_2, and pH.

In our investigative unit, cardiac output is measured using a dye dilution method. Indocyanine green dye is injected into the central venous catheter and sampled from the arterial site. Measurements of plasma volume are also facilitated by the use of the central venous and arterial catheters. A tracer dose of radioactive iodinated serum albumin (I^{125}) is injected through the central venous catheter and samples of arterial blood are collected at 15, 25, and 35 minutes after injection of the radioactive material for scintillation counting. The volume in which the tracer has been diluted may then be calculated.

An indwelling urinary catheter is routinely inserted to facilitate measurement of urinary volume, particularly in response to the fluid challenge which has now assumed so major a role in patient management. Assessment of renal function is further enhanced by measurement of urine and plasma osmolality.

TREATMENT

Maintenance of effective circulating blood volume and of effective pulmonary gas exchange are the keys to successful management.

INTRAVENOUS FLUID

Selection of fluids

Colloid solutions, especially 5% human resum albumin, are preferred for initial treatment. Since electrolyte and crystalloid solutions, by their dilutional effects, are likely to decrease the colloid osmotic pressure of plasma, they are less likely to sustain an increase in intravascular volume. Expansion of intravascular volume appears to be particularly helpful in the early stages of fluid repletion when deficits in intravascular volume are likely to be most profound. We advise infusion of up to one liter of 5% albumin solution as part of the initial treatment. Subsequently, intravenous infusion of one liter aliquots of 10% glucose solution is alternated with one liter aliquots of 0.45% saline in 5% glucose solution. The 10% glucose solution also serves as an osmotic diuretic, like mannitol, but has the advantage of providing glucose and thereby prevents starvation acidosis. The administration of low molecular weight dextran offers no advantage over albumin solutions, and when given in volumes in excess of one liter, may impair blood coagulation. Since the primary blood volume deficit is due to a reduction in plasma volume and not to a deficiency in red cell mass, there is no indication for infusion of red blood cells. Blood transfusions are indicated only for complications in which there is massive blood loss.

Method of fluid administration

A reference value for the central venous pressure is established during a 10-minute observation period. The fluid is then infused, usually into a peripheral vein, at a rate of 20 ml per min., while at the same time central venous pressure is observed on a continuous basis. If the CVP increases by more than 5 cm of water above the initial pressure, the infusion is discontinued. If the CVP does not exceed the control value by more than 2 cm water at the end of 10 minutes, or if it declines to within that range over a second 10-minute observation period, an additional aliquot of 200 ml of fluid is administered over 10 minutes. The process is then repeated. This method of fluid challenge tests the competence of the heart to accept the volumes presented to it (Weil *et al.*, 1965). After the initial 400–600 ml fluid challenge, intravenous fluid is administered at rates ranging from 300 ml to 700 ml per hr., guided both by changes in CVP and urine flow. A progressive increase in CVP indicates overloading, and indicates the need for a reduction in the volumes of fluid that are being infused.

Barbiturate excretion

Administration of large amounts of fluid intravenously serves the dual purpose of augmenting the plasma volume with a consequent increase in cardiac output and blood pressure, and promoting a forced diuresis. Barbiturate clearance varies directly with the rate of urinary flow (Bunn and Lubash, 1965; Setter *et al.*, 1966). When the serum level of long- or intermediate-acting barbiturates is greater than 4 mg%, much larger amounts of barbiturate may be recovered from the urine (Linton *et al.*, 1967). Moreover, it has been demonstrated by chromatographic analysis that the excretion product recovered from the urine is the active drug (Bunn and Lubash, 1965).

Alkalinization of the urine

Passive renal tubular reabsorption of barbiturate is decreased by reducing the concentration of the diffusable or non-ionized form of the drug. Increasing the volume of urine by the administration of diuretics is one means of reducing the concentration of the diffusable drug, and thereby increasing its excretion. Another method of increasing excretion of barbiturate is to increase the ionized or non-diffusable form of the drug. In alkaline filtrate, a larger portion of the barbiturate is ionized, and the amount of barbiturate available for reabsorption is thereby reduced (Waddell and Butler, 1957; Lassen, 1960; Mollaret *et al.*, 1959; Myschetzky and Lassen, 1963). However, alkalinization of the urine is not a uniformly effective therapeutic technique because of the disassociation constants of individual barbiturates (Robinson *et al.*, 1967). When the pK value is relatively low as it is in the case of phenobarbital (pK 7.2), alkalinization may be useful (Lassen, 1960; Mollaret *et al.*, 1959; Myschetzky and Lassen, 1963; Robinson *et al.*, 1967; Monsallier *et al.*, 1967). However, when the pK value is relatively high as it is with secobarbital (pK of 7.9), alkalinization does not significantly increase excretion of ionized metabolite.

Diuretic therapy

With the availability of highly potent diuretic agents, and especially furosemide and ethacrynic acid, forced diuresis or so-called 'endogenous dialysis' has been widely adopted for routine therapy. Linton *et al.* (1967) suggest that the diuretic is used to increase urine flow so that, except for the initial load of 2 liters of fluid, urine flow keeps pace with volume infused. These investigators concluded that relatively large amounts of phenobarbital are removed by forced diuresis, and that this shortens the duration of coma and hence lowers the mortality rate. Forced diuresis is also regarded as therapeutically indicated in patients with poisoning due to intermediate-acting barbiturates (Bunn and Lubash, 1965; Setter *et al.*, 1966; Henderson and Merrill, 1966). Although osmolar diuresis by infusion of hypertonic solutions of mannitol was widely used (Cirksena *et al.*, 1964), it is now known that it offers no special advantage over glucose as an osmolar diuretic, and it may have detrimental effects in causing cellular dehydration (Morgan *et al.*, 1968).

The removal of barbiturate is the primary objective of forced diuresis. However, in patients in whom renal function has been previously impaired, or in those in whom excessively high levels of barbiturate are encountered (serum barbiturate of more than 20 mg%) hemodialysis or peritoneal dialysis may be employed (Robinson *et al.*, 1967; Leonards and Sunshine, 1953; Kyle *et al.*, 1953; Schreiner, 1958; Lubash *et al.*, 1962).

Vasoactive drugs

Adrenergic drugs

An increase in both blood pressure and cardiac output occurs when metaraminol (Aramine) or levarterenol (Levophed) are used in moderate doses to increase systolic pressure to a level of approximately 90 mm Hg. When larger doses are used and systolic pressure is increased to 'normal' levels, cardiac output usually diminishes. The increase in cardiac output and arterial pressure with moderate doses of metaraminol or levarterenol is attributable to joint alpha and beta adrenergic receptor stimulation. Beta adrenergic effect enhances myocardial contractility; alpha adrenergic effect primarily increases arterial constriction. When larger amounts of metaraminol or levarterenol are administered to raise arterial pressure to levels which approximate those prior to shock, this is accomplished by a disproportionate alpha adrenergic action, resulting in an increased workload on the heart, marked arterial constriction and venoconstriction, a decrease in venous return of blood to the heart, and a consequent decrease in cardiac output (Shubin and Weil, 1965).

The effect of metaraminol and levarterenol on blood volume is also of major concern. Protracted use of these drugs leads to an egress of intravascular fluid because they increase capillary hydrostatic pressure. Hence, they potentiate hypovolemia which in itself is a major mechanism accounting for the initial shock state (Kaltreider et al., 1942; Finnerty et al., 1958; Spoerel et al., 1964). Under these circumstances, even larger doses of the vasoactive drug will be needed to maintain 'normal' blood pressure levels. The problem is compounded during acidosis, when the blood pressure response to metaraminol and levarterenol is further decreased (Weil et al., 1958).

In our own series of 33 patients, we found 10 deaths among patients who had been treated with these vasoactive drugs, but not a single fatality among patients who were not so treated. Although patients treated with vasoactive drugs had a slightly lower arterial pressure initially, the striking disparity in survival is not fully explained by the difference in severity of shock. For these reasons, we disadvise the routine use of vasoactive drugs for therapy of circulatory failure when it is associated with barbiturate poisoning. Only in exceptional cases, as in an elderly patient with severe coronary heart disease, would we be inclined to administer vasoactive drugs on a temporary basis to increase systolic pressure to approximately 90 mm Hg to favor adequacy of coronary blood flow. However, as soon as volume has been repleted, therapy with vasoactive drugs would be discontinued.

Beta adrenergic drugs, such as isoproterenol (Isuprel), and alpha adrenergic receptor blocking agents, such as phenoxybenzamine (Dibenzyline) and phentolamine (Regitine), are also reserved for special indications. These drugs increase the capacity of the vascular bed. If they are administered prior to fluid, the disproportion between the vascular volume and size of the vascular bed is increased, and a sharp decline in arterial pressure and cardiac output may be noted. Restitution of plasma volume properly precedes treatment with these agents. In a small minority of patients who fail to improve after fluid challenge, and in whom limitations in cardiac competence are reflected in increased central venous pressure, isoproterenol may have beneficial effects. After infusion of isoproterenol in amounts ranging from 3 to 30 mcg per minute, central venous pressure is likely to decrease and concurrently an increase in blood pressure, cardiac output, and urine flow is observed. However, isoproterenol increases the requirement for myocardial oxygen and hence coronary blood flow (Weil and Shubin, 1969), and by its chronotropic action may greatly increase heart rate and myocardial irritability.

Digitalis

When barbiturate intoxication is severe, myocardial metabolism may be adversely affected, resulting in congestive heart failure (Farah and Maresh, 1948; Boniface and Brown, 1953; Vick et al., 1957; Goldberg et al., 1961). This is manifested by elevations of CVP, usually to levels in excess of 20 cm water, prior to or after infusion of less than one liter of fluid. However, CVP of between 12 and 20 cm of water is not necessarily an indication of this type of heart failure. The use of fluid challenge, as described earlier (Weil *et al.*, 1965), will help in the clinical differentation. When initially observed, the reduction in intravascular volume and consequent lowering of cardiac output and arterial pressure accounts for a significant decline in coronary blood flow. As the vascular space is filled during infusion, both cardiac output and coronary artery flow are increased. With more adequate coronary perfusion, myocardial function improves with a consequent reduction in central venous pressure. This is the paradoxical decline in CVP which is observed during fluid challenge. It is only for those patients in whom expansion of fluid volume causes a disproportionate increase in CVP that we advise treatment with digitalis glycoside. In our own unit lanoxin is preferred and is given intravenously in an initial dose of 0.5 mg. This is followed by an additional one to four doses, each of 0.25 mg, to reduce central venous pressure to a normal range.

RESPIRATORY MANAGEMENT

Airway

Prompt insertion of an oropharyngeal airway and suctioning of the oropharynx and trachea precede all other treatment in the comatose patient (Weil and Shubin, 1969). If gastric content is returned in the tracheal aspirate, extensive irrigation and tracheobronchial lavage are mandatory. The aspirate is routinely submitted for bacterial culture. Repetitive suctioning of the tracheobronchial passage, to prevent accumulation of secretions and atelectasis, is best performed with sterile disposable catheters which are discarded after each use.

The common practice of lavaging the stomach in order to remove residual barbiturate is potentially hazardous. If the patient vomits during the course of the lavage, disastrous flooding of the airway with gastric contents is likely to lead to life-threatening aspiration pneumonia. The gastric tube is first inserted and gastric contents are removed. An endotracheal tube is then inserted and the tracheal cuff is inflated. Only then, when the bronchi have been protected, is gastric lavage undertaken in the comatose patient. Periodic deflation of the endotracheal cuff, usually for a period of at least five minutes every hour, prevents pressure ischemic necrosis of the tracheal mucosa. Before the cuff is deflated, the contents of the oropharynx are thoroughly suctioned to prevent seepage of oropharyngeal secretions into the lungs.

The endotracheal tube is removed after spontaneous ventilation is restored. However, it may be left in place for at least three days, although we find that it is rarely needed for more than 48 hours. When mechanical or medical complications indicate the need of protracted intubation, a tracheostomy is advised.

The endotracheal tube is carefully secured, not only to prevent its accidental removal, but also to prevent advancement beyond the carina with occlusion of the main stem bronchus of one lung. This is likely to occur when the position of the patient in the bed is changed as a part of the nursing care, or when the patient reacts to the suction catheter. A sudden deterioration in the respiratory and cardiac status of the intubated patient brings this possibility immediately to mind. Asymmetry of movement of the chest wall and the absence of breath sounds over one lung serve as reliable physical signs which establish the diagnosis. Confirmation by X-ray entails an unwarranted delay. Prompt withdrawal of the tip of the endotracheal tube to a position above the carina is curative of this complication.

VENTILATION AND GAS EXCHANGE

In our series, progressive respiratory failure accounted for deterioration in the hemodynamic status of a majority of the fatal cases. We are convinced that physical signs fail us in assessing the adequacy of gas exchange. Only by repetitive measurements of arterial blood gases and pH can we establish the severity of ventilatory failure and response to respiratory therapy. Even when the patient appears to be ventilating adequately, hypoxia and hypercarbia may be so marked as to be immediately life-threatening. Hypoxia, with a reduction in partial pressure of oxygen in arterial blood (PO_2) to levels of less than 55 mm Hg (normal 80–100 mm Hg), and oxygen saturation to less than 90 % (normal 94 % or more), complicates the course of most of these patients. The arterial oxygen tension may be markedly reduced, but a corresponding decrease in the mixed venous oxygen content is not necessarily found. Since there is a large amount of peripheral arteriovenous shunting, little oxygen may be extracted during peripheral circulation. Decreased cellular metabolism is also implicated. The metabolic rate and hence the oxygen consumption are often profoundly reduced, and this is reflected in the low body temperature of these patients, which sometimes declines to less than 33°C.

If the arterial PO_2 is reduced to a level of less than 80 mm Hg or the arterial oxygen saturation to less than 94%, oxygen therapy is employed. The common practice of administering 100% oxygen on a continuous basis, however, invites further difficulty. 'Oxygen toxicity' following exposure to the 100% oxygen leads to a reduction in alveolar surface tension and atelectasis. Hence, oxygen may also potentiate the respiratory defect. When the arterial PO_2 is reduced, inhaled oxygen concentration is increased in a stepwise manner. Oxygen is first delivered in a concentration of 40%, using either a pressure-limited or volume-limited ventilator. Arterial blood samples are then taken and arterial PO_2 and oxygen saturation are again measured. If the oxygen has not increased to a normal range, then oxygen content of inhaled gas is increased by 10–20 % increments. Measurements of arterial PO_2 and oxygen saturation are repeated at intervals of two to four hours to guide oxygen therapy.

Carbon dioxide retention and respiratory acidosis are due to alveolar hypoventilation, which is in turn due to the reduced or absent stimulus to breathing. A reduction in minute volume to less than 4 liters is presumptive evidence of alveolar hypoventilation (Matthew and Lawson, 1966). The estimate of expected alveolar ventilation is based on body surface area. If the partial pressure of carbon dioxide in arterial blood (PCO_2) exceeds 55 mm Hg, an increase in alveolar ventilation is needed to reverse respiratory acidosis. The actual tidal volume which is delivered is repetitively measured with a suitable spirometer in the outflow line of the ventilator. If airway resistance is increased or pulmonary compliance reduced, the pressure delivered by the ventilator must be adjusted so as to maintain adequate alveolar ventilation. If compliance is reduced, delivery of an adequate tidal volume may require ventilator pressures in excess of 45 cm water, in which case use of a volume-limited ventilator may be required in place of a pressure-limited ventilator. By measuring tidal volume on a breath-to-breath basis, changes in blood gases may be anticipated and subsequently confirmed by periodic sampling of arterial blood.

The combined effects of metabolic acidosis due to perfusion failure and the respiratory acidosis of ventilatory failure account for unexpected but clinically dangerous cardiac arrhythmias. The reversal of the respiratory component of acidosis with restoration of pH towards normal is likely to terminate the arrhythmia and obviate the need for therapy with antiarrhythmic drugs.

RESPIRATORY INFECTION

Both gram negative and gram positive bacteria are likely to infect the respiratory tract in patients who are in coma and shock (Lewin *et al.*, 1970). More recently, gram negative organisms have predominated. In our own series, more than 40% of the patients had documented pulmonary infection, with gram negative organisms recovered almost twice as often as gram positive bacteria. The clinical course of these patients is characterized by a progressive reduction in arterial PO_2 despite delivery of increasing concentration of oxygen. Pulmonary compliance is progressively reduced and increasing ventilator pressure is required to deliver even a marginal tidal volume. The X-ray of the chest shows evidence of infiltration, often diffuse and resembling that due to congestive heart failure.

We recognize no indication for routine administration of antibiotics in the case of patients who maintain spontaneous ventilation after barbiturate intoxication. However, there is great likelihood of pulmonary infection in the most critically ill patients who have had ventilatory failure and shock. Specimens for bacteriological culture and sensitivity studies of the tracheal aspirate and blood are secured prior to instituting antibiotic therapy. However, we disadvise the 24 to 48 hour delay for identification of organisms and their sensitivity to antibiotics. A gram stain of the tracheal aspirate provides a clue as to the organism and a guide in the selection of an appropriate antibiotic. An awareness of current bacterial sensitivities within the individual hospital environment also is a major consideration in the choice of antibiotic. When gram positive organisms, particularly staphylococcus aureus, are suspected, methicillin is the drug of choice. When a gram negative infection seems most likely, gentamicin combined with chloramphenicol is initially selected by us. As soon as culture and sensitivity studies are available, antibiotic therapy is adjusted accordingly.

SUMMARY

Shock due to barbiturate poisoning is almost invariably associated with deep coma and severe impairment of respiration. Hypotension and a reduction in cardiac output are attributable to a disproportion between vascular capacity and volume. The blood volume is reduced and not adequate for the expanded capacity of the intravascular fluid space.

Treatment is directed primarily to restoration of an effective plasma volume. Large volumes of fluid are administered, guided by central venous pressure measurements. The fluid challenge is beneficial, not only in reversing the hemodynamic defect, but in promoting diuresis and excretion of barbiturate. Alkalinization of the urine and administration of a diuretic further enhance phenobarbital excretion. Peritoneal and hemodialysis are reserved for exceptional patients with impaired renal function.

Endotracheal intubation facilitates bronchial aspiration and mechanical ventilation for delivery of effective tidal volumes. The concentration of oxygen in the inhaled gas is modified on the basis of arterial PO_2. The tidal volume and respiratory rate required to reverse respiratory acidosis are established on basis of arterial blood PCO_2 and pH. Meticulous and aseptic airway care and appropriate antibiotic therapy are essential aspects of treatment because of the high incidence of pulmonary infection which constitutes the major cause of late deaths.

ACKNOWLEDGEMENTS

The investigations which form the basis of this presentation were supported by grants from The John A. Hartford Foundation, Inc., New York, and by the United States Public Health Service research grants HE 05570 and GM 16462 from the National Heart Institute and grant HS 00238 from the National Center for Health Services Research and Development.

REFERENCES

BERMAN, L. B., JEGHERS, H. J., SCHREINER, G. E., and PALLOTTA, A. J. (1956), Hemodialysis, an effective therapy for acute barbiturate poisoning. *J. Amer. med. Ass.*, 161, 820.

BONIFACE, K. J. and BROWN, J. M. (1953), Quantitative evaluation of cardiovascular-stimulant drugs in barbiturate depression of heart of dogs. *Anesthesiology*, 14, 23.

BUNN, H. F. and LUBASH, G. D (1965), A controlled study of induced diuresis in barbiturate intoxication. *Ann. intern. Med.*, 62, 246.

CIRKSENA, W. J., BASTIAN, R. C., MALLOY, J. P., and BARRY, K. G. (1964), Use of mannitol in exogenous and endogenous intoxication. *New Engl. J. Med.*, 270, 161.

FARAH, A. and MARESH, G. (1948), Determination of therapeutic, irregularity and lethal doses of cardiac glycosides in heart-lung preparation of dog. *J. Pharmacol. exp. Ther.*, 92, 32.

FINNERTY, F. A., BUCHOLZ, J. H. and GUILLANDEAU, R. L. (1958), The blood volumes and plasma protein during levarterenol-induced hypertension. *J. clin. Invest.*, 37, 425.

GOLDBERG, A. H., MALING, H. M., GAFFNEY, T. E. and WILLIAMS, M. A. (1961), The effect of digoxin pre-treatment on heart contractile force during thiopental infusion in dogs. *Anesthesiology*, 22, 974.

HENDERSON, L. W. and MERRILL, J. P. (1966), Treatment of barbiturate intoxication. *Ann. intern. Med.*, 64, 876.

JOLY, H. R. and WEIL, M. H. (1969), Temperature of the great toe as an indication of the severity of shock. *Circulation*, 39, 131.

KALTREIDER, N. L., MENEELY, G. R., and ALLEN, J. R. (1942), Effect of epinephrine on volume of blood. *J. clin. Invest.*, 21, 339.

KYLE, L. H., JEGHERS, H., WALSH, W. P., DOOLAN, P. D., WISHINSKY, H., and PALOTTA, A. (1953), The application of hemodialysis to the treatment of barbiturate poisoning. *J. clin. Invest.*, 32, 364.

LASSEN, N. A. (1960), Treatment of severe acute barbiturate poisoning by forced diuresis and alkalinization of the urine. *Lancet*, 2, 338.

LEONARDS, J. R. and SUNSHINE, I. (1953), Removal of barbiturates from blood by the artificial kidney. *Fed. Proc.*, 12, 237.

LEWIN, I., WEIL, M. H., SHUBIN, H., and SHERWIN, R. (1970), Pulmonary failure associated with clinical shock states. *J. Trauma* (in press)

LINTON, A. L., LUKE, R. G., and BRIGGS, J. D. (1967), Methods of forced diuresis and its application in barbiturate poisoning. *Lancet*, 2, 377.

LUBASH, G. D., FERRARI, M. J., SCHERR, L., and RUBIN, A. L. (1962), Sedative overdose and the role of hemodialysis. *Arch. intern. Med.*, 110, 884.

MATTHEW, H. and LAWSON, A. A. H. (1966), Acute barbiturate poisoning – a review of two years experience. *Quart. J. Med.*, New Series XXXV, 140, 539.

MOLLARET, P., RAPIN, M., POCIDALO, J. J., and MONSALLIER, J. F. (1959), Le traitement de l'intoxication barbiturique aigue; l'epuration par l'alcalinisation plasmatique et urinaire. *Presse méd.*, 67, 1435.

MONSALLIER, J. F., POCIDALO, J. J., and VACHON, F. (1967), Le traitement de l'intoxication barbiturique aigue. *Presse méd.*, 75, 2031.

MORGAN, A. G., BENNETT, J. M., and POLAK, A. (1968), Mannitol retention during diuretic treatment of barbiturate and salicylate overdosage. *Quart. J. Med.*, New Series, 37, 589.

MYSCHETZKY, A. and LASSEN, N. A. (1963), Urea induced osmotic diuresis and alkalinization of urine in acute barbiturate intoxication *J. Amer. med. Ass.*, 185, 116.

ROBINSON, R. R., HAYES, C. P. JR., and GUNNELLS, J. C. JR. (1967), Treatment of acute barbiturate intoxication. *Mod. Treatm.*, 4, 679.

SCHREINER, G. E. (1958), The role of hemodialysis (artificial kidney) in acute poisoning. *Arch. intern. Med.*, 102, 896.

SETTER, J. G., MAHER, J. F., and SCHREINER, G. E. (1966), Barbiturate intoxication: evaluation of therapy including dialysis in a large series selectively referred because of severity. *Arch. intern. Med.*, 62, 224.

SHUBIN, H. and WEIL, M. H. (1963), Acute elevation of serum transaminase and lactic dehydrogenase during circulatory shock. *Amer. J. Cardiol.*, 11, 327.

SHUBIN, H. and WEIL, M. H. (1965), The mechanism of shock following suicidal doses of barbiturates, narcotics and tranquilizing drugs, with observations on the effects of treatment. *Amer. J. Med.*, 38, 853.

SHUBIN, H. and WEIL, M. H. (1970), Shock associated with barbiturate intoxication. *J. Amer. med. Ass.* (in press)

SPOEREL, W. E., SELENY, F. L., and WILLIAMSON, R. D. (1964), Shock caused by continuous infusion of metaraminol bitartrate. *J. Canad. med. Ass.*, 90, 349.

VICK, R. L., KAHN, J. G., and ACHESON, G. H. (1957), Effects of dihydroouabain, dihydrodigoxin and dihydrodigitoxin on heart-lung preparation of dog. *J. Pharmacol. exp. Ther.*, 121, 330.

WADDELL, W. J. and BUTLER, T. C. (1957), The distribution and excretion of phenobarbital. *J. clin. Invest.*, 36, 1217.

WEIL, M. H., HOULE, D. B., BROWN, E. B., CAMPBELL, G. S. and HEATH, C. (1958), Vasopressor agents: influence of acidosis on cardiac and vascular responsiveness. *Calif. J. Med.*, 88, 437.

WEIL, M. H., SHUBIN, H. and ROSOFF, L. (1965), Fluid repletion in circulatory shock: central venous pressure and other practical guides. *J. Amer. med. Ass.*, 192, 668.

WEIL, M. H. and SHUBIN, H. (Ed) (1967), *Diagnosis and Treatment of Shock*, pp. 64 and 274. Williams and Wilkins, Baltimore.

WEIL, M. H. and SHUBIN, H. (1969), Isoproterenol for the treatment of circulatory shock. *Ann. intern. Med.*, 70, 638.

WEIL, M. H. and SHUBIN, H. (1969), The 'VIP' approach to the bedside management of shock. *J. Amer. med. Ass.*, 207, 337.

10. *the electroencephalogram in acute barbiturate poisoning*

Ijaz Haider

Recent progress in the field of experimental and clinical psychopharmacology has made available a large number of psychotropic drugs for the treatment of psychiatric disorders. At the same time incidence of self-poisoning is also rising and accounts for almost 10% of all acute medical admissions to certain general hospitals (Matthew, 1966). Figures of yearly admissions of poisoned patients to the Poisoning Treatment Centre of the Royal Infirmary of Edinburgh (Matthew and Lawson, 1970) showed a sharp rise from 120 admissions in 1948 to 1067 in 1968.

The epidemic nature of acute non-fatal poisoning has been highlighted in a recent publication (Central and Scottish Health Services Councils, 1968). An important factor in the increase of acute drug poisoning is the ready availability of drugs. According to Ministry of Health Report (1961) the amount of prescribed barbiturates doubled in England and Wales between 1953 and 1959 to about 1.5 g per head per annum, since which time the rate of increase has slowed (Ministry of Health, 1964), yet admissions of patients suffering from acute barbiturate poisoning have continued to rise. In the U.S.A. a production of 2.4 g of barbiturates per head was quoted for 1948 (Isbell *et al.*, 1950). In Czechoslovakia the prescription of barbiturates doubled between 1958 and 1965 (Vondracek *et al.*, 1968). In Australia hypnotic drugs constituted 13.2% of all prescriptions in 1966 (Commonwealth Director-General of Health, 1966). In Britain in 1962 hypnotics represented about 10% of all prescriptions (Ministry of Health, 1964). Overdosage of barbiturates is the commonest cause of acute poisoning due to drugs. Statistics for Britain indicate that approximately one half of the total annual mortality due to drug poisoning results from acute overdosage of barbiturates. Barbiturate poisoning results in prolonged unconsciousness accompanied by numerous alterations in vital autonomic functioning. The introduction of new methods of management, however, has meant that the duration of coma has gradually become less important.

The majority of patients with acute barbiturate poisoning are conscious or merely drowsy on admission, about one-third being unconscious (Matthew *et al.*, 1969). Many reports (*Brit. med. J.*, 1964; Matthew and Lawson, 1966; Kennedy *et al.*, 1969) have been published describing the clinical signs and symptoms and management of cases of acute barbiturate poisoning. Little work, however, has been done on the effects of overdose of barbiturates on brain functioning during acute poisoning.

REVIEW OF THE LITERATURE

Isolated EEG studies of coma patients were recorded in the early literature, *e.g.*, by Berger (1932). Gibbs *et al.* (1937) were the first to comment that marked slowing was characteristic of a variety of comatose states. Davis and Davis (1939) believed that the delta activity in coma was analogous to the delta of deep sleep, an opinion with which Strauss *et al.* (1952) later concurred. In the study of delirium Romano and Engel (1944) observed a general correlation between the degree of disturbance of consciousness and the degree and character of the EEG slowing, regardless of the aetiology of the comatose state. However, exceptions to the rule of delta slowing in coma have been reported (Fischgold and Bounes, 1946; Loeb and Poggio, 1953; Gastaut, 1954; Whelan *et al.*, 1955; Lundervold *et al.*, 1956; and Kaada *et al.*, 1961). In line with the investigation of Bancaud *et al.* (1955) and of Dell (1957) on cerebral lesions with and without disturbances of consciousness, Mathis *et al.* (1957) proposed that reactivity in comatose states was an important prognostic sign. Lennox and Petersen (1958) found a good correlation between clinical severity and EEG changes in patients with carbon monoxide poisoning. Pampiglione (1962) reported on 20 children with cardiac arrest and considered subsequent early EEGs to be of prognostic value. Loeb (1958) failed to find the EEG a reliable index of coma depth. He also described a variety of EEG patterns in 25 selected coma patients with verified brain lesions and concluded that generalized slowing was not to be found in this type of coma and that there was no definite relationship between the degree of coma and the types of EEG change.

The most exhaustive study of coma was reported by Fischgold and Mathis (1959); they studied 155 patients, roughly one-third of whom had coma due to trauma and one-third due to space-occupying lesions; only three cases were of toxic or metabolic origin. They described four stages of coma from both the clinical and the electrical viewpoints. On their scheme the EEG in Stage I shows a mixture of alpha, theta and some monophasic frontal or focal delta activity, and with alerting stimuli usually some initial blocking; patients can be aroused and when alerted have no loss of cephalic reflexes. In Stage II, the EEG shows delta activity which alternates with flattened and faster rhythms during periods of cardiac and respiratory slowing; alerting stimuli rarely cause blocking, but more often accentuate the delta activity (at times some alpha and theta may appear or a delta focus may become apparent). Only motor or monosyllabic verbal responses to stimuli can be obtained. In Stage III the EEG tends to become flat and is rarely affected by any arousal stimuli. All contact is lost, all cephalic reflexes disappear, vegetative derangements ensue and at times a state of decerebrate rigidity exists. In Stage IV the EEG is isoelectric and in this stage life has to be supported by artificial respiration. The prognosis, they reported, is progressively graver as one proceeds down the scale of coma – from 25% mortality in Stage I to 100% in Stage IV. As for differentiating coma from other states, they concluded that there were no electrical properties specific for coma and 'still less for a determined aetiology'.

Jouvet (1959) described Stage IV isoelectric comas of traumatic origin in four patients who were trephined; he found electrical silence in the thalamus as well as in the scalp recording. He felt that efforts to maintain life with artificial respiration for more than 24 hours were hopeless if the EEG remained isoelectric, a sentiment with which Schwab *et al.* (1962) concurred. On the other hand, Bental and Leibowitz (1961) published a case of possible encephalitis in which the EEG was flat for weeks, yet the patient ultimately recovered. Loeb *et al.* (1959) emphasized that considerable care must be exercised in assessing a flat record in a coma patient; with stimulation (*e.g.*, mechanical opening and closing of eyelids), some reactivity and a normal-appearing alpha rhythm may be demonstrated, particularly when the lesion is in the upper two-thirds of the pons.

Silverman (1963) in a retrospective study reviewed the EEG of 184 patients in relation to coma depth and the EEG. He divided clinical and electrical findings into four stages of coma identical with those of Fischgold and Mathis (1959). Out of twelve cases of drug intoxication seven were Stage I, one Stage II, and four Stage III. He concluded that study of the electrical responses to external stimuli, as well as the appearance of sleep-state potentials, gave a reasonable electrical indication of coma depth. In Stage I coma reactivity and sleep approached the normal; in Stage II both reactivity and sleep became distorted; in Stages III to IV both reactivity and sleep disappeared and the record tended to become monorhythmic and finally isoelectric. It was further concluded that a marked discrepancy between the clinical and electrical signs of deep coma suggests a brain stem lesion with a relatively intact cortex. He added that the finding of a barbiturate fast type of EEG record or of a mixed fast-theta record was suggestive of barbiturate or other sedative drug poisoning.

An isoelectric EEG in a patient with deep coma has become a problem in recent years with the greater success of resuscitation teams and with the greater efficiency in maintaining circulation and respiration in intensive care units. As surgeons and immunologists have made advances in organ transplantation, patients in irreversible coma become the main source of donor organs. Obviously the patient must be certifiably dead before organs can be transplanted, yet the organs must not have undergone degeneration. This has raised questions regarding the truth and certifiability of death and the exact time of death. With respect to the latter, there are two alternatives, either to await the cessation of the heart after the withdrawal of mechanical aids, or to declare the patient dead before such withdrawal once the irreversibility of the coma is established. Exceptions to the rule of cerebral death with isoelectric EEGs have been reported in the literature.

It has been shown (Opitz and Schneider, 1950) that in animals during experimentally produced anoxia the EEG becomes progressively lower in amplitude until it reaches zero potential, and if this anoxic state is allowed to persist for more than approximately four minutes, the brain and the EEG will not recover their function (Schneider, 1961 a and b); and in dogs Spoerel (1962) found a time of from three to five minutes from onset of ischaemia to irreversible EEG electrical silence. Under experimental conditions normal cardiac and respiratory function is usually maintained, so that perfusion of the brain with normally oxygenated blood follows immediately on cessation of anoxia; these conditions do not usually occur in clinical situations.

The changes observed in the human EEG during anoxia have been described by many investigators. Gronquist et al. (1952), Bellville and Howland (1957) and Brechner et al. (1961) have described fast (16–25 cps) low-voltage activity ('file pattern') in otherwise severely depressed or flat records. Bellville et al. (1955) noted slowing within 4 seconds of cerebral ischaemia in a patient undergoing cardiac surgery. Thies-Puppel and Wieners (1961) studied 30 patients undergoing cardiac surgery during hypothermia, and found that the interval between onset of ischaemia and disappearance of all electrical activity of the brain varied from 12–60 seconds. Return of EEG activity occurred between 30 seconds and 4 minutes after restoration of blood flow when ischaemia had been less than 7 minutes and up to 25 minutes after over 8 minutes of ischaemia. Brechner et al. (1961) noted that the EEG reappeared and became normal within minutes after cardiac arrest of only 2 minutes.

Hockaday et al. (1965) reported EEG changes in 39 comatose patients who had suffered cardiac arrest (26) or who had apnoea (13). The EEGs were classified into five grades, each with two subdivisions (a and b):

Grade 1 (within normal limits)
   a. Alpha rhythm.
   b. Predominant alpha with rare theta.
Grade 2 (mildly abnormal)
   a. Predominant theta, with rare alpha.
   b. Predominant theta, with some delta.
Grade 3 (moderately abnormal)
   a. Delta, mixed with theta and rare alpha.
   b. Predominant delta, with no other activity.
Grade 4 (severely abnormal)
   a. Diffuse delta, with brief isoelectric intervals.
   b. Scattered delta in some leads only with absence of activity in other leads.
Grade 5 (extremely abnormal)
   a. A nearly flat record.
   b. No EEG at all.

This system of classification consisting of ten types of EEG abnormality (five grades each with two subdivisions) was therefore used in a selected group of patients of acute cerebral anoxia. The anoxia was in every case sufficiently severe so that early recovery of consciousness failed to occur and the emergency EEG was obtained to establish whether the brain was alive and, if so, whether clinical recovery would follow.

Only six of the 39 patients survived. Patients with records of Grades IV and V (26) had a nearly hopeless prognosis as only one (Grade VI) survived. Patients with EEGs of Grade I, who invariably were conscious at the time of recording, carried an excellent prognosis for full recovery. Records of Grades II and III were of less certain prognostic value as only one of three of Grade II and three of nine of Grade III survived. Their overall accuracy of prognosis was 83%. They concluded that the EEG can be of considerable help in establishing death in the presence of a restored heart-beat, and suggested that further attention be given to the definition of death.

It has also been known experimentally and clinically that anaesthetics produce periods of isoelectric activity in the EEG. The intravenous administration of amylobarbitone, pentobarbitone, barbitone and thiopentone initially induced 18–20 cps fast activity, beginning in the frontal areas and gradually spreading over the whole cortex, associated with slight clouding of consciousness or euphoria. With further administration, 3–4 cps activity appears usually at the time of loss of consciousness (Cohn and Katzenelbogen, 1942; Brazier and Finesinger, 1945). Swank and Foley (1948) have studied the electroencephalographic changes during progressive sodium amylobarbitone narcosis in dogs. In light narcosis, the record was dominated by periodic bursts of 10 cps sharp waves; gradual slowing of the brain waves, with concomitant amplitude increase, was seen during moderate narcosis and the appearance of periods of electrical silence in the EEG during sleep narcosis. These periods of suppression were one to five seconds long at first. They became longer as the narcosis deepened and finally, just before death, continuous suppression was present. They reported that in all instances the cortex became electrically inactive, continuously, before the breathing and the heart stopped.

Kiersey et al. (1951) studied the EEG patterns after thiopentone sodium anaesthesia in patients undergoing surgical treatment for varicose veins of the legs. They classified the EEG changes into five patterns. The first pattern (fast) was characterized by high-amplitude, fast, spiky activity of mixed frequencies varying between 10 and 30 cps with the predominant frequency near 20 cps. During this pattern consciousness, though dulled, was retained in the early phases. The second pattern (complex) consisted of many frequencies of predominantly slower wave forms of very irregular contour and random occurrence. Superimposed on these slower waves and occupying the intervals between them was a faster activity at about 10 cps, rather spiky in character and irregular in amplitude. This second pattern was accompanied by loss of consciousness and reduced reflex activity. Withdrawal reaction to painful stimuli was abolished. The third pattern was characterized by a progressive suppression of cortical activity taking the form of short periods of relative quiescence which separated bursts of activity. In this pattern the periods of inactivity did not exceed 3 seconds in length. As the third pattern appeared, reduction of respiratory minute volume became more marked. The fourth pattern differed from the third in respect of duration of the periods of cortical inactivity, which were defined as lasting between 3 and

10 seconds. The amplitude of the waves in the period of activity was slightly less than in the third pattern, but the frequency characteristics remained unaltered. In the fifth pattern periods of inactivity did not appear more frequently than once every 10 seconds and there was further reduction in the amplitude of the components to below 25 mV. The frequency of the waves was the same as that found in the active phase of the fourth pattern. There was marked respiratory depression, possibly requiring a respirator. The pupils retained some reaction to light.

The investigations reported so far are based either on retrospective studies or on EEG recordings for a short time. The reports on EEG changes, particularly regarding the significance of flat records in cases of coma, are conflicting (Jouvet, 1959; Loeb, 1958; Bental and Leibowitz, 1961), possibly because in all these studies EEG recordings were done only for short periods. The existing literature does not contain any report of continuous EEG recording of comatose patients from the time of admission to hospital until their recovery from coma.

The published reports (Fischgold and Mathis, 1959; Chatrian et al., 1963) reveal a lack of correlation between the clinical and electrical signs of depth of coma. Moreover, most studies have been done on patients with organic brain disease, including head-injury, and little is known about drug-induced coma.

Wulff (1950) studied 26 patients suffering from acute barbiturate poisoning. EEG records were taken daily until the patients either recovered consciousness or died. In one case cortical activity was absent. In the most severely poisoned patients, periods of absent cortical activity (blackouts) of a few seconds to several minutes duration were observed. Most of these cases died, but the blackouts disappeared before death. Neither variations in blood pressure (from subnormal to normal) nor oxygen therapy had any effect on the blackouts. The author suggested that the presence of blackouts indicated an unfavourable prognosis. However, Warter et al. (1963) reported a case of phenobarbitone overdose who had respiratory arrest and almost complete absence of electrical activity of the brain; following artificial respiration and alkaline diuretic treatment, the patient emerged from the coma and recovery took place without sequelae. Mellerio (1964) studied 33 cases of acute barbiturate intoxication with periods of EEG silence lasting up to 52 sec. Twenty-two cases were caused by barbiturates with rapid elimination; eight by barbiturates with slow elimination; three by unidentified barbiturates. The majority of these patients recovered.

Mantz et al. (1965) reported six cases of severe barbiturate coma with episodes of 5–180 sec. of EEG flattening interrupted by paroxysmal, high voltage bursts. All the six cases recovered, and the authors emphasized that a well-conducted reanimation programme 'can succeed in intoxications classically considered mortal'. Bird and Plum (1968) reported a case of acute barbiturate poisoning who had an isoelectric EEG record for 23 hours, but who recovered after five days of coma.

Sament and Huott (1969) from the Massachusetts General Hospital have reported EEG changes in 26 cases of acute barbiturate poisoning. Seven of 26 cases died, including every one of their six cases who had completely isoelectric records (Stage VI).

The remaining death was a patient who had an isoelectric record with bursts of sharp activity (Stage V). Their Stages I–III were associated with drowsiness or confusion and Stages IV–VI with coma. The authors could not distinguish clinically the three Stages (IV–VI) associated with coma, but found a correlation between these EEG changes and complications. Cardiac arrest occurred only during Stage VI, whereas respiratory failure occurred during Stages III–VI, and the authors emphasized, 'if these complications can be prevented, all cases of barbiturate intoxication are potentially reversible'.

The management of a patient who has taken an overdose of a psychotropic drug must be based on the clinical assessment of the patient, with the assistance of a toxicologist. However, the existing literature shows that EEG studies have been entirely based on sampling, using short runs of EEGs, usually without consideration of any other variables. Some attempts have been made to correlate the degree of abnormality of EEG and the clinical level of consciousness. As far as long-term EEG monitoring is concerned, this has been almost exclusively used in sleep research and then rarely carried on for more than 10–12 hours at a time. Therefore an investigation was undertaken to study the EEG changes in patients suffering from acute barbiturate poisoning by means of the continuous EEG monitoring technique.

PATIENTS AND METHODS

The investigation was carried out at the Edinburgh Regional Poisoning Treatment Centre, which serves a population of about half a million in Edinburgh and the surrounding district, and has an admission rate of over 1000 per annum. All adult cases of acute drug poisoning are admitted, regardless of the severity of the poisoning. The number of admissions has doubled in the past five years, and in 1968 there were 1067 admissions (634 women and 433 men). The unit has seven-day laboratory support for the qualitative and quantitative estimation of commonly involved poisons. The organization and day to day functioning of the unit has been described in detail by Matthew et al. (1969).

On admission each patient was examined by one of the ward physicians to assess the clinical level of consciousness and graded* into one of the four grades (Matthew and Lawson, 1966).

The level of unconsciousness and progress of the patient while under care was based on repeated clinical evaluation and regular sampling of such physiological variables as temperature, pulse rate, blood pressure, and respiration. This was supported by supplementary investigations where possible, such as estimation of the blood levels of the toxic drug, assessment of serum electrolyte levels, and blood gases.

---

* The clinical grade of coma is not to be confused with the EEG grading. To enable easy distinction, the clinical grade will be designated by Arabic numerals and the EEG grade by Roman numerals.

The clinical examination included assessment of the presence of any co-existing disease which would have made the patient more vulnerable to the toxic effects of the drug.

Silver cup-electrodes were filled with electrode jelly and were attached to the scalp with collodion, in positions Fz, Cz, Pz, F_4, C_4, P_4, F_3, C_3 and P_3 of the inter-national '10/20' system of electrode placement (Fig. 1). A central montage with the following channels was used in most of the cases studied:

Channel 1 – F_Z–Cz
         2 – C_Z–P_Z
         3 – F_Z–F_4
         4 – F_Z–F_3
         5 – C_Z–C_4
         6 – C_Z–C_3
         7 – P_Z–P_4
         8 – P_Z–P_3

It proved to be advantageous as this allowed the patient's head to be kept on the side, an important principle in the management of unconscious patients. Each electrode had four inches of wire and was connected to the headbox by means of a longer connecting lead (Fig. 2). This procedure allowed freedom to disconnect the patient from the machine for nursing care, physiotherapy, or when the patient became restless at about the time of regaining consciousness. The EEG machine used was

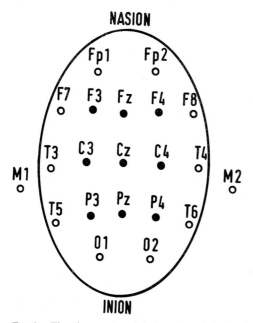

Fig. 1. The placement and designation of the 19 electrodes of the international 10/20 system and of two additional electrodes on each mastoid process. A central montage involving the electrode positions with dark dots was found useful and was used in most of the cases.

a fully portable 16-channel Elema-Schonander Mingograph. It is specially modified for continuous recording and is capable of running from batteries as well as from the mains supply. Therefore, it was possible to move the machine to the bedside of the patient. The machine was run at a constant speed of 1.5 cm per second, producing 4,000 sheets of recorded paper over the 24-hour period. As a routine procedure the machine was calibrated at 1 cm per 100 mV, time constant = 0.3 sec. and high frequency filters = 0. Precautions were taken to ensure an artefact-free record.

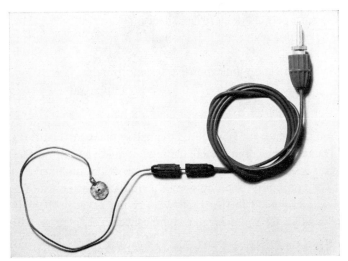

Fig. 2.   Each silver disc-electrode with 4 inches of wire (left) was connected to the head box by means of a longer connecting lead (right). This procedure made it possible to disconnect the patient from the EEG machine when required.

In each patient recordings were made continuously throughout the period of unconsciousness till the patient either recovered or died. After recovery recordings were usually made twice daily and a pre-discharge full montage EEG was recorded.

On recovery from coma, when patients were medically fit to be discharged from the hospital, a battery of psychological tests was administered to the first 20 patients in the hope of detecting any possible organic brain damage. At intervals of one, three, and nine months after discharge from hospital, the first 20 patients for follow-up examination were again administered psychometric tests and EEG, while in a further 15 cases only EEG examination was repeated. As no evidence of residual brain damage was found in these patients, the follow-up procedure was discontinued.

ANALYSIS OF THE RECORD

As no internationally agreed method of scoring coma records is available, a system of classifying these records had to be established. After recording the first few records, the following system of classification was found useful, and these criteria were employed in scoring all the records. An EEG was classified as follows*:

Grade I: Alpha rhythm or predominant alpha rhythm, with beta or some rare theta waves.

Grade II: Predominant theta rhythm, with some alpha, beta and low voltage delta activity.

Grade III: Predominant low/high voltage delta activity mixed with some theta waves.

Grade IV: Delta activity with or without brief isoelectric intervals.

Grade V: Suppression burst activity, namely where 5–10 cps activity of several seconds duration alternated with periods of electrical silence.

Grade VI: Near silence, but with isolated and low voltage 3–7 cps waves occurring singly or in bursts of half a second.

Grade VII: An isoelectric record totally unresponsive to any stimuli.

STATISTICAL METHODS

A rank correlation method (Kendall, 1955) was used to analyse the data. This is the correlation statistic 'tau'. The technique used for calculating tau involved contingency tables and hence there were a great many tied ranks. The value of tau obtained had therefore to be corrected for continuity, thereby giving a unit normal deviate (z). The significance of this z was evaluated in the usual way, giving exact probability values. For example, z values of 1.64 and 2.33 give significance levels of $p = 0.05$ and $p = 0.01$ respectively.

PATIENTS

Fifty patients, 15 men and 35 women, were studied (Table 1). All patients recovered.

TABLE 1

Sex distribution and barbiturate ingested in 50 patients

Barbiturate preparation	Number of patients		
	Male	Female	Total
Phenobarbitone	5	8	13
Barbitone	1	1	2
Amylobarbitone	2	6	8
Butobarbitone	1	3	4
Quinalbarbitone	2	5	7
Pentobarbitone	3	3	6
Cyclobarbitone	—	3	3
Tuinal[1]	1	6	7
Total	15	35	50

[1] Combination of equal parts of quinalbarbitone and amylobarbitone.

* Note that Roman numerals are used for the EEG grade of coma.

Three of the patients had a cardiac arrest of less than 90 sec., but were resuscitated, and serial electrocardiogram showed no evidence of myocardial damage. Ten patients required assisted ventilation, of whom four needed the respirator for less than 5 hours, five for 6–12 hours and one patient for 13 hours. Three patients were treated with forced alkaline diuresis and the remainder were given intensive supportive therapy as described by Matthew and Lawson (1966).

EEG CHANGES AS OBSERVED IN THE RECORD

A normal EEG record (Fig. 3) contains rhythmic activity in the range of 9–11 cps. The EEG changes after an overdose of barbiturates vary from drug-induced fast activity (Fig. 4) at about 16–24 cps to complete electrical silence.

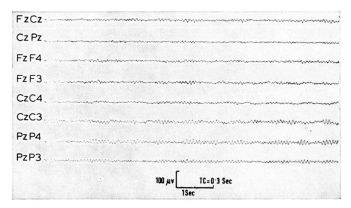

Fig. 3. Normal record. The background rhythmic activity shows alpha rhythm, dominated at about 9–10 cps.

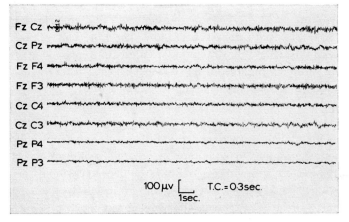

Fig. 4. Barbiturate-induced fast EEG activity. This excerpt shows barbiturate-induced fast activity at about 18–22 cps, in a patient with pentobarbitone poisoning.

The findings from the initial EEG recording for patients in each barbiturate preparation are tabulated in Table 2. These grades do not take account of subsequent deterioration or improvement in the EEG record. Twenty of 50 patients were Grades V–VII; all the seven cases of quinalbarbitone poisoning were in this 'deep' coma range. In contrast the majority of patients who took phenobarbitone (12 of 13) were Grades II–IV; only one case was Grade V.

TABLE 2

EEG grade of coma and various barbiturate preparations ingested by 50 patients

Barbiturate preparation	EEG grade of coma							
	I	II	III	IV	V	VI	VII	Total
Phenobarbitone	—	5	4	3	1	—	—	13
Barbitone	—	1	—	—	—	—	1	2
Amylobarbitone	—	1	2	3	1	1	—	8
Butobarbitone	—	—	—	3	—	—	1	4
Quinalbarbitone	—	—	—	—	2	2	3	7
Pentobarbitone	—	—	—	3	1	2	—	6
Cyclobarbitone	—	—	1	1	—	1	—	3
Tuinal*	—	1	1	1	3	1	—	7
Total	—	8	8	14	8	7	5	50

* Combination of equal parts of quinalbarbitone and amylobarbitone.

Complete electrical silence or isoelectric record lasting up to 28 hours was observed in eight cases. In five of these it was seen in the initial record, whereas in the remaining three it was observed some time after the beginning of the initial recording. Of the five patients who had isoelectric records on initial recording, three had taken quinalbarbitone, one butobarbitone, and one barbitone. The EEG changes observed during the recovery of these patients are illustrated (Figs. 5, 6 and 7) by the representative cases.

In cases of long-acting drugs such as phenobarbitone the EEG abnormalities were not severe, but EEG and clinical recovery were slow. The EEG changes seen during the recovery of these patients are illustrated by a representative case (Fig. 8). During recovery, the record showed 'spontaneous shifts' (Fig. 8e), when faster frequencies of several seconds duration with abundant superimposed drug-induced fast activity would alternate with slow-wave activity with less marked superimposed drug-induced fast activity. Patients were more responsive clinically during the faster activity phase and much less so during the slow-wave activity period. These spontaneous shifts were also seen in barbitone poisoning. In addition, these patients showed a great improvement both in EEG record and clinical condition on repeated stimulation, but when left undisturbed they would become deeper again; consequently, there was a tendency of these patients to relapse into coma after having responded to a vocal command, which was taken as a guide to the time when the patient regained consciousness.

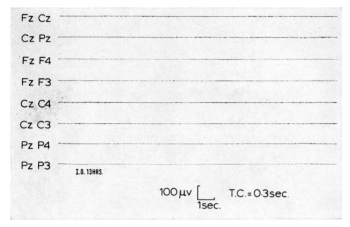

Fig. 5a. EEG in acute barbiturate (butobarbitone) poisoning. Totally flat record (complete electrical silence) 13 hrs after ingestion of large quantities of butobarbitone tablets. Classified as Grade VII. Female, 54 years old. Deeply unconscious and unresponsive to all stimuli. Pulse 92 per min; rectal temperature 31.0°C and serum butobarbitone concentration 7.0 mg%.

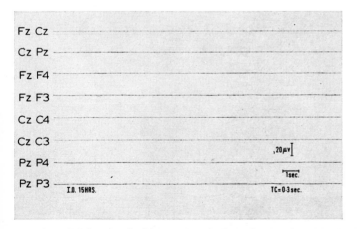

Fig. 5b. EEG in acute barbiturate (butobarbitone) poisoning. After 15 hours of coma record was still isoelectric and recording done on maximum amplification (20 mV per cm) revealed no change. Classification of coma: Grade VII. Rectal temperature 30.6°C and serum butobarbitone level 6.8 mg%.

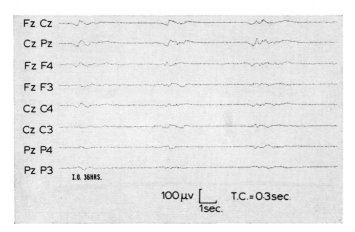

Fig. 5c. EEG in acute barbiturate (butobarbitone) poisoning. After 36 hours of coma the EEG tracings contained suppression–burst activity (Grade V), 5–10 cps activity of 3–4 seconds duration would alternate with electrical silence. Clinically she was deeply unconscious and unresponsive to all stimuli. Rectal temperature 36.4°C and serum butobarbitone level 6.2 mg%.

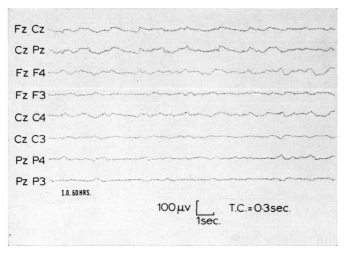

Fig. 5d. EEG in acute barbiturate (butobarbitone) poisoning. Sixty hours after lapsing into coma the EEG record revealed continuous slow-wave activity at ½–2 cps. Classified as Grade IV. Clinically she made a minimal response to maximal painful stimulation. Rectal temperature 38.2°C and serum butobarbitone concentration 4.0 mg%.

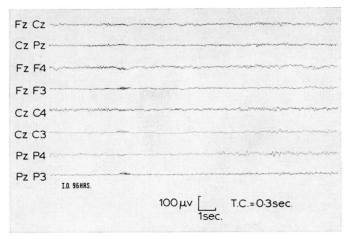

Fig. 5e. EEG in acute barbiturate (butobarbitone) poisoning. Ninety-six hours after ingestion of the drug her EEG tracing showed predominantly 6–8 cps activity with some 4–6 cps activity. Classified as Grade II. Muscle artefact was present. Patient was conscious but drowsy and confused. Rectal temperature 37.0°C and serum butobarbitone 1.5 mg%.

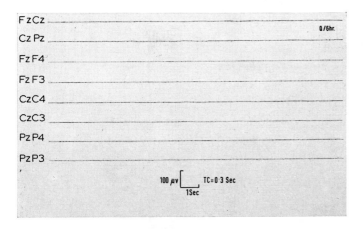

Fig. 6a. EEG in quinalbarbitone poisoning. A flat record (complete electrical silence or an isoelectric record), six hours after ingestion of large quantities of quinalbarbitone tablets. Classified as Grade VII. Patient GF, male, 32 years old. Deeply unconscious and unresponsive to all stimuli. Blood pressure 70/45 mm; pulse 92 per minute; rectal temperature 35.5°C and barbiturate level in the blood 1.9 mg% as quinalbarbitone.

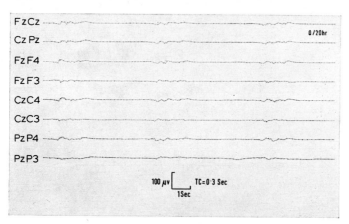

Fig. 6b. EEG in quinalbarbitone poisoning. After 20 hours of coma suppression–burst activity was observed in the EEG tracings, namely where 5–8 cps activity of 3–5 sec duration would alternate with periods of electrical silence. Classified as Grade V. Clinically the patient was deeply unconscious and unresponsive to all stimuli. Rectal temperature 37.8°C and serum quinalbarbitone concentration 1.9 mg%.

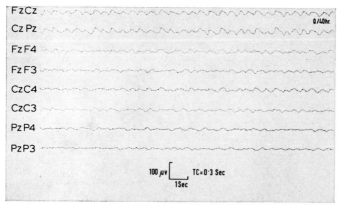

Fig. 6c. EEG in quinalbarbitone poisoning. Forty hours after lapsing into coma his EEG record showed continuous slow wave activity at ½–2 cps. Classified as Grade IV. Clinically he made minimal response to a maximal stimulation of the sternum with the knuckles; rectal temperature was 38.3°C and serum quinalbarbitone 1.1 mg%.

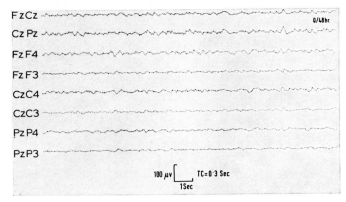

Fig. 6d.   EEG in quinalbarbitone poisoning. Forty-eight hours after drug ingestion his EEG record contained predominant low/high voltage 2–4 cps activity mixed with which was some 4–6 cps activity. Classified as Grade III. Clinically he responded to painful stimulation. Rectal temperature was 37.8°C and serum quinalbarbitone level 0.8 mg%.

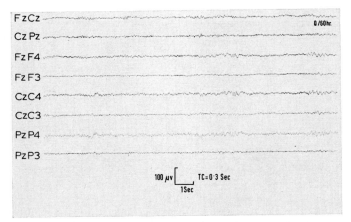

Fig. 6e.   EEG in quinalbarbitone poisoning. After 60 hours of coma the EEG record revealed 8–10 cps activity with some 4–6 cps activity. Rectal temperature was 37.2°C and serum quinalbarbitone 0.4 mg%.

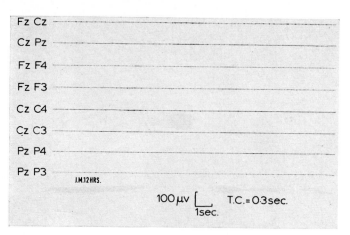

Fig. 7a. EEG in acute barbiturate (barbitone) poisoning. Totally flat record (isoelectric record) 12 hours after the ingestion of large quantities of sodium barbitone tablets. Classified as Grade VII. Female, 64 years old. Clinically the patient was deeply unconscious and unresponsive to all stimuli. Blood pressure 75/50 mm Hg; pulse 84 per min; rectal temperature 34.1°C and serum barbitone level 70 mg%.

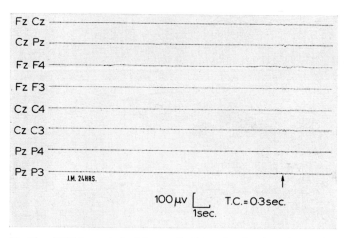

Fig. 7b. EEG in acute barbiturate (barbitone) poisoning. Twenty-four hours after ingestion of the drug her EEG record for the first time showed an isolated burst of 3–7 cps activity marked with the arrow. Classified as Grade VI. Clinically she remained unchanged. Blood pressure 80/60 mm Hg; pulse 76 per min; rectal temperature 33.0°C and serum barbitone concentration 65 mg%.

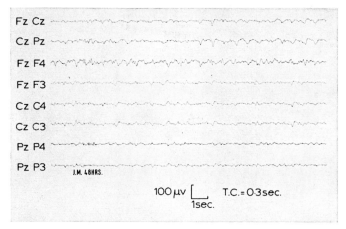

Fig. 7c. EEG in acute barbiturate (barbitone) poisoning. After 48 hours of coma her EEG tracings contained 2–3 cps activity more marked in the top three channels and low-voltage 4–6 cps activity in the lower five channels. Clinically she was unconscious but responded to stimulation of the sternum with the knuckles. Blood pressure 85/65 mm Hg; pulse 72 per min; rectal temperature 35.5°C and serum barbitone 42 mg%.

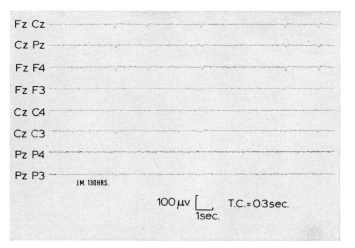

Fig. 7d. EEG in acute barbiturate (barbitone) poisoning. One hundred and thirty hours after the overdose the EEG record during wakefulness revealed a generalized flatness with prominent blinks. The background activity consisted of low-voltage 7–10 cps activity. Her serum barbitone level was 9.5 mg%.

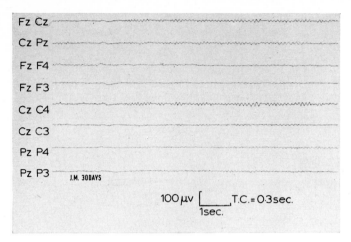

Fig. 7e.   EEG in acute barbiture (barbitone) poisoning. The EEG record one month after the overdose was normal. It contained alpha rhythm at 9–11 cps.

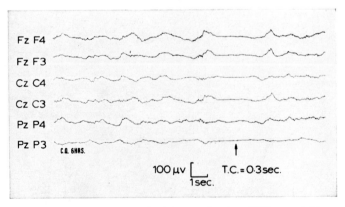

Fig. *8a.*   EEG in acute phenobarbitone poisoning. EEG record 6 hours after the ingestion of large
quantities of phenobarbitone tablets contained background ½–1 cps activity with superimposed 9–10
cps fast activity. Separating the slow waves is an area of flattening marked with an arrow. Female, 28
years old. Clinically she was deeply unconscious, making no response to sternal stimulation. Blood
pressure 100/60 mm Hg; pulse 80 per min; rectal temperature 37.0°C and serum phenobarbitone level
9.0 mg%.

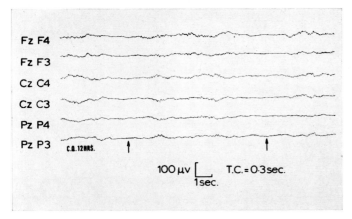

Fig. 8b. EEG in acute phenobarbitone poisoning. Twelve hours after the overdose the EEG trac-ings revealed bursts of ½–1 cps activity with superimposed 9–10 cps fast activity. Alternating with these slow waves were areas of less activity of 2–4 sec duration, thus showing a deterioration in the condition of the patient as judged from the record of electrical activity of the brain. Clinically the patient remained unchanged. Blood pressure 90/50 mm Hg; pulse 75 per min; rectal temperature 37.2°C and serum phenobarbitone level 9.2 mg%.

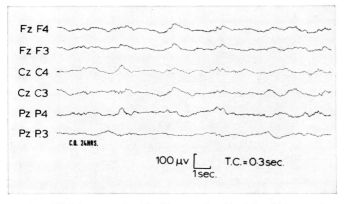

Fig. 8c. EEG in acute phenobarbitone poisoning. After 24 hours of coma this excerpt shows contin-uous slow wave activity at ½–1 cps. Clinically the patient's condition remained the same and no clinical response was noticeable on sternal stimulation. Blood pressure 85/55 mm Hg; pulse 78 per min; rectal temperature 37.2°C and serum phenobarbitone level 9.4 mg%.

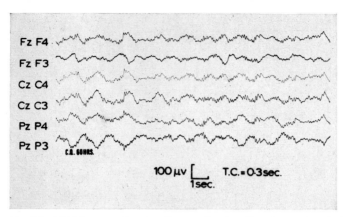

Fig. 8d. EEG in acute phenobarbitone poisoning. Sixty hours after the ingestion of the phenobarbitone tablets her EEG record contained ½–2 cps slow-wave activity, with superimposed 10–12 cps fast activity. Clinically she was unconscious but responded to maximal stimulation of the sternum with the knuckles. Blood pressure 85/60 mm Hg; pulse 70 per min; rectal temperature 37.1°C and serum phenobarbitone level 9.6 mg%.

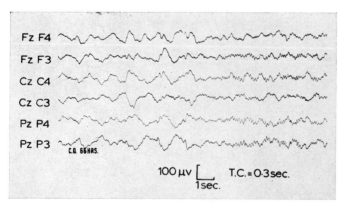

Fig. 8e. EEG in acute phenobarbitone poisoning. After 66 hours of coma the patient's record showed 'spontaneous shifts', i.e. alternating periods of slow waves and faster frequencies appeared spontaneously. High-voltage slow waves at ½–1 cps with little superimposed fast activity gave way to 1–4 cps activity with abundant superimposed fast activity. Blood pressure 95/65 mm Hg; rectal temperature 37.1°C and serum phenobarbitone level 9.7 mg%.

EEG findings were related to the clinical assessment of depth of coma. EEG Grades I and II were associated with consciousness or drowsiness; with Grades III and IV patients were unconscious but responded to stimulation of the sternum with the knuckles. Grade V to VII were associated with deep coma and these three Grades could not be distinguished clinically. During these grades, clinically patients were in deep coma and unresponsive to all stimuli, and an improvement or deterioration in the electrocerebral activity was the only reliable index of change in the condition of the patient.

A change in the electrical activity always preceded the change in the clinical condition of the patient. For many hours the patient might not show any observable change in the clinical condition, whereas EEG activity would continue to indicate a change in either direction. In this respect it was also observed that, if a patient was stimulated and no clinical response was obtained, a noticeable response in the electrical activity was always present.

In two cases (one of barbitone and the other of butobarbitone), changes in EEG activity were also indicative of the effectiveness of an active regime employed, as patients were deeply unconscious and unresponsive to stimuli. No clinical response was observed throughout the period of forced alkaline diuresis but an improvement in EEG record was a useful guide in assessing the effectiveness of the active regime.

CLINICAL GRADE OF COMA

Most of the patients (12 of 13) who had taken phenobarbitone were Grades 1 and 2, whereas the majority of the patients having taken other barbiturate preparations were Grades 3 and 4. For example, 6 of the 7 who had taken quinalbarbitone and 5 of the 6 who had taken pentobarbitone were Grade 4. All the patients who had taken butobarbitone, quinalbarbitone or pentobarbitone were Grades 3 and 4. The correlation between clinical assessment of depth of coma and the EEG depth of coma was significant ($p = 0.002$).

TEMPERATURE ON ADMISSION

Seventeen of 50 patients were hypothermic. Patients who had taken an overdose of medium- or short-acting barbiturate seemed especially liable to hypothermia with a temperature below 35.6°C. Six out of the 13 patients who had taken either quinalbarbitone or pentobarbitone were hypothermic, whereas 11 of the remaining 37 patients were hypothermic. This difference, however, is not significant ($X^2 = 0.5$; $df = 1$). The majority of phenobarbitone cases (11 of 13) had a temperature in the range of 35.6 and 37.8°C. A significant correlation was found between temperature and the EEG grade of coma ($p = 0.007$).

BLOOD BARBITURATE LEVELS

Of the 15 patients who took long-acting barbiturates (phenobarbitone or barbitone), 11 had a blood drug level of more than 8.0 mg%. One patient in the barbitone group had a record level of 70.0 mg%. Blood drug levels of the long-acting barbiturates and EEG grade were significantly correlated (p = 0.007). In 17 of the 35 cases who took medium- and short-acting barbiturates the serum levels were 2.9 mg% or less. Five of the 35 cases had a serum level of more than 5.0 mg%. In one case (of amylo-barbitone) the level of drug in the blood was not estimated.

TOTAL DURATION OF COMA

Twenty-five of 50 were in coma for 25 to 72 hours, 38% less than 25 hours and 12% more than 72 hours. Only two patients (both from the phenobarbitone group) were in coma for more than 96 hours. The correlation between the total period of unconsciousness and the EEG grade of coma was significant (p = 0.001).

DISCUSSION

As outlined in the introduction, previous investigations of drug-induced coma (Wulff, 1950; Silverman, 1963; Mantz et al., 1965) have described the EEG changes varying from drug-induced fast activity to slowing and general flattening of the electroencephalogram in acute barbiturate poisoning, but these reports dealt with only small series of cases compared with the present study and did not employ continuous EEG monitoring. The results of the present investigation offer strong confirmation of the few previous case reports (Warter et al., 1963; Bird and Plum, 1968) that flat EEG records in cases of barbiturate intoxication are quite compatible with eventual recovery. The use of the term 'flat' record in previous reports (Mellerio, 1964; Mantz et al., 1965) is difficult to interpret, owing to the use of only short periods of EEG sampling. The continuous EEG monitoring technique employed in this study confirmed the presence of very prolonged periods of isoelectric record in the cases reported here. In the investigations mentioned above the recording sensitivity used was only that customary in routine clinical recordings and it was this that was used in determining electrocerebral silence. The use of stimulation and increased amplification in the present study made it possible to show that the EEG records were completely isoelectric.

EEG monitoring proved at times superior to clinical observation and of great help in assessing a change in the condition of those patients who were deeply comatose and unresponsive to all stimuli. The absence of EEG reactivity was observed during the initial period of massive toxaemia, of vegetative disturbance, and deep comatose state; reactivity appeared at a later period, after a fall in the concentration of the drug, disappearance of vegetative disturbance, and lightening of coma depth. The EEG Grades V–VII were associated with deep coma and could not be distinguished clinically, whereas the EEG provided evidence of beginning improvement from, for example, Grade VII to Grade V. In this respect the present investigation confirms the findings of Sament and Huott (1969). An improvement in the electrical activity always preceded the clinical signs of improvement. For many hours a patient may not show any notable change in the clinical condition, whereas EEG activity will continue to show steady improvement (Haider et al., 1968). Another area in which EEG monitoring proved to be useful was in the assessment of the effectiveness of some active regime adopted, such as forced alkaline diuresis. Other investigators (Brazier and Finesinger, 1945; Swank and Foley, 1948; Kiersey et al., 1951; Sament and Huott, 1969) have shown that the EEG is the best single measure of the depth of barbiturate narcosis and that it is superior, in this respect, to clinical or biochemical testing. These studies were performed experimentally on animals and also during thiopentone anaesthesia in man. The present study allows the same conclusions for acute barbiturate poisoning in man.

Non-parametric tests were able to establish significant correlations between the EEG grades of coma and other parameters. A significant positive correlation between the EEG grade of coma and the clinical assessment of depth of coma was found even though EEG grading was based on entirely different criteria. A direct correlation between EEG grades and blood drug levels of long-acting barbiturates and total duration of unconsciousness was found. But a significant negative correlation between the temperature and EEG grade was found. This implies that hypothermia was associated with EEG Grades IV–VII. Patients who had taken medium- or short-acting barbiturates were especially liable to hypothermia. As far as is known no previous investigation of these inter-relationships has been reported. If the EEG is to be used to monitor coma it is plain that body temperature especially must always be taken into account.

In a Poisoning Treatment Centre the EEG is a useful adjunct to the standard equipment, improving care and supervision during the period the drug is being metabolized or eliminated. EEGs with long periods of electrical silence, in spite of being serious, are not incompatible with total recovery. This discovery constitutes the most important contribution during past years in the domain of EEG monitoring of unconscious patients.

The value of the EEG for monitoring coma is abundantly clear, but its routine clinical use must be admitted to have limitations because it throws heavy demands on skilled labour and involves complex and bulky equipment producing miles and miles of recorded paper. It must be thought too expensive and intricate for use in routine monitoring. However, the present study suggests that a simple and less expensive device for continuous monitoring, such as the cerebral function monitor described by Maynard et al. (1969), could be a valuable aid to the clinician in making decisions about the treatment of comatose patients and in assessing the probability of survival.

REFERENCES

BANCAUD, J., HACAEN, H., and LAIRY, G. C. (1955), Modifications de la reactivité EEG, troubles des fonctions symboliques et troubles confusionnels dans les lesions hemispheriques localisées. *Electroenceph. clin. Neurophysiol.*, 7, 179.

BELLVILLE, J. W., ARTUSION, J. F., and GLENN, F. (1955), The electroencephalogram in cardiac arrest. *J. Amer. med. Ass.*, 157, 508.

BELLVILLE, J. W. and HOWLAND, W. S. (1957), Prognosis after severe hypoxia in man. *Anesthesiology*, 18, 389.

BENTAL, E. and LEIBOWITZ, U. (1961), Flat electroencephalograms during 78 days in a case of 'encephalitis'. *Electroenceph. clin. Neurophysiol.*, 13, 457.

BERGER, H. (1932), Über das Elektroenkephalogramm des Menschen IV. *Arch. Psychiat. Nervenkr.*, 97, 6.

BIRD, T. D., and PLUM, F. (1968), Recovery from barbiturate overdose coma with a prolonged isoelectric electroencephalogram. *Neurology (Minneap.)*, 18, 456.

BRAZIER, M. A. B., and FINESINGER, J. E. (1945), Action of barbiturates on the central cortex (electroencephalographic studies. *Arch. Neurol. Psychiat. (Chic.)*, 53, 51.

BRECHNER, V. L., BETHUNE, R. W. M., KAVAN, E. M., BAUER, R. O., PHILLIPS, R. E., and DILLON, J. B. (1961), The EEG effect of arrested circulation in the normothermic human and dog. *Anaesth. Amalg. Curr. Res.*, 4, 1.

British Medical Journal (1964), Treatment of Acute Poisoning I and II. *Brit. med. J.*, 2, 927; 993.

Central and Scottish Health Services Councils (1968), *Hospital Treatment of Acute Poisoning*. HMSO, London.

CHATRIAN, G. E., WHITE, L. E. JR., and DALY, D. (1963), Sleep EEG patterns in certain comatose states following head-injury. *Electroenceph. clin. Neurophysiol.*, 15, 145.

COHN, R., and KATZENELBOGEN, S. (1942), Electroencephalographic changes induced by intravenous sodium amytal. *Proc. Soc. exp. Biol. Med. (N.Y.)*, 49, 560.

Commonwealth Director-General of Health (1966), Annual Report, 1965–1966, Canberra.

DAVIS, P. A. and DAVIS, H. (1939), The electrical activity of the brain: its relation to physiologic states and to states of impaired consciousness. *Res. Publ. Ass. nerv. ment. Dis.*, 19, 50.

DELL, M. G. (1957), Electro-encephalogramme et syndrome frontal. *Electroenceph. clin. Neurophysiol.*, 9, 505.

FISCHGOLD, H., and BOUNES, G. (1946), Exploration electroencephalographique des états comateux. *Sem. Hop. (Paris)*, 22, 1245.

FISCHGOLD, H., and MATHIS, P. (1959), Obnubilations, comas et stupeurs. *Electroenceph. clin. Neurophysiol. Suppl.*, 11, 126.

GASTAUT, H. (1954), The brain stem and cerebral electrogenesis in relation to consciousness. In: E. A. Adrian, E. Bremer, and H. Jasper (Ed), *Brain mechanisms and consciousness*, 249. Blackwell, Oxford.

GIBBS, F. A., GIBBS, E. L., and LENNOX, W. G. (1937), Effect on the electroencephalogram of certain drugs which influence nervous activity. *Arch. intern. Med.*, 60, 154.

GRONQUIST, Y. K. J., SELDON, T. H., and HAULCONER, A., JR. (1952), Prognostic significance of electroencephalographic changes. *Ann. Chir. Gynaec. Fenn.*, 41, 149.

HAIDER, I., OSWALD, I., and MATTHEW, H. (1968), EEG signs of death. *Brit. med. J.*, 3, 314.

HOCKADAY, J. M., POTTS, F., EPSTEIN, E., BONAZZI, A., and SCHWAB, R. S. (1965), Electroencephalographic changes in acute cerebral anoxia from cardiac or respiratory arrest. *Electroenceph. clin. Neurophysiol.*, 18, 575.

ISBELL, H., ALTSCHUL, S., KORNETSKY, C. H., EISENMAN, A. J., FLANARY, H. G., and FRASER, H. F. (1950), Chronic barbiturate intoxication. *Arch. Neurol. Psychiat. (Chic.)*, 64, 1.

JOUVET, M. (1959), Diagnostic electro-sous-corticographique de la mort du système nerveux central au cours de certain comas. *Electroenceph. clin. Neurophysiol.*, 18, 805.

KAADA, B. R., HARKMARK, W., and STOKKE, O. (1961), Deep coma associated with desynchronisation in the EEG. *Electroenceph. clin. Neurophysiol.*, 13, 785.

KENDALL, M. G. (1955), *Rank Correlation Methods*, 2nd Ed. Griffin, London.

KENNEDY, C, BRIGGS, J. D., YOUNG, N., LINDSAY, R. M., LUKE, R. G., and CAMPBELL, D. (1969), Successful treatment of three cases of very severe barbiturate poisoning. *Lancet*, 17, 995.

KIERSEY, D. H., BICKFORD, R. G., and FAULCONER, A. (1951), Electro-encephalographic patterns produced by thiopentone sodium during surgical operations. Descriptions and classifications. *Brit. J. Anaesth.*, 23, 141.

LENNOX, M. A. and PETERSON, P. B. (1958), Electroencephalographic findings in acute carbon monoxide poisoning. *Electroenceph. clin. Neurophysiol.*, 10, 63.

LOEB, C., and POGGIO, G. (1953), Electroencephalograms in a case with ponto-mesencephalic haemorrhage. *Electroenceph. clin. Neurophysiol.*, 5, 295.

LOEB, C. (1958), Electroencephalographic changes during the state of coma. *Electroencephal. clin. Neurophysiol.*, 10, 589.

LOEB, C., ROSADINI, G., and POGGIO, G. F. (1959), Electroencephalograms during coma; normal and borderline records in 5 patients. *Neurology (Minneap.)*, 9, 610.

LUNDERVOLD, A., HAUGE, T., and LOKEN, A. C. (1956), Unusual EEG in unconscious patient with brain stem atrophy. *Electroenceph. clin. Neurophysiol.*, 8, 665.

MANTZ, J. M., KURTZ, D., OTTENI, J. C., and ROHMER, F. (1965), EEG aspects of six cases of severe barbiturate coma. *Electroenceph. clin. Neurophysiol.*, 18, 424.

MATHIS, P., TORUBIA, A., and FISCHGOLD, H. (1957), Réactivité periodicite et correlation cortico-cardio-respiratoire dans le coma. In: H. Fischgold and H. Gastaut (Ed) *Conditionnement et réactivité en electroencéphalographie. Electroenceph. clin. Neurophysiol. Suppl.* 6, 453.

MATTHEW, H. (1966), Poisoning by medicaments. *Brit. med. J.*, 2, 278.

MATTHEW, H., and LAWSON, A. A. H. (1966), Acute barbiturate poisoning – a review of two years experience. *Quart, J. Med.*, 35, 539.

MATTHEW, H., and LAWSON, A. A. H. (1967), *Treatment of common acute poisoning.* Livingstone, Edinburgh.

MATTHEW, H., PROUDFOOT, A. T., BROWN, S. S., and AITKEN, R. C. B. (1969), Acute poisoning: Organisation and work-load of a treatment centre. *Brit. med. J.*, 3, 489.

MAYNARD, D., PRIOR, P. F. and SCOTT, D. F. (1969), Device for continuous monitoring of cerebral activity in resuscitated patients. *Brit. med. J.*, 4, 545.

MELLERIO, F. (1964), *L'électroencéphalographie dans les intoxications aigues.* Masson, Paris.

Ministry of Health and Department of Health for Scotland (1961), Drug Addiction, Report of inter-departmental committee. HMSO, London.

Ministry of Health (1964), *Recent National Health Prescribing Trends.* HMSO. London.

OPITZ, E., and SCHNEIDER, M. (1950), Über die Sauerstoffversorgung des Gehirns und den Mechanismus von Mangelwirkungen. *Ergebn. Physiol.*, 46, 126.

PAMPIGLIONE, G. (1962), Electroencephalographic studies after cardiorespiratory resuscitation. *Proc. roy. Soc. Med.*, 55, 653.

ROMANO, J., and ENGEL, G. L. (1944), Delirium I., Electroencephalographic data. *Arch. Neurol. Psychiat. (Chic.)*, 51, 536.

SAMENT, S., and HUOTT, A. D. (1969), The EEG in acute barbiturate intoxication, with particular reference to isoelectric EEGs. *Electroenceph. clin. Neurophysiol.*, 27, 695.

SCHNEIDER, M. (1961a), Critical blood pressure in the cerebral circulation. In: J. P. Schade and W. H. McMenemey (Ed) *Selective vulnerability of the brain in hypoxaemia,* 7. Davis, Philadelphia.

SCHNEIDER, M. (1961b), Survival and revival in the brain in anoxia and ischemia. In: H. Gastaut and J. S. Meyer (Ed) *Cerebral anoxia and the encephalogram,* 134. Thomas, Illinois.

SCHWAB, R. A., POTTS, F. and BONAZZI, A. (1962), EEG as an aid in determining death in the presence of cardiac activity. *Electroenceph. clin. Neurophysiol.*, 15, 147.

SILVERMAN, D. (1963), Retrospective study of the EEG in coma. *Electroenceph. clin. Neurophysiol.*, 15, 486.

SPOEREL, W. E. (1962), The electroencephalogram after cardiac arrest. *J. Can. anaesth. Soc.*, 9, 479.

STRAUSS, H., OSTOW, M., and GREENSTEIN, L. (1952), *Diagnostic electroencephalography,* 292. Grune and Stratton, New York.

SWANK, R. L., and FOLEY, J. M. (1948), Respiratory, electroencephalographic and blood gas changes in progressive barbiturate narcosis in dogs. *J. Pharmacol.*, 92, 381.

THIES-PUPPEL, H., and WIENERS, K. (1961), Survival time and latency of recovery of EEG during heart surgery in hypothermia. In: H. Gastaut and J. S. Meyer (Ed) *Central anoxia and the electroencephalogram,* 279. Thomas, Springfield, Ill.

VONDRACEK, V., PROKUPEK, J., FISCHER, R., and AHRENBERGOVA, M. (1968), *Recent patterns of addiction in Czechoslovakia.* Brit. J. Psychiat., 114, 285.

WARTER, J., MANTZ, J. M., METAIS, P., HAMMANN, B., and KURTZ, D. (1963), Coma prolongé par intoxication massive au phénobarbital (25 mg). Apnée prolongee (4 jours) – respiration artificielle. *Guerison Pr. Med.* 71, 1409.

WHELAN, J. L., WEBSTER, J. E., and GURDJIAN, E. S. (1955), Serial electroencephalography in recent head-injuries with attention to photic stimulation. *Electroenceph. clin. Neurophysiol.*, 7, 495.

WULFF, M. H. (1950), Electroencephalographic investigations in acute barbiturate poisoning. *Electroenceph. clin. Neurophysiol.*, 2, 111.

11. medical management of acute barbiturate poisoning

A. A. H. Lawson and A. T. Proudfoot

In almost all developed countries of the world, acute poisoning is a serious and increasing medical and social problem. In major hospitals throughout Britain, patients suffering from acute poisoning constitute between 10% and 25% of all acute medical admissions (Curry, 1965; Ellis *et al.*, 1966; Jones, 1969). Though many psychotropic drugs and other hypnotics have recently gained popularity in self-poisoning episodes, barbiturates remain the drugs most commonly consumed in overdosage, as found at the Regional Poisoning Treatment Centre, Edinburgh, in 1968 (Table 1).

TABLE 1

Number of occasions on which poisons were encountered in 1968
(From Matthew *et al.*, 1969)

Poison	No.	%
Barbiturates	340	26
Aspirin preparations	182	14
Benzodiazepines	153	12
Mandrax	126	10
Tricyclic antidepressants	74	6
Other hypnotics	55	4
Carbon monoxide	58	4
Phenothiazines	46	3
Miscellaneous	270	21

In the course of the past 30 years the emphasis in the basic aims of medical treatment has changed (Ibsen, 1966). Between 1930 and 1950 the main objective was to achieve precision in diagnosis and to give direct and specific treatment for each condition. In the field of clinical toxicology, and acute barbiturate overdosage in particular, this led to the use of vigorous gastric aspiration and lavage and to efforts to provide 'antidotes' to the poisoning.

Intensive analeptic drug therapy was widely advocated (Koppanyi and Fazekas, 1950) and enjoyed great popularity, particularly following the introduction of bemegride as a specific antidote to barbiturates (Shulman *et al.*, 1955; Shaw, 1955). The clinical response to bemegride was transient and repeated doses were required. Analeptics, however, did not reduce the high mortality from barbiturate poisoning (Clemmesen and Nilsson, 1961; Setter *et al.*, 1966) and their use was associated with a high incidence of serious side effects which included cardiac arrhythmias (Reed *et al.*, 1952; Dobos *et al.*, 1961), convulsions (Kjaer-Larsen, 1956; Roche *et al.*, 1950) and visual hallucinations and psychoses (Kjaer-Larsen, 1956; Louw and Sonne, 1956; Myschetzky, 1961). Despite these serious disadvantages, it was some years before it became clear that bemegride was not a specific antidote to barbiturates and analeptic therapy finally fell from favour. The claims for the efficacy of analeptics have been critically reviewed by Mark (1967).

The major breakthrough in the treatment of barbiturate poisoning was the development of effective supportive therapy initially by Kirkegaard (1949) and Nilsson (1951) and later by Clemmesen and Nilsson (1961). This treatment, the 'Scandinavian Method', was established only with difficulty and those who continued to favour analeptic therapy criticized it severely (Koppanyi and Fazekas, 1950). The general principles of supportive therapy propounded by Clemmesen and Nilsson (1961) are now accepted by authorities in the field of clinical toxicology and form the basic approach to the treatment of all types of poisoning. The original 'Scandinavian Method' has undergone modifications (Matthew and Lawson, 1970) with further reduction in the mortality from acute barbiturate poisoning (Table 2). This modified form of intensive supportive therapy has in our experience proved to be highly successful (Matthew *et al.*, 1969) and we consider it to be the most effective regimen at the present time.

TABLE 2

Stages in the development of modern treatment of acute barbiturate poisoning

Year	Regimen of treatment	Mortality (%)
1945	Treatment of shock	25
1948	Methods to maintain a clear airway	15
1949	Special treatment centres	10
1950	Avoidance of analeptic treatment	5
1966	Modern intensive supportive therapy	<1

DIAGNOSIS OF ACUTE BARBITURATE POISONING

Often there is such strong circumstantial evidence that the diagnosis of acute barbiturate poisoning is quite clear. The majority of adults have indulged in self-poisoning in which the motive is to draw attention to some intolerable situation rather than self-destruction. Under these circumstances patients who are conscious will usually provide the information that an overdose has been taken. The latter may also be clear from the suicide notes left by some patients. Difficulties in diagnosis arise when the patient is unconscious. It is useful to remember under these circumstances that in patients below the age of 50, apart from trauma and head-injury in particular, the commonest cause of loss of consciousness is acute poisoning. Even in older patients this is frequently the diagnosis.

When the patient is unconscious, relatives and friends should be closely questioned to determine where and when the patient was last seen conscious, his state of mind at that time, and whether he had given any warning of attempting suicide. The latter is of some value since Kessel (1965) has shown that 34% of poisoned patients had given some warning of their intention. Many of these patients may have made similar attempts in the past (Matthew et al., 1969). Every effort must be made to obtain as much information as possible about the type of poisoning, the amount taken and the time of ingestion. This is frequently overlooked and as a result much valuable time may be wasted in waiting for laboratory support for the diagnosis. A considerable amount of useful information may be obtained from the tablet-containers or from telephone calls to the patient's family doctor or to the pharmacist who dispensed the medicines. It is also of importance to determine whether alcohol or drugs which might potentiate the effects of barbiturates were available or were ingested simultaneously.

Few poisonings produce diagnostic features, and the doctor is left with the differential diagnosis of unconsciousness. In the case of acute barbiturate poisoning a useful diagnostic feature is the presence of bullae, which occur frequently in the interdigital clefts of fingers and toes and on other areas exposed to relatively minor pressure. These lesions occur in approximately 6% of all patients with barbiturate poisoning (Beveridge and Lawson, 1965) and it is considered that they are due to a toxic effect of the drug on the epidermis with pressure being simply a factor in the localization of the blisters (See Chapter 7, 'The Skin in Acute Barbiturate Poisoning').

Acute barbiturate intoxication characteristically produces depression of the central nervous system with loss of muscle tone, diminished limb reflexes and loss of the cough and gag reflexes. Carroll (1969), however, has reported four young adults who had focal neurological signs during acute barbiturate overdosage. These signs recovered completely in every case but the exclusion of head-injury, cerebro-vascular accidents and hypoglycaemia was necessary while the patients were unconscious.

When the diagnosis of acute barbiturate poisoning is in doubt after due consideration of the history, circumstances, and clinical features, confirmation of the diagnosis is always possible by chemical analysis either of plasma or urine. A useful and rapid method of quantitative barbiturate estimation in small volumes of blood was described by Curry (1964). This method was modified slightly and used as a ward side-room test on 127 occasions by Clow and Smith (1967). Each estimation was completed in 10–15 minutes using simple apparatus. Though primidone and glutethimide gave positive results a reliable qualitative result for barbiturates was obtained in all cases and acceptable quantitative results were obtained in over 50%. More definitive methods of analysis have been described by Broughton (1956), but this method also measured metabolites to some extent and further modifications have been introduced. At present the most convenient method of chemical estimation is that of Wright and Johns (1953). These last mentioned methods may be used for the assay of barbiturates in blood and urine.

ASSESSMENT OF THE SEVERITY OF POISONING

The initial assessment of the patient is of paramount importance, not only to gain a base-line knowledge of the patient's condition from which his progress may be judged, but also to decide upon the measures required to preserve life.

The major impact of acute barbiturate poisoning is on the central nervous system with impairment of the level of consciousness and depression of respiration. Cardiovascular function may also be markedly impaired, which is partly due to a direct toxic effect on the myocardium and peripheral vasculature and partly a result of depression of the cardiovascular centre in the brain. The resulting hypotension may be severe and, if prolonged, may lead to renal damage. In severe cases there is also depression of the thermal regulatory mechanism with subsequent hypothermia. Clinical assessment in every case is, therefore, directed at determining the magnitude of disturbance of these vital functions. Though physical examination must be rapid it must also be complete so that coincident disease which may influence management is detected at an early stage.

Several schemes have been devised to assess the severity of poisoning. Some of these (Reed et al., 1952; Baker, 1969) attempt to cover the patient's overall clinical state, and in addition to depression of consciousness they take into consideration the presence or absence of respiratory depression and hypotension. Such schemes are complicated and we have found them of little practical value. Moreover, other neurological features of barbiturate poisoning such as changes in the size and reactivity of the pupils and in the state of the limb reflexes are so variable as to be more confusing than helpful.

Depression of consciousness is the most constant manifestation of barbiturate poisoning and is, therefore, the most useful single parameter in assessment of the severity of poisoning. The degree of impairment of consciousness is readily determined from the response of the patient to painful stimuli. By this means four grades of severity of poisoning are distinguished (Matthew and Lawson, 1966):

Grade I: the patient is drowsy or asleep, but can be roused to respond to vocal commands;

Grade II: the patient is unconscious but responds to minimally painful stimuli;
Grade III: the patient is unconscious and responds only to maximally painful stimuli;
Grade IV: the patient is unconscious and makes no response to painful stimuli.

Painful stimuli may be applied in a variety of ways, but a satisfactory and safe maximum stimulus is to rub the patient's sternum with the knuckles of the clenched fist. This method of assessing the severity of poisoning has the benefit of being simple and readily and rapidly reproducible so that any change is easily determined. The assessment of respiratory function, hypotension, and hypothermia is discussed below.

A frequent misconception is that the severity of acute barbiturate poisoning is assessed most accurately by measurement of blood barbiturate levels. Those who adhere to this view ignore the question of drug tolerance, which is a most important factor and one extremely common with barbiturates. These drugs are used so commonly for the treatment of insomnia and epilepsy that patients frequently have quite high blood barbiturate levels and yet show remarkably little in the way of sedative effects. The problem of tolerance and variation in response to sedative drugs has been reviewed by Richards and Taylor (1956) who showed that the response to barbiturates in experimental animals could vary by as much as 50%. They also showed that individual animals could demonstrate different effects with the same dose of drugs given on different occasions. Similarly, we have found that patients who have taken more than one overdose of the drugs have presented with different degrees of coma, despite identical blood barbiturate levels. There are several studies in animals (Kinsey, 1940a; 1940b; 1940c; Gruber and Keyser, 1946), and in humans (Isbell et al., 1950; Brodie et al., 1951), which have also demonstrated the development of tolerance to barbiturates. In support of this, we have encountered patients with blood levels of medium- and long-acting barbiturates well in excess of 'potentially fatal levels' (Berman et al., 1956) and yet the patients were only drowsy. Hadden et al. (1969) showed that the duration of coma in drug addicts is shorter than in those not addicted.

It is our strong conviction that the assessment of the patient with acute barbiturate poisoning must be based primarily on clinical criteria and that the blood barbiturate level should never take precedence (Maher and Schreiner, 1965). A further objection to the use of blood levels for the assessment of the severity of this poisoning is the considerable difficulty of devising a standard method of chemical assay. The commonly used method (Broughton, 1956) in fact measures non-toxic barbiturate metabolites as well as the active drug. Misleading high results may therefore be obtained, particularly when urine is being analysed.

INTENSIVE SUPPORTIVE THERAPY

The basic therapeutic regime may be discussed under the headings of emergency treatment and general care.

In practice, emergency treatment is concerned with the management of respiratory failure, circulatory failure, and the prevention of further absorption of the poison. It is particularly important that the simpler measures are instituted as early as possible even before the patient is transferred to hospital.

Respiratory failure

This is a common sequel of acute barbiturate poisoning and arises because of major airway obstruction or drug-induced respiratory centre depression or a combination of both.

Care of the airway Scrupulous maintenance of a clear airway is the first essential when dealing with unconscious patients. The mouth and fauces must be carefully examined and any debris removed using either a swab wrapped round a finger or a suction apparatus. Aspiration of the pharynx by a catheter introduced through the nostrils is not recommended, as trauma to the nasal epithelium can cause profuse haemorrhage which may pass post-nasally and make care of the airway more difficult. An oro-pharyngeal airway of appropriate size (size 3 for an adult of average build) should then be inserted to prevent the tongue from falling backwards and obstructing the airway. The patient must be nursed at all times in the semi-prone position to lessen the ever-present risk of aspiration of secretions or vomitus into the respiratory tract. At this stage the neck should be kept extended in order to increase the anteroposterior diameter of the larynx. Regular aspiration of pharyngeal secretions should be carried out particularly before the patient is turned from lying on one side to the other.

In more deeply unconscious patients (Grades III and IV) the cough reflex is usually absent and under these circumstances a cuffed endotracheal tube should be inserted. By this means not only is the patency of the airway ensured but regular bronchial toilet and assisted ventilation are facilitated. The cuff of the tube should be deflated for ten minutes every two hours and adequate humidification of the inspired air is essential if encrustation of the inside of the tube or even complete obstruction is to be prevented (Lindholm, 1969). Again regular bronchial toilet is essential, the frequency of which is determined by the quantity of secretions. When the patient is intubated the head should be slightly flexed to avoid distortion of the curve of the endotracheal tube and undue pressure on the larynx (Bergström, 1962).

The use of endotracheal intubation is not without hazard (Lewis and Swerdlow, 1964; Lindholm, 1969) and there has been particular concern about laryngeal damage after prolonged intubation (Tonkin and Harrison, 1966; Harrison and Tonkin, 1968). Bergström (1962) demonstrated laryngeal ulceration after as little as 16½ hours intubation and for this reason Leegaard (1960), Bergström *et al.* (1962) and Bergström (1966) stated that the duration of intubation should not exceed 24 hours. In contrast, Clemmesen and Nilsson (1961) suggested that intubation was acceptable up to 96 hours and after a recent survey Tonkin and Harrison (1966) proposed a maximum duration of 48 hours. A decision about the optimum duration of endotracheal intubation must be based on a knowledge of the short- and long-term complications of this technique compared with those of tracheostomy.

Complications of endotracheal intubation commonly occur around the time of intubation or extubation, the commonest being intubation of the right main bronchus. Bergström (1962) reported intubation of the right main bronchus in 10% of his poisoned patients, but this complication need not have serious consequences, provided it is recognized and rectified soon after intubation, before collapse of the left lung takes place. We agree that the only reliable method of determining the position of the tube is a chest radiograph.

Obstruction of the endotracheal tube by inspissated secretions is the most treacherous of complications as it arises insidiously and, unless promptly treated, the patient may die. This complication is the result of inadequate humidification of the inspired air and poor bronchial toilet. Constant surveillance of the intubated patient is mandatory and the nursing staff must report any difficulty in performing bronchial toilet or the development of cyanosis or increased respiratory effort.

Laryngeal oedema and stridor after extubation have in our experience only occurred in young women, the sex and age group in which one is most anxious to avoid tracheostomy. It seems likely that the small size of the female larynx with the resulting technical difficulties of intubation predisposes to this complication (Tonkin and Harrison, 1966) and in the last five years we have encountered two young women in whom the stridor was so severe as to necessitate emergency tracheostomy. This has also been reported by Milthers (1963). Tonkin and Harrison (1966) suggested that a high fluid intake, as in forced diuresis, also predisposed to post-extubation laryngeal oedema, but this has not been a factor in our experience. Nilsson (1951) documented the possible fatal outcome if prompt attention is not given to this complication.

Tonkin and Harrison (1966) based their conclusions regarding the duration of intubation on patients' symptoms and laryngoscopic examination following prolonged intubation. Though sore throats and hoarseness commonly occur and may indicate quite severe laryngeal damage, they settle rapidly and seem of little importance in a context of severe poisoning. Milthers (1963) reported no complications of intubation in any of 46 poisoned patients intubated for periods of 5 to 164 hours. Three of the eight tracheostomies in that series, however, were performed on account of laryngeal oedema. Pedersen and Petersen (1965) did not encounter serious complications even after long-standing intubation in 84 patients. Long-term follow-up studies of 120 patients after prolonged intubation revealed no more than mild residual sore throat or hoarseness in seven cases, all of whom had no abnormality on laryngoscopy (Tonkin and Harrison, 1966). Similarly, Nilsson (1951), Elbrond (1964) and Lindholm (1969) found few instances of serious long-term damage after follow-up for long periods. Thus, though there is no doubt that severe laryngeal damage may be delayed and present difficult therapeutic problems (Harrison and Tonkin, 1965; 1967), the incidence of such complications is very small. In the majority of patients, therefore, laryngeal ulceration and oedema must heal readily (Lindholm, 1969).

The tracheostomy rate in reported series of poisoned patients varies considerably. In our experience the duration of intubation and anxiety about possible laryngeal damage have been the most common indications for tracheostomy. These were the main reasons for the 44% tracheostomy rate reported by Bergström (1962), but difficulty in bronchial suction or the presence of respiratory obstruction and cyanosis despite intubation were also important. Neither Tonkin and Harrison (1966) nor we have performed tracheostomy for the latter reasons, though suction was more difficult through an endotracheal tube than a tracheostomy tube.

Several surveys of tracheostomy (Kuner and Goldman, 1967; Deverall, 1967) show a mortality of about 3% associated with the complications, quite apart from the underlying disease necessitating the operation. Since this mortality is of the same order of magnitude as the incidence of severe laryngeal damage following prolonged intubation, we can find little justification for abandoning prolonged endotracheal intubation in favour of early tracheostomy in the management of poisoned patients.

Assessment of ventilation   Once the patency of the airway has been ensured an objective assessment of the adequacy of ventilation should be obtained. Ideally, this means arterial puncture and measurement of blood pH, pCO_2, pO_2, and standard bicarbonate. Venous and capillary blood samples are inadequate in patients who are peripherally vasoconstricted and hypothermic. Unfortunately, analysis of arterial blood gases is not universally available at short notice and a simpler method of assessment is desirable. The pCO_2 may be measured by the rebreathing method of Campbell and Howell (1962).

In our experience and that of Baker (1969) measurement of the respiratory minute volume has been most useful. We have used a Wright's spirometer, which is not highly accurate, particularly at low flow rates, but has the great advantage of being simple to use. If the minute volume is less than four litres, significant respiratory impairment is almost certainly present and arterial blood gas analysis should be undertaken immediately. Further treatment depends on the results obtained.

Because metabolism is depressed by barbiturate and hypothermia, carbon dioxide production is reduced and the pCO_2 is not as commonly raised as might be expected (Sykes *et al.*, 1969). Kirby and McNicol (1966) showed that arterial pCO_2 exceeded 45 mm Hg in 30% of a group of patients with moderately severe barbiturate poisoning. On the other hand, significant hypoxia was present more often than could be suspected from clinical examination, with 10% of patients having an arterial oxygen saturation below 55%.

When the pO_2 is reduced but above 60 mm Hg and the pCO_2 lies between 40 and 50 mm Hg, oxygen therapy should be administered using initially a 24% Ventimask with an oxygen flow rate of 4 lit/min. The arterial blood gases should be repeated after 30 min, and if there is no further rise in pCO_2 a 28% Ventimask may then be used. Careful and continued monitoring of the arterial blood gases is necessary until the patient's condition becomes satisfactory.

Respiratory failure may be assumed if the pO_2 falls below 60 mm Hg and/or the pCO_2 is greater than 50 mm Hg. Under these circumstances assisted ventilation using a mechanical respirator is necessary.

Circulatory failure

Clinical assessment of peripheral circulatory failure in acute barbiturate poisoning is often difficult since the usual features of shock are prevented from appearing because of the nervous system depression and hypothermia. Under these circumstances tissue perfusion is best assessed by measuring the urinary output and this should be done in all severe cases. In practice, however, shock may be assumed to exist if the systolic blood pressure falls below 90 mm Hg in patients over the age of 50 years, or below 80 mm Hg in younger patients.

Shock in poisoned patients should not be treated till a clear airway has been established and hypoxia corrected. These measures alone will frequently correct shock (Reed *et al.*, 1952). Oxygen therapy is indicated for all patients in whom there has been a sustained fall in blood pressure, and acidaemia, which may contribute to the 'shocked' state, should be sought by measurement of arterial blood pH, pCO_2, and standard bicarbonate. Depending on these results, assisted respiration or intravenous infusion of sodium bicarbonate should be undertaken.

The exact mechanism of circulatory failure in acute barbiturate poisoning remains unknown (see Chapter 8, 'Shock in Acute Barbiturate Poisoning'). It has, however, been studied in detail by Shubin and Weil (1965), who showed that, apart from a direct depressant effect of barbiturates on the myocardium, the main causative factor was increased capillary permeability with exudation of fluid into the extra-cellular space with resulting reduction of the circulating blood volume and cardiac output. They also suggested that there was marked venous pooling, particularly in the lower limbs where the venous valves were considered to become incompetent. If severe, diminution of cardiac output and hypotension may result in acute renal tubular necrosis or cerebral ischaemia or thrombosis. For these reasons the pulse and blood pressure must be monitored constantly and treatment instituted without delay.

There has been considerable discussion about the most appropriate form of treatment for circulatory failure in poisoned patients. In the light of what is known of the aetiology of shock, the first step in management is to elevate the foot of the bed. By this means we have successfully treated 78% of 143 hypotensive patients poisoned with a variety of drugs in the last two years.

If the blood pressure does not rise satisfactorily following elevation of the foot of the bed, more specific treatment becomes necessary. Clemmesen and Nilsson (1961) recommended the use of plasma expanders rather than vasopressor agents, and Shubin and Weil (1965) produced further evidence to support this. The main risk of vasopressor drugs is excessive constriction of the renal arterioles, which may result in acute renal tubular necrosis. Considering the suggested mechanism of circulatory failure in acute barbiturate poisoning, it would seem logical to give intravenous infusions to re-establish the circulating blood volume, but, although the circulating blood volume is diminished, these patients are seldom dehydrated. In fact, they have tissue fluid excess. If the circulating blood volume is, therefore, reconstituted in the stage of severe poisoning with substances such as plasma expanders or whole blood, it is possible that with reversal of the mechanisms of circulatory failure during the period of re-covery the patient may develop circulatory overload with cardiac failure and acute pulmonary oedema. In practice, we have found that if elevation of the lower limbs is ineffective in raising the blood pressure, metaraminol 2.5 mg should be given intra-venously and followed after an interval of 20 min. by double this dose if the desired effect is not obtained. Care should be taken not to elevate the systolic blood pressure above 100 mm Hg since above this level metaraminol produces a net reduction in cardiac output and intense constriction of the renal arterioles, and it is under these circumstances that renal damage is likely. If the systolic blood pressure does not rise above 100 mm Hg it has been shown that the urinary flow increases (Weil, 1957; Haugen and Roden, 1959) and previous studies (Matthew and Lawson, 1966) indi-cated a very low incidence of renal failure in a large series of patients with acute bar-biturate poisoning treated in this way.

This regimen of metaraminol is, therefore, simple and has been effective in 63 % of patients whose hypotension was not corrected by elevation of the foot of the bed.

In a small proportion of poisoned patients attempts to increase the venous return and two injections of metaraminol fail to correct hypotension. In these cases no further vasopressor agents should be given and the intravascular volume should be expanded using either plasma or low-molecular weight dextran. Several litres may have to be infused and the central venous pressure should be monitored in every case.

Prevention of further absorption of poison

This may be achieved by inducing vomiting or performing gastric lavage. In view of the danger of inhalation of gastric content, vomiting should only be induced if the patient is lying on his side with his head dependent; children should be placed in the 'spanking' position. As good a stimulus to emesis as any is the old-fashioned one of introducing a finger or spoon handle into the patient's pharynx. Various drugs have also been widely recommended as emetics, especially in children. These include apo-morphine, syrup of ipecacuanha and various copper preparations. The latter two substances tend to be rather uncertain in their effects and sometimes rather slow in action. The emetine content of the ipecacuanha may be absorbed and itself produce undesirable toxic effects. Apomorphine is also dangerous insofar as it may induce protracted vomiting and may exacerbate hypotension. It is true that the effects of apomorphine may be counteracted by an injection of nalorphine, but in general these preparations are not recommended.

In hospital, the removal of poison from the stomach is most satisfactorily achieved by gastric aspiration and lavage. The dangers associated with this procedure are inadequately recognized and its limitations are not fully appreciated. Vomiting and inhalation of gastric content are frequent complications in inexperienced or careless hands. Gastric aspiration and lavage should, therefore, only be carried out if the patient has an adequate cough reflex or is sufficiently unconscious to permit protection of the lungs by cuffed endotracheal intubation. The position of the patient is most important; he should be placed in the head-down position and maintained on his left side throughout the procedure. In view of the ever-present danger of inhalation, suction apparatus must be available and ready for immediate use at all times. An adequate size of tube such as a Jacques stomach tube (30 English gauge) must be used and this is lubricated and introduced through the mouth. This tube is of sufficient calibre to make it extremely unlikely that it will enter the patient's trachea. It is, therefore, technically easy to insert and has the added advantage that removal of semi-solid food particles is possible. Before lavage is commenced stomach content should be aspirated either by lowering the end of the tube and making use of gravity or by actual suction using a Dakin's syringe. Lavage is then carried out with 300 ml aliquots of lukewarm water (38°C) and continued until the returning fluid is clear. In children, appropriate sizes of tubes and volumes of water should, of course, be used.

It is generally accepted that gastric aspiration and lavage may be of value in barbiturate poisoning when carried out within four hours of ingestion of the overdose or in deeply unconscious patients whose stomachs are narcotized by the drugs (Matthew et al., 1966). The quantity of barbiturate recovered by this means is extremely variable but there is no doubt that on occasions substantial amounts are obtained with benefit to the patient.

GENERAL CARE

General care of the patient poisoned with barbiturates includes the management of hypothermia, correction of water and electrolyte imbalance, treatment of infection and general nursing care.

Hypothermia

The treatment of hypothermia is controversial largely as a result of insufficient knowledge of the precise mechanisms which operate as a result of severe reduction in body temperature. Hypothermia is a common finding in acute barbiturate poisoning and is conventionally regarded as present when the rectal temperature falls below 36°C. Low reading rectal thermometers must be used routinely if this diagnosis is not to be overlooked. The great majority of patients with acute barbiturate poisoning are only moderately hypothermic with temperatures between 30 and 36°C. At these levels, other things being equal, normal body metabolism can be maintained. The management of these patients is, therefore, relatively simple and should be directed primarily at prevention of further heat loss by nursing the patient in an environmental temperature between 26.4 and 29.4°C (Hockaday, 1969). The patient is usually covered with warm blankets but it is important, if accidents are to be avoided, that electric blankets and hotwater bottles are not used. If hypothermia has been prolonged, and particularly if it is associated with hypotension, hydrocortisone 100 mg should be administered intravenously at six-hourly intervals (Duguid et al., 1961; Mitchell et al., 1959; Matthew and Lawson, 1970). It is also usual to give a broad spectrum antibiotic, preferably intravenously.

Occasionally, severe hypothermia with a rectal temperature below 30°C is present. As a result metabolism becomes very sluggish and further heat loss will result unless active reheating is instituted. Several methods are available but the rate at which re-warming is carried out must be governed by the age of the patient and the duration of hypothermia. If hypothermia is reasonably recent and the patient is in a young age group it is generally agreed that rapid re-warming is indicated (Burton and Edholm, 1955; Lee and Ames, 1965; Keatinge, 1969). This may be satisfactorily carried out using a warm water bath at 40°C. On the other hand, if the hypothermia is of considerable duration or if the patient is in the older age group, rapid surface warming may induce serious cardiac arrhythmias and severe and irreversible peripheral circulatory failure (Adolph, 1950; Duguid et al., 1961; Hockaday, 1969). For these patients it is necessary to provide heat centrally and various techniques have been used. Lash et al. (1967) used repeated peritoneal dialysis using warm fluid. Blades and Pierpoint (1954) irrigated the pleural sac, and perfusion of the mediastinum was employed by Linton and Ledingham (1966). Haemodialysis using warm dialysis fluid has been used by Lee and Ames (1965) and Cooper (1968), but it did not prove to be highly successful. A further method which has proved very successful and can produce rapid re-warming is the immersion of one forearm in water at 43°C with the patient otherwise wrapped in blankets and kept in a warm environment. This method has been claimed (Cooper, 1968) to achieve elevation of the body temperature by as much as 3°C every hour and it would seem from the reports that it is effective and has the great advantage of being technically very simple. At the present time it would seem to be the method of choice.

Many patients with severe hypothermia appear cyanosed, but it should be remembered that these patients may be extremely sensitive to procedures such as bladder catheterization or endotracheal intubation, both of which may provoke cardiac arrest. It is most important, therefore, that respiratory intensive care is carried out only in those cases in which arterial blood gas analysis gives a clear indication.

In otherwise young and healthy patients, the prognosis is generally favourable, but elderly patients tolerate hypothermia very poorly and the mortality is high in this age group.

Water and electrolyte balance

Treatment to maintain water and electrolyte balance in patients with acute barbiturate poisoning should simply follow conventional lines of assessment and treatment. It is often possible to correct dehydration by increasing oral fluids if the patient is sufficiently conscious to drink and has no nausea or vomiting. If the patient is unconscious for longer than 12 hours, however, intravenous infusion of 0.5 lit normal saline and 1 lit 5% dextrose in rotation is usually all that is necessary. The rate of infusion can be judged simply on clinical assessment of the patient and careful measurement of urinary output. Particular care must be taken when the patient is hypothermic since marked polyuria may occur during the re-warming phase.

Electrolyte supplements may be added according to the results of plasma electrolyte levels. Cooper (1968), however, stressed that in severely hypothermic patients, measurement of plasma electrolytes should be performed on arterial blood, as stagnation of venous blood in these cases may produce erroneous results.

Antibiotic therapy

When there is clinical or laboratory support for a diagnosis of infection in patients with acute barbiturate poisoning there can be no argument but that a suitable antibiotic must be given without delay and in adequate dosage. There is considerable controversy, however, about the use of prophylactic antibiotics in patients unconscious as a result of poisoning. Many believe that all patients unconscious from whatever cause should be given prophylactic treatment in this way, but there is considerable evidence that prophylactic antibiotics are of little or no value in unconscious patients and that this treatment may even be harmful (Petersdorf *et al.*, 1957; Mackintosh and Matthew, 1965). If sufficient care is given to the toilet of the mouth and airway together with frequent turning of the patient and physiotherapy the incidence of respiratory infection is low and prophylactic antibiotics are unnecessary (Henderson and Merrill, 1966; Matthew and Lawson, 1970; Hadden *et al.*, 1969).

Nursing care

From this description of the regimen of intensive supportive therapy it will have become clear that nursing care must be of a very high standard. Indeed, the success of this form of treatment largely depends on the skill of the nursing attendants. Patients must be turned half-hourly to prevent the occurrence of skin pressure sores and at each turning full passive movements of all limbs together with percussion of the chest must be performed. Maintenance of the patency of the airway with careful, sterile catheterization of endotracheal and tracheostomy tubes is a vital part of nursing care.

In the great majority of patients with acute barbiturate poisoning it is unnecessary to employ the highly dangerous procedure of bladder catheterization. In deeply unconscious patients with this condition incontinence of urine in the absence of gross bladder distension is often a good prognostic sign that the patient will soon recover consciousness. It is usually possible, with judicious positioning of receptacles or the use of Paul's tubing in males, to avoid frequent wetting of the bed-clothes, but even if this does occur, with the frequency of nursing care required, it should not present a major problem. Only if the bladder becomes grossly distended and simple hand pressure does not readily provoke urine flow should bladder catheterization be performed (Matthew and Lawson, 1970).

The eyes should be protected by instilling methyl cellulose drops into the conjunctival sac and taping the eyelids to prevent exposure keratitis.

THE RETURN TO CONSCIOUSNESS

In this centre barbiturates have been found to be responsible for the greatest number of deep comas (Table 3) and also for the majority of the longest comas (Table 4). The duration of coma in individual cases of barbiturate poisoning cannot be predicted with any accuracy. Alcoholics and drug addicts have been shown to have shorter periods of coma than normal individuals, while those suffering from other medical conditions or liver and renal disease have longer periods of coma (Hadden et al., 1969).

TABLE 3

Depth of coma and drug ingested in 222 unconscious patients
(From Matthew et al., 1969)

	Coma Grade		
Drug	Grade II	Grade III	Grade IV
Barbiturates	41	42	27
Mandrax	15	14	4
Others	45	30	4
Total	101	86	35

TABLE 4

Duration of coma and drugs ingested in 220 patients (From Matthew et al., 1969)

Duration (hr)	Barbiturates	Mandrax	Others	Total
< 12	64	25	66	155
13–18	8	4	9	21
19–24	7	—	3	10
25–48	20	—	1	21
49–72	4	1	—	5
73–96	5	2	—	7
97+	—	1	—	1

Return to consciousness is associated with a return of reflex activity and increasing responsiveness to painful stimuli. Intubated patients can be seen to gag upon their endotracheal tube and those being ventilated struggle against the respirator. Positive pressure ventilation should be discontinued as soon as the patient makes adequate respiratory efforts. It is our practice to disconnect the patient from the ventilator for a period of up to three minutes. If spontaneous respiration commences, its adequacy can be assessed as before; otherwise, ventilation must be continued for a further period of time.

Endotracheal tubes should also be removed as soon as the patient begins to gag or cough on the tube or make movements of the head. Removal of the tube at this stage may reduce the incidence of serious laryngeal damage.

During the return to consciousness body temperature rises from hypothermic levels and patients frequently show an irregular pyrexia up to 39°C. This pyrexia commonly persists while the patient is unconscious; it usually cannot be explained on the basis of infection and is not necessarily a reason for antibiotic therapy. Within 24 hours of recovering consciousness the temperature returns to normal.

Attention has recently been drawn to elevation of serum enzymes in acute poisoning (Brown et al., 1969). Patients unconscious as a result of sedative drug poisoning including barbiturate poisoning may show marked rises in creatine kinase levels and less dramatic elevation of serum levels of aspartate transaminase and hydroxybutyrate dehydrogenase. Isoenzyme studies show that the creatine kinase probably derived from skeletal muscle. Presumably, there is some degree of muscle necrosis which if extensive may provide a basis for the ischaemic contractures and muscle calcification which occasionally complicate acute barbiturate poisoning (Clark and Sumerling, 1966; Howse and Seddon, 1966). It is important to appreciate that the elevated serum enzymes do not necessarily indicate myocardial damage.

During recovery from acute barbiturate poisoning a small minority of patients become violent and abusive as a result of confusion and disorientation. It is frequently necessary to restrain patients in this state and a small dose of chlorpromazine (e.g., 50 mg intramuscularly) is usually sufficient to sedate the patient and permit calm emergence to full consciousness. In some patients, especially those habituated to barbiturates, fits may occur during the period of recovery; these are best treated by diazepam (Valium) 10 mg intravenously.

CONCLUSIONS

When the Scandinavian method of supportive therapy was introduced it was widely criticized as being a policy of 'therapeutic nihilism' (Koppanyi and Fazekas, 1950). The regimen of treatment which has been described is a development from the original form promoted by Clemmesen and Nilsson (1961). Far from being nihilistic, intensive supportive therapy requires a high standard of medical and particularly nursing care.

Its use as the basic approach to all forms of sedative poisoning and to barbiturate poisoning in particular has been more than justified by the very low mortality in various series (Clemmesen and Nilsson, 1961; Matthew and Lawson, 1966; Baker, 1969; Burston, 1969; Matthew et al., 1969).

The wide use of specialized techniques such as forced diuresis, peritoneal dialysis and haemodialysis has been advocated by several authors (Lee and Ames, 1965; Setter et al., 1966; Linton et al., 1967). Though undoubtedly these methods have a role in the treatment of severe poisoning by long-acting barbiturates (Lassen, 1960; Myschetsky and Lassen, 1963; Linton et al., 1967; Mawer and Lee, 1968; Kennedy et al., 1969; Raeburn et al., 1969), it is now clear that they are required in no more than 5% of patients poisoned by barbiturates. In particular, they have been shown to be of no value in poisoning by quinalbarbitone, amylobarbitone and pentobarbitone (Mawer and Lee, 1968; Hadden et al., 1969).

In our experience also, apart from a very few carefully selected cases, the use of these highly sophisticated techniques is unnecessary, particularly when the cost in terms of money and manpower is considered together with the dangers to the patients inherent in their use. Intensive supportive therapy must form the basis of treatment in every case and if properly applied will be all that is necessary for the successful management of the vast majority of patients with acute barbiturate poisoning.

REFERENCES

ADOLPH, E. F. (1950), Oxygen consumption of hypothermic rats and acclimatization to cold. Amer. J. Physiol., 161, 359.
BAKER, A. B. (1969), Early treatment of the unconscious patient suffering from drug overdose. Med. J. Aust., 1, 497.
BERGSTRÖM, J. (1962), Laryngologic aspects of the treatment of acute barbiturate poisoning. Acta oto-laryng. (Stockh.), 54, Suppl. 173, 1.
BERGSTRÖM, J. (1966), Intubation and tracheotomy in barbiturate poisoning. Int. Anesth. Clin., 4, No. 2, 323.
BERGSTRÖM, J., MOBERG, A. and ORELL, S. R. (1962), On the pathogenesis of laryngeal injuries following prolonged intubation. Acta oto-laryng. (Stockh.), 55, 342.
BERMAN, L. B., JEGHERS, H. J., SCHREINER, G. E. and PALLOTTA, A. J. (1956), Hemodialysis, an effective therapy for acute barbiturate poisoning. J. Amer. med. Ass., 161, 820.
BEVERIDGE, G. W. and LAWSON, A. A. H. (1965), Occurrence of bullous lesions in acute barbiturate intoxication. Brit. med. J., 1, 835.
BLADES, B. and PIERPOINT, H. C. (1954), A simple method for inducing hypothermia. Ann. Surg., 140, 557.
BRODIE, B. B., MARK, L. C., LIEF, P. A., BERNSTEIN, E. and PAPPER, E. M. (1951), Acute tolerance to thiopental. J. Pharmacol. exp. Ther., 102, 215.
BROUGHTON, P. M. G. (1956), A rapid ultraviolet spectrophotometric method for the detection, estimation and identification of barbiturates in biological material. Biochem. J., 63, 207.
BROWN, S. S., PROUDFOOT, A. T., RAEBURN, J. A. and WRIGHT, N. (1969), Elevation of serum enzyme levels in acute poisoning. Proc. VIIth Int. Congr. Clin. Chem. (in press).
BURSTON, G. R. (1969), Severe self-poisoning in Sunderland. Brit. med. J., 1, 679.
BURTON, A. C. and EDHOLM, O. G. (1955), Man in a cold environment: physiological and pathological effects of exposure to low temperatures. Monographs of the Physiol. Soc., 2. Arnold, London.

CAMPBELL, E. J. M. and HOWELL, J. B. L. (1962), Rebreathing method for measurement of mixed venous pCO_2. *Brit. med. J.*, 2, 630.

CARROLL, B. J. (1969), Barbiturate overdosage: presentation with focal neurological signs. *Med. J. Aust.*, 1, 1133.

CLARK, J. G. and SUMERLING, M. D. (1966), Muscle necrosis and calcification in acute renal failure due to barbiturate intoxication. *Brit. med. J.*, 2, 214.

CLEMMESEN, C. and NILSSON, E. (1961), Therapeutic trends in the treatment of barbiturate poisoning. *Clin. Pharmacol. Ther.*, 2, 220.

CLOW, W. M. and SMITH, A. C. A. (1967), Rapid quantitative barbiturate estimation: a critical study of a bedside method. *Scot. med. J.*, 12, 307.

COOPER, K. E. (1968), Temperature regulation and its disorders. In: D. N. Baron *et al.* (Ed) *Recent Advances in Medicine*, p. 333. Churchill, London.

CURRY, A. S. (1964), Rapid quantitative barbiturate estimation. *Brit. med. J.*, 1, 354.

CURRY, A. S. (1965), Systematic toxicological analysis. Symposium – *Identification of Drugs and Poisons*, p. 46. Pharmaceutical Society of Great Britain. Unwin, Surrey.

DEVERALL, P. B. (1967), Tracheal stricture following tracheostomy. *Thorax*, 22, 572.

DOBOS, J. K., PHILLIPS, J. and COVO, G. A. (1961), Acute barbiturate intoxication. *J. Amer. med. Ass.*, 176, 268.

DUGUID, H., SIMPSON, R. G. and STOWERS, J. M. (1961), Accidental hypothermia. *Lancet*, 2, 1213.

ELBROND, O. (1964), Laryngeal damage following prolonged intubation. A follow-up investigation. *Dan. med. Bull.*, 11, 134.

ELLIS, G. G., COMISH, K. A. and HEWER, R. L. (1966), Attempted suicide in Leicester. *Practitioner*, 196, 557.

GRUBER, C. M. and KEYSER, G. F. (1946), A study on the development of tolerance and cross tolerance to barbiturates in experimental animals. *J. Pharmacol. exp. Ther.*, 86, 186.

HADDEN, J., JOHNSON, K., SMITH, S., PRICE, L. and GIARDINA, E. (1969), Acute barbiturate intoxication. Concepts of management. *J. Amer. med. Ass.*, 209, 893.

HARRISON, G. A. and TONKIN, J. P. (1965), Laryngeal complications of prolonged endotracheal intubation. *Med. J. Aust.*, 2, 709.

HARRISON, G. A. and TONKIN, J. P. (1967), Some serious laryngeal complications of prolonged endotracheal intubation. *Med. J. Aust.*, 1, 605.

HARRISON, G. A. and TONKIN, J. P. (1968), Prolonged (therapeutic) endotracheal intubation. *Brit. J. Anaesth.*, 40, 241.

HAUGEN, H. M. and RODEN, J. S. (1959), Septic abortion with adrenal shock. *Obstet. and Gynec.*, 14, 184.

HENDERSON, L. W. and MERRILL, J. P. (1966), Treatment of barbiturate intoxication. *Ann. intern. Med.*, 64, 876.

HOCKADAY, T. D. R. (1969), Accidental hypothermia. *Brit. J., hosp. Med.*, 2, 1083.

HOWSE, A. J. G. and SEDDON, H. (1966), Ischaemic contracture of muscle associated with carbon monoxide barbiturate poisoning. *Brit. med. J.*, 1, 192.

IBSEN, B. (1966), Intensive therapy: background and development. *Int. Anesth. Clin.*, 4, No. 2, 277.

ISBELL, H., ALTSCHUL, S., KORNETSKY, C. H., EISENMAN, A. J., FLANARY, H. G., and FRASER, H. F. (1950), Chronic barbiturate intoxication. *Arch. Neurol. Psychiat. (Chic.)*, 64, 1.

JONES, D. I. R. (1969), Self-poisoning with drugs. A view from a general medical unit. *Practitioner*, 203, 73.

KEATINGE, W. R. (1969), *Survival in Cold Water*. Blackwell, Oxford.

KENNEDY, A. C., LINDSAY, R. M., BRIGGS, J. D., LUKE, R. G., YOUNG, N., and CAMPBELL, D. (1969), Successful treatment of three cases of very severe barbiturate poisoning. *Lancet*, 1, 995.

KESSEL, N. (1965), Self-poisoning. *Brit. med. J.*, 2, 1265 and 1336.

KINSEY, V. E. (1940a), Use of sodium pentobarbital for repeated anesthesia in the rabbit. *J. Amer. pharm. Ass.*, 29, 292.

KINSEY, V. E. (1940b), The use of sodium pentobarbital for repeated anesthesia in the guinea pig. *J. Amer. pharm. Ass.*, 29, 342.

KINSEY, V. E. (1940c), Use of sodium pentobarbital for repeated anesthesia in the white rat. *J. Amer. pharm. Ass.*, 29, 387.

KIRBY, B. J. and MCNICOL, M. W. (1966), personal communication to A. J. Levi. In: D. N. Baron *et al.* (Ed) *Recent Advances in Medicine*, 1968, p. 107. Churchill, London.

KIRKEGAARD, A. (1949), Severe acute barbiturate poisoning. *Ugeskr. Laeg.*, 111, 356.

KJAER-LARSEN, J. (1956), Delirious psychosis and convulsions due to Megimide. *Lancet*, II, 967.

KOPPANYI, T. and FAZEKAS, J. F. (1950), Acute barbiturate poisoning. Analysis and evaluation of current therapy. *Amer. J. med. Sci.*, 220, 559.

KUNER, J. and GOLDMAN, A. (1967), Prolonged nasotracheal intubation in adults versus tracheostomy. *Dis. Chest.*, 51, 270.

LASH, R. F., BURDETTE, J. A. and OZDIL, T. (1967), Accidental profound hypothermia and barbiturate intoxication. *J. Amer. med. Ass.*, 201, 269.

LASSEN, N. A. (1960), Treatment of severe acute barbiturate poisoning by forced diuresis and alkalinization of the urine. *Lancet*, II, 338.

LEE, H. A. and AMES, A. C. (1965), Haemodialysis in severe barbiturate poisoning. *Brit. med. J.*, 1, 1217.

LEEGAARD, T. (1960), in discussion. *Acta oto-laryng. (Stockh.)*, Suppl., 158, 102.

LEWIS, R. N. and SWERDLOW, M. (1964), Hazards of endotracheal anaesthesia. *Brit. J. Anaesth.*, 36, 504.

LINDHOLM, C. E. (1969), Prolonged endotracheal intubation. *Acta anaesth. scand.*, Suppl. 33.

LINTON, A. L. and LEDINGHAM, I. M. (1966), Severe hypothermia with barbiturate intoxication. *Lancet*, 1, 24.

LINTON, A. L., LUKE, R. G. and BRIGGS, J. D. (1967), Methods of forced diuresis and its application in barbiturate poisoning. *Lancet*, 2, 377.

LOUW, A. and SONNE, L. M. (1956), Megimide in the treatment of barbituric acid poisoning. *Lancet*, II, 961.

MACKINTOSH, T. F. and MATTHEW, H. (1965), Do unconscious poisoned patients need prophylactic penicillin? *Lancet*, I, 1252.

MAHER, J. F. and SCHREINER, G. E. (1965), The clinical dialysis of poisons. *Trans. Amer. Soc. artif. intern. Org.*, 11, 349.

MARK, L. C. (1967), Analeptics: changing concepts, declining status. *Amer. J. med. Sci.*, 254, 296.

MATTHEW, H. and LAWSON, A. A. H. (1966), Acute barbiturate poisoning – a review of two years experience. *Quart. J. Med.*, 35, 539.

MATTHEW, H. and LAWSON, A. A. H. (1970), *Treatment of Common Acute Poisonings*. Livingstone, Edinburgh.

MATTHEW, H., MACKINTOSH, T. F., TOMPSETT, S. L. and CAMERON, J. C. (1966), Gastric aspiration and lavage in acute poisoning. *Brit. med. J.*, 1, 1333.

MATTHEW, H., PROUDFOOT, A. T., BROWN, S. S. and AITKEN, R. C. B. (1969), Acute poisoning: organization and work-load of a treatment centre. *Brit. med. J.*, 3, 489.

MAWER, G. E. and LEE, H. A. (1968), Value of forced diuresis in acute barbiturate poisoning. *Brit. med. J.*, 2, 790.

MILTHERS, E. (1963), Respiratory embarrassment in narcotic poisoning. *Dan. med. Bull.*, 10, 109.

MITCHELL, J. R. A., SURRIDGE, D. H. C. and WILLISON, R. G. (1959), Hypothermia after chlorpromazine in myxoedematous patients. *Brit. med. J.*, 2, 932.

MYSCHETZKY, A. (1961), The significance of Megimide in the treatment of acute barbiturate poisoning. *Dan. med. Bull.*, 8, 33.

MYSCHETZKY, A. and LASSEN, N. A. (1963), Osmotic diuresis and alkalinization of the urine in the treatment of severe acute barbiturate intoxication. *Dan. med. Bull.*, 10, 104.

NILSSON, E. (1951), On treatment of barbiturate poisoning. *Acta med. scand.*, Suppl. 253.

PEDERSEN, B. S. and PETERSEN, P. N. (1965), A resuscitation centre for acute poisoning. *Dan. med. Bull.*, 12, 145.

PETERSDORF, R. G., CURTIN, J. A., HOEPRICH, P. D., PEELER, R. N. and BENNET, I. L. (1957), A study of antibiotic prophylaxis in unconscious patients. *New Engl. J. Med.*, 257, 1001.

RAEBURN, J. A., CAMERON, J. C. and MATTHEW, H. (1969), Severe barbiturate poisoning. Contrasts in management. *Clin. Toxicol.*, 2, 133.

REED, C. E., DRIGGS, M. F. and FOOTE, C. C. (1952), Acute barbiturate intoxication: a study of 300 cases based on a physiologic system of classification of the severity of the intoxication. *Ann. intern. Med.*, 37, 290.

RICHARDS, R. K. and TAYLOR, J. D. (1956), Some factors influencing distribution, metabolism and action of barbiturates: a review. *Anesthesiology*, 17, 414.

ROCHE, M., WYNNE, L. C. and Haskins, D. M. (1950), Therapy of acute barbiturate poisoning: report of three cases. *Ann. intern. Med.*, 33, 73.

SETTER, J. G., MAHER, J. F. and SCHREINER, G. E. (1966), Barbiturate intoxication. Evaluation of therapy including dialysis in a large series selectively referred because of severity. *Arch. intern. Med.*, 117, 224.

SHAW, F. H. (1955), Further experiences with Megimide – a barbiturate antagonist. *Med. J. Aust.*, 2, 889.

SHUBIN, H. and WEIL, M. H. (1965), The mechanism of shock following suicidal doses of barbiturates, narcotics and tranquilizer drugs, with observations on the effects of treatment. *Amer. J. Med.*, 38, 853.

SHULMAN, A., SHAW, F. H., CASS, N. M. and WHYTE, H. M. (1955), A new treatment of barbiturate intoxication. *Brit. med. J.*, 1, 1238.

SYKES, M. K., MCNICOL, M. W. and CAMPBELL, E. J. M. (1969), *Respiratory Failure*, p. 211. Blackwell, Oxford.

TONKIN, J. P. and HARRISON, G. A. (1966), The effect on the larynx of prolonged endotracheal intubation. *Med. J. Aust.*, 2, 581.

WEIL, M. H. (1957), Current concepts on the management of shock. *Circulation*, 16, 1097.

WRIGHT, J. T. and JOHNS, R. G. S. (1953), A study of barbiturate intoxication by an ultraviolet spectrophotometric technique. *J. clin. Path.*, 6, 78.

12. forced diuresis in treatment of acute barbiturate poisoning

A. Myschetzky and N. A. Lassen

An increased rate of elimination of barbiturates may be effected either by enhancing the urinary excretion or by haemodialysis, peritoneal dialysis, or exchange transfusion. This chapter summarizes ten years' experience with forced diuresis as active treatment in the 50 most severely poisoned patients out of the 500 patients suffering from acute barbiturate poisoning admitted each year to the Poisoning Treatment Centre, Copenhagen.

The treatment is based on urea-induced osmotic diuresis and alkalinization of the urine, resulting in a 24-hour urinary output of approximately 12 litres of urine with a pH of 8. The duration of the period of unconsciousness can thereby be reduced to about one-third for several of the long-acting barbiturates (Lassen, 1960; Myschetzky and Lassen, 1963). The therapeutic advantage of this shortening of coma – e.g., from six days to two days – must be weighed against the complications of the therapy and against its technical difficulties. This chapter will give special attention to these problems in order to render possible a realistic evaluation of the indications for this therapy.

It must be emphasized that active therapy plays a distinctly secondary role to general supportive treatment, i.e., control of respiration (in some cases assisted ventilation), fluid administration, chemotherapy of secondary infections, and avoidance of gastric lavage and of analeptic drugs (Lassen, 1960). Fig. 1 illustrates the effect of the introduction of the various components of supportive treatment. Mortality fell from 20 to 5%. Adding diuretic treatment has only resulted in a further small drop to 0.9%.

METHOD OF TREATMENT

Before starting forced diuresis the patient must not be in a state of severe circulatory shock; the blood pressure must be above 90 mm Hg, perhaps even a little higher in elderly, habitually hypertensive patients. The patient must be well hydrated, but not

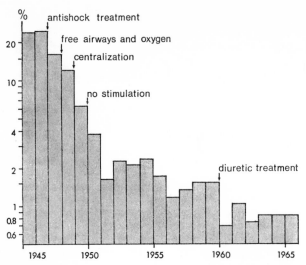

Fig. 1.   Mortality rate in Copenhagen from acute narcotic poisoning.

overloaded; *i.e.*, overt cardiac failure as evidenced by pulmonary vascular engorgement must not be present. Respiratory insufficiency (determination of arterial pH, pCO_2, O_2 saturation, and standard bicarbonate) must be corrected by assisted ventilation. Renal function must be adequate as shown by spontaneous diuresis and a serum creatinine value not above 2.5 to 3.0 mg per 100 ml. Obviously the serum barbiturate should be of such a level that a coma duration of more than 72 hours can be expected if no active treatment is given. As will be shown, a combination of laboratory findings and clinical signs must be present before forced diuresis is used.

TYPES OF BARBITURATES

Forced diuresis is mainly indicated in severe cases of poisoning with long-acting barbiturates. Preparations of this type most widely used as hypnotics in Copenhagen and consequently also used as means of self-poisoning are allyl-isopropyl-barbituric acid (aprobarbital), diethyl-barbituric acid (barbitone – especially in combination with equal amounts of aprobarbital), and phenyl-ethyl-barbituric acid (phenobarbitone). In poisoning by these drugs forced diuresis is very effective and a high proportion of the barbiturate ingested can be found in the urine. The barbiturate levels indicating that forced diuresis might be used depend on the particular preparation ingested and the possible degree of habituation in the individual patient. The mean serum levels at which patients wake up are 3.5 mg per 100 ml for aprobarbital, about 10 mg per 100 ml for barbitone, and about 8 mg per 100 ml for phenobarbitone, individual variation being widest in the two latter-mentioned preparations. From this it will be evident that measurement of the serum barbiturate level is only of value when it is supplemented by a determination of the type of barbiturate concerned.

We usually only institute forced diuresis in patients who are severely poisoned and who have serum levels greater than 10 mg per 100 ml for aprobarbital and 15 mg per 100 ml for barbitone and phenobarbitone. Patients habituated to the drug, and only in light coma (still reacting to pain), are not actively treated in spite of serum concentrations exceeding these limits.

FLUIDS USED FOR DIURETIC TREATMENT

UREA SOLUTION

The diuretic agent used is purified urea, which is available in a concentration of 50% in isotonic saline. The solution is sterilized by filtration and can be stored at 4°C for several months. Mannitol can also be used but, if it is, it is more difficult to maintain the fluid balance during treatment lasting several days. It is of practical value that with urea it is easy to obtain daily measurement of the osmotic load by blood urea determinations.

The urea solution is added in suitable amounts to the hourly fluid load. Several such hourly fluid loads, e.g., six, are prepared at a time in order to facilitate practical management.

ELECTROLYTE SOLUTION

Lactate is preferred to bicarbonate as the alkalinizing agent because the glucose containing electrolyte solution cannot be autoclaved if its pH is too high. The solution we use is hypotonic, each litre containing 40 mEq sodium lactate, 12 mEq sodium chloride, 12 mEq potassium chloride and 18 g glucose.

This standard solution is available in bottles of 600 ml and of 400 ml, corresponding to the hourly fluid loads most commonly used.

INDUCTION OF THERAPY

INITIAL PERIOD

Three hundred ml of electrolyte solution and 80 ml of urea solution are given per hour for 4 hours. If diuresis does not exceed 350 ml per hour at the end of this 4-hour period, treatment must be discontinued or modified.

Such a failure of diuretic response is rarely encountered but may signify dehydration or marked hypoxia possibly due to atelectasis or other pulmonary complication. Diuretic treatment can usually be continued cautiously, e.g., by keeping the fluid input equal to the urinary output in the preceding hour and keeping the load of urea at 10 to 15 g per hour. If a steady diuretic response results, a fixed hourly fluid volume is used. A complete failure of diuretic response signifies acute renal failure, and treatment is stopped.

STEADY INFUSION PERIOD

Six hundred ml of electrolyte solution and 30 ml of urea solution are given per hour. After about 4 hours it is often possible to reduce the amount of urea solution to 20 or even to 10 ml per hour, without fluid retention. In patients in whom the diuretic response to this treatment is sluggish – diuresis failing to reach about 600 ml per hour despite a urea load resulting in blood urea levels up to 400 mg per 100 ml – modified treatment is given. An hourly infusion of only 400 ml of electrolyte solution plus 20 to 30 ml of urea solution is used in such cases.

The blood urea concentration is in practice not allowed to exceed 400 mg per 100 ml. Fluid retention must not exceed 1 litre in 24 hours. If signs of overloading occur in the form of engorgement of the neck veins or hilar congestion on the chest X-ray, frusemide (Lasix) 40 mg in the vein is indicated. Serum sodium values exceeding 150 mEq/l are occasionally seen and can be readily corrected by substituting for the electrolyte infusion fluid a 2.5% glucose solution. In rare instances, slightly subnormal serum concentrations of sodium or potassium are found. This is easily corrected by appropriate addition to the infusion fluid. To counteract hypocalcaemia, 1 g (10 ml of a 10% solution) of calcium levulinate is injected intravenously every eight hours. In general, we have been impressed by the ability of the body to maintain fluid and electrolyte balance. On many occasions we have followed the urinary concentrations of electrolytes, and usually they match those infused even when we use an infusion fluid differing somewhat from the above-described standard solution. The kidney evidently maintains some degree of control of the plasma composition, *i.e.*, it is not so much the therapist as the patient who in the usual case is 'responsible' for balance being maintained.

TERMINATION OF TREATMENT

When the patient has regained consciousness, the infusion of urea is discontinued. In order to prevent a fluid deficit, the infusion of electrolyte solution is continued for eight hours. Patients with an hourly diuresis of about 600 ml during treatment are given 400 ml electrolyte solution for four hours, followed by 200 ml hourly for the next four hours. For patients with a diuresis of about 400 ml the corresponding fluid volumes given are 300 and 150 ml.

CLINICAL RESULTS

In the Poisoning Treatment Centre at Copenhagen forced diuresis has been given to more than 500 patients with barbiturate poisoning during the last ten years. Out of these, 122 patients were unconscious for more than 72 hours. In two instances diuretic treatment was continued for ten days.

The maximum amounts of barbiturate excreted in the urine were aprobarbital 4.5 g, barbitone 11.3 g, and phenobarbitone 18 g.

EFFICACY OF TREATMENT IN ACCELERATING BARBITURATE ELIMINATION

Figs. 2 and 3 demonstrate the accelerated elimination resulting from forced diuresis. They show the rate of elimination expressed as the percentage decrease of the serum barbiturate concentration per 24 hours as compared with that of non-treated controls having comparable serum levels.

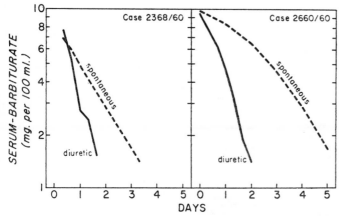

Fig. 2. Allyl-isopropyl barbiturate. The two graphs each illustrate the elimination in the same patient on two different admissions.

By comparing the elimination rate with and without treatment, the effect of diuretic treatment in reducing the duration of coma can be calculated. On the average, duration of coma was reduced to one-third. This reduction has been depicted graphically in Fig. 4. The calculations are based on the elimination rates obtained, as previously mentioned, in the postabsorption phase (Myschetzky and Lassen, 1963). Hence the calculated reduction of duration of coma applies to this phase only. During continued drug absorption from the intestinal tract, the effect of diuretic treatment is that of keeping the blood concentration of the drug at a lower level, thereby reducing the depth of coma.

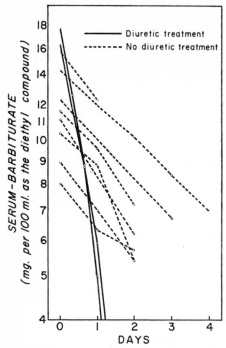

Fig. 3. Effect of diuretic treatment in combined diethyl- and allyl-isopropyl barbiturate poisoning.

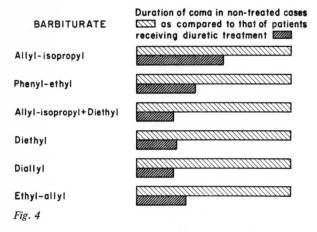

Fig. 4

COMPLICATIONS OF TREATMENT

We have studied the incidence of complications in 42 consecutive cases given diuretic treatment in 1969. Defining a complication as a factor clearly harmful to the patient's health at a general or local level, we looked for:

1. *Gross overhydration* to the point of severe pulmonary engorgement or oedema. This occurred in one case, an 82-year-old man with a mixed aprobarbital and barbi-

tone intoxication. He had electrocardiographic signs of heart disease (atrial fibrillation) and a moderate degree of hypoventilation (pCO$_2$ approx. 50 mm Hg) not treated with artificial ventilation. After 3½ days of uninterrupted diuretic treatment X-ray signs of fluid retention in the lungs were manifest and the diuresis failed to match the input rate of 630 ml/hr. Retention of 2–3 litres of fluid had occurred during the last 24 hours. The patient died in a state of hypotension without overt signs of pulmonary oedema. Autopsy was not performed.

2. *Cases with very high serum urea levels.* Only in one case did we suspect that urea retention as already defined may have been a complication.

This was in a 77-year-old woman with a combined aprobarbital and barbitone intoxication (max. concentration 21.5 mg per 100 ml as barbitone). The serum creatinine level was 1.5 mg per 100 ml. Disregarding serum urea values of 800 to 1000 mg per 100 ml, the hourly load of urea was inappropriately kept at 15 mg (= 30 ml)/hr. After 3½ days of treatment including artificial ventilation, the patient died in a state of hypotensive shock, despite administration of fluids and pressor amines.

Cardiac arrest had occurred in another hospital before admission, an additional complication. At autopsy only moderate fluid retention in the lungs was found and the brain showed gross signs of anoxia including oedema, small haemorrhages and cellular degeneration. One cannot exclude, nevertheless, that the very high urea levels contributed to the fatal outcome.

3. *Cases where diuretic treatment had to be stopped* because of failing urinary response or electrolyte derangement. This did not occur in our series. In particular, haemodialysis was not required to correct water-electrolyte-urea imbalance in any patient.

4. *Evaluation of the remaining three fatal cases of the five* occurring in the series of 42 patients. None of these patients died as a result of complications arising from the diuretic treatment. One died suddenly of cardiac arrest and the other two died after regaining consciousness and cessation of diuretic treatment.

5. *Other complications.* Phlebitis occurred in the arms or legs where infusion had been given, and sepsis originated from thrombi in the infusion catheter or from the urinary tract due to the bladder catheter.

This type of complication could only be suspected in one case, that of a 79-year-old man with mixed aprobarbital and barbitone (max. level 23.4 mg per 100 ml as barbital). After 32 hours of uneventful diuretic treatment he woke up. During the convalescent period he had a low-grade fever for five days and clinical signs of urinary infection, successfully treated by chemotherapy.

In conclusion, severe complications due to diuretic treatment were of decisive clinical importance only in the 82-year-old man first mentioned.

CLINICAL ADVANTAGES OF USING DIURETIC TREATMENT

The question of whether an overall gain is achieved by diuretic treatment can only be answered indirectly, as no properly controlled series has been reported. A reduction in mortality due to all types of poisoning was seen in Copenhagen after the introduction of diuretic treatment in 1960 and barbiturates are still the dominant cause of poisoning (60% of all cases). This at least suggests that some real gain has been made.

We have analyzed two consecutive series of barbiturate intoxication in some detail: in 1957–1958, 1,401 cases, and in 1962–1963, 1,398 cases. For the sake of brevity they will be referred to as the 1958 series and the 1963 series respectively. The general supportive treatment given was practically the same in the two groups.

The serum concentrations above the levels indicated in Table 1 were accepted for starting diuretic treatment.

TABLE 1

Drugs and minimum levels in serum accepted for starting diuretic treatment

Allyl-isopropyl-barbituric acid	10 mg/100 ml
(Aprobarbital, Numal, Allypropymal)	
Diethyl-barbituric acid	15 mg/100 ml
(Barbitone, Veronal, Diemal)	
Barbitone and aprobarbital equal amounts	15 mg/ 100 ml
(Noctifen, Somnifen, Hypofen)	
Phenyl-ethyl-barbituric acid	15 mg/100 ml
(Phenobarbitone, Luminal, Fenemal)	
Diallyl-barbituric acid	10 mg/100 ml
(Allobarbital, Dial, Diallymal)	
Ethyl-allyl-barbituric acid	15 mg/100 ml
(Dormin, Æthallymal)	

Table 2 concerns patients admitted to the Poisoning Treatment Centre suffering from barbiturate poisoning and demonstrates a reduction in mortality from 14.2% to 6.2%, as well as a reduced incidence of pulmonary complications and of patients needing tracheostomy (this is usually considered to be indicated after 72 hours of oral intubation).

TABLE 2

Series	No. of cases	Pneumonia	Atelectasis	Tracheos-tomy	Fatal cases	Mortality %
1958	113	30	38	16	16	14.2
1963	96*	10	13	10	6	6.2

* Of this group only 64 were given diuretic treatment – it being considered unnecessary in the remaining 32 patients showing a light level of unconsciousness as a consequence of habituation to barbiturates before the acute poisoning.

The clinical course in the two series as a whole reflects the same tendency. The total mortality of the 1958 series was 3.5% as compared with 2.4% in the 1963 series.* If the deaths in the above-mentioned subgroups with the severest intoxications are subtracted there is almost the same mortality for the remaining approximately 93% of the cases in the two series (2.6% in 1958 *versus* 2.1% in 1963).

With respect to pulmonary complications the two series were comparable. Tracheostomy was more frequent (14 in 1963 compared with 7 in 1958) in the large groups comprising all patients with serum barbiturate concentrations below the critical levels. This reflects a somewhat more active attitude towards this intervention in 1963 as compared to 1958. Hence it lends credence to the conclusion, suggested by the above data, that a true reduction in tracheostomy frequency results from diuretic treatment.

DISCUSSION

Forced diuresis influences the two crucial factors of barbiturate intoxication: the drug concentration in the body, and the duration of the poisoning. Hence one cannot doubt *a priori* its beneficial action. The clinical value of the treatment depends, nevertheless, on a number of factors which we have tried to evaluate in this study.

First the simplicity and low cost of the treatment must be emphasized. Comparison should be made with one alternative mode of active treatment, haemodialysis. With the efficiency obtained in most centres a comparable rate of elimination using haemodialysis would necessitate eight hours of dialysis daily for two to three days (Myschetzky and Lassen, 1963).

The decision regarding the value of diuretic treatment is, therefore, the gain *versus* loss argument. Our clinical observations suggest that the gains far outbalance the risks.

The complications encountered have all been due to factors which could be observed quantitatively and counteracted by proper measures. We have also been looking for side effects in the sense of apparently unavoidable adverse reactions. For a time it seemed that patients receiving diuretic treatment had a higher incidence of post-intoxication seizures and withdrawal psychosis. An analysis of the clinical material presented above did not, however, support this impression, as such symptoms were found in 28 of 113 cases in 1958 as compared with 20 of 98 cases in the 1963 series.

As emphasized, diuretic treatment is only indicated in the severest cases of intoxication with long-acting barbiturates.

It is also stressed that diuretic treatment is only of secondary importance in the handling of severe acute barbiturate poisoning. At the outset, general supportive treatment must be instituted according to conventional principles and only in the 10% of severest cases should diuretic treatment be considered.

* These figures only concern barbiturate poisoning cases, whereas the data in Fig. 1 (showing different figures for mortality) concern the total number of poisoning cases comprising all types of intoxication.

It is obvious that forced diuresis is impracticable and contra-indicated if the patient is in a state of severe shock with gross impairment of cardiac and/or renal function. Hence it is necessary to determine whether any patients in our series, with high barbiturate levels, died from their poisoning before the contra-indications had been corrected.

In our last series of approximately 700 patients treated for barbiturate poisoning in 1969, four patients died without receiving diuretic treatment. One patient had a cardiac arrest immediately on arrival in the ward and although routine treatment with external cardiac massage and sodium bicarbonate intravenously restored cardiac function to normal for 20 minutes, there were three more episodes of cardiac asystole, the last one not being responsive to treatment. One patient died from pulmonary embolism a few hours after admission during otherwise uneventful supportive treatment. One patient with barbiturate poisoning of moderate severity was severely hypoxic on admission due to aspiration of gastric contents either at home or during transport to the hospital. The treatment of the poisoning was uncomplicated, but the patient died from anoxic brain damage one month after admission without regaining consciousness. Only one patient of the four mentioned had a barbiturate level justifying forced diuresis, 15.8 mg per 100 ml of barbitone, but this patient remained in a condition of shock in spite of supportive treatment until death seven hours after admission.

In no instance was haemodialysis indicated and a review of the cases did not change this opinion, as all patients receiving forced diuresis had adequate renal function and responded well to the procedure.

In conclusion, we maintain that forced diuresis in the manner explained here is a definite advance in the treatment of severe barbiturate poisoning with long-acting barbiturates.

It should be mentioned that the procedure is also of value in patients poisoned by lithium compounds and by salicylates. The latter poisoning, in contrast with what obtains in many other countries, is extremely rare in Denmark.

REFERENCES

LASSEN, N. A. (1960), Treatment of severe acute barbiturate poisoning by forced diuresis and alkalinization of urine. *Lancet*, II, 338.
MYSCHETZKY, A. and LASSEN, N. A. (1963), Urea-induced, osmotic diuresis and alkalinization of urine in acute barbiturate intoxication. *J. Amer. med. Ass.*, 185, 936.

13. *the role of peritoneal and haemodialysis treatment*

H. A. Lee

Any claim for the need or effectiveness of dialysis treatment of acute barbiturate poisoning must be viewed against the background of excellent results obtained with conservative treatment not employing methods designed to increase the rate of elimination of the intoxicating drug. Thus Ferguson and Grace in 1961 reported a mortality of 1% in a series of 95 patients, whilst later Baker (1969), in a series of 553 patients in coma from a variety of poisons, had a mortality rate of 0.74%. In a review dealing with 776 cases of acute barbiturate poisoning, Matthew and Lawson (1966) achieved a mortality rate of only 0.8%. Later, Matthew (1969) reported a series of 2,041 patients, covering a period from 1967 to 1968, in which the mortality had been reduced further to 0.6%. In this impressive series, the mainstay of therapy had been intensive supportive therapy without active treatment unless very clearly indicated. However, small as these mortality figures may be, they must be considered in the context of the large number of barbiturate poisoning cases admitted to hospital each year. It should also be noted that in the United Kingdom some 2,000 people per year die from this type of poisoning, the majority however outside hospital.

If only the more serious cases of barbiturate poisoning are considered, that is, corresponding to Grades III and IV coma cases (Reed, 1952), then the mortality figures are more striking. Thus a mortality rate of around 8% is seen in some series (Matthew and Lawson, 1966; Henderson and Merrill, 1966; Myschetszky and Lassen, 1963) but has reached as high as 12.4% in one series (Setter *et al.*, 1966).

About 5% of all barbiturate poisoning cases are likely to fall in the severe category and to require intensive eliminative measures, such as forced diuresis, or some other dialytic therapy, if recovery is to be achieved (Lancet, 1967). It is amongst this group that dialysis procedures may be life-saving. That dialysis is effective and has a role to play in this situation is undoubted. The main problem has been in defining the precise indications for peritoneal or haemodialysis treatment in a clinical situation that does not permit of a controlled trial. It is clear from the literature on the subject that the enthusiasm of groups for one form of treatment or another has more often dictated the demand for dialysis than adherence to any particular set of criteria, and thus the need for dialysis treatment has been difficult to interpret.

In the interpretation of any animal experiments in this field, the important obser-vations of Richards and Taylor (1956) should be recalled. They showed how the response to a given dose of barbiturate in experimental animals could vary by as much as 50% and that individual animals would respond in a different way to the same dose of drug given on different occasions. A similar theme was referred to in another experiment quoted by Merrill (1967), in which a dog was cross-transfused with another after having been rendered unconscious with pentobarbitone. The blood levels in the two dogs were eventually the same and yet one dog was asleep and the other was awake. This immediately reminds one of the difficulty of deter-mining what significance to place on serum barbiturate level alone in the poisoned patient. Koppanyi and Linegar (1942), in cross-circulation experiments between barbiturate-poisoned dogs and normal partners, found that after one hour of cross-circulation the test animals recovered in an average time of 27 min compared with a recovery time of 29 hr for controlled animals in which the same dose of barbiturate had been given but without cross-circulation. It is noteworthy that these authors actually alluded to the fact that it would be possible to devise some apparatus for clearing the blood of barbiturate and thus possibly shortening coma duration.

Alwall et al. (1952) reported their findings on barbiturate intoxication in rabbits. These animals were divided into three groups and all were poisoned with equal doses of phenobarbitone and then treated, respectively, with forced diuresis, ultra-filtration of the blood and haemodialysis. The rabbits which were dialysed had the shortest recovery times with the greatest and most rapid decrease in blood barbiturate levels. This therapeutic efficacy was almost matched in the group of rabbits whose blood was ultra-filtered. Both methods proved superior to forced diuresis.

The value of haemodialysis in dogs poisoned with barbitone was reported by Pallotta et al. (1952). They found that about 40% of the administered dose could be removed in the dialysate and that coma duration was shortened. Sunshine and Leonards (1954) reported their observations in groups of dogs poisoned with pheno-barbitone, pentobarbitone and amylobarbitone, and haemodialysed with a Skeggs-Leonards apparatus. The experimental animals were compared with the controlled animals in regard to fall in barbiturate levels, recovery times and mortality rates. All the test animals showed a significant reduction in blood barbiturate levels during dialysis. It was also noted that there were varying degrees of clinical response, the most striking improvement occurring in that group which had been poisoned with phenobarbitone. The mean recovery rates for barbiturate in the dialysate were 40% for the phenobarbitone group, 20% for the pentobarbitone group and 35% for the amylobarbitone group.

It is well recognised in the management of acute renal failure that haemodialysis is more efficient than peritoneal dialysis (Boen, 1961; Lee et al., 1964). Thus, peritoneal dialysis has not received as much attention as haemodialysis in experimental animal work in this field, though such investigations as have been done have been aimed at improving the efficiency of drug removal by peritoneal dialysis. Knochel *et al.* (1963) observed that the addition of THAM [Tris (hydroxymethyl) amino-methane] to peritoneal dialysate doubled the removal of phenobarbitone and amylobarbitone and increased ten-fold the quinalbarbitone extraction in experimental dogs. Since all barbiturates are weak acids known to permeate cell membranes more easily when undissociated rather than when ionised, these experiments suggested that intra-peritoneal THAM which diffuses, but slowly, across membranes, might act as a hydrogen ion acceptor for faster diffusing weak acids or their salts. Thus, by lowering the hydrogen ion concentration of the dialysate, the non-ionised barbiturate that diffuses across the peritoneal membrane is promptly ionised, thus maintaining a high concentration gradient for the diffusion of the non-ionised form. These observations were extended in further dog experiments by Nahas *et al.* (1964). Firstly, they noted that peritoneal dialysate containing 100 mM/l of THAM did not result in inflammatory reactions of the omentum. They then compared the effectiveness of three types of peritoneal dialysate in extracting pentobarbitone and phenobarbitone. It was found that peritoneal dialysate containing THAM trebled the extraction rates of both drugs.

PERITONEAL DIALYSIS

The value of peritoneal dialysis in the management of acute renal failure has been well defined (Boen, 1961; Burns *et al.*, 1962) but its place in the management of acute barbiturate intoxication is less clear. There are but a few sporadic reports of its use in this situation in the literature, which undoubtedly reflects on the poorer efficiency of peritoneal dialysis compared with haemodialysis for the removal of poisons. Now that modern conservative measures are so effective in the general management of barbiturate intoxications together with the judicious use of forced alkaline diuresis (Bloomer, 1967; Mawer and Lee, 1968), if some further eliminative treatment is required, then a high efficiency dialysis procedure, such as haemodialysis rather than peritoneal dialysis, would seem indicated. Indeed, Burns *et al.* (1962), when reviewing the then current status of peritoneal dialysis, stated clearly that haemodialysis was the method of choice in patients being treated for acute intoxications with potentially dialysable poisons.

Where some additional rapid eliminative therapy is required, it should have a high confidence rating with regard to reliability, implementation and effectiveness. It is worth recalling that in one series of patients treated by peritoneal dialysis for acute renal failure (Maxwell *et al.*, 1959) six patients (7.3%) could not be effectively treated by this method because of technical difficulties. Elsewhere, in a series of acute barbiturate poisoning patients treated with peritoneal dialysis, an impressive list of complications resulting from this treatment was reported.

It has been clearly shown that the incidence of pulmonary complications rises sharply with the length of coma in acute barbiturate poisoning (Hadden *et al.*, 1969). Henderson and Merrill (1966) alluded to the fact that intermittent elevation of the diaphragm during peritoneal dialysis might increase the incidence of pulmonary complications in this situation. This was confirmed by Berlyne *et al.* (1966), who stressed the importance of pulmonary complications occurring during peritoneal dialysis and suggested modifications in the technique to overcome this. Again it should be stressed that the dialysis cycling times as used in the management of acute renal failure, *i.e.*, one litre per half hour or every hour, are insufficient in the treatment of barbiturate intoxication. The equilibration time for barbiturates has been shown to be closer to 90–120 min (Berman and Vogelsang, 1964; Bloomer, 1965).

The use of peritoneal dialysis in the management of acute barbiturate intoxication was first reported by Maxwell *et al.* (1959). They described a 34-year-old male who had ingested 6 g of a mixture of quinal- and amylobarbitone, who was in grade IV coma and who required a tracheostomy and peritoneal dialysis. In this case peritoneal dialysis was continued for 30 hours, but after a mere six hours of dialysis deep pain sensation returned, bringing seriously into question the role played by peritoneal dialysis in this particular case.

In 1964 Berman and Vogelsang reported their findings with peritoneal dialysis in four adult cases of acute barbiturate intoxication. This report deals primarily with the mechanics of dialysis and is not concerned with the effects of peritoneal dialysis on the clinical course of the patients who were treated, since dialysis was brief and variable. Two types of dialysate were compared: the normal one as used in acute renal failure and another containing 5% albumin. They found that equilibration between plasma and dialysate was barely reached at 60 min per exchange and that for pentobarbitone it may require a two-hour equilibration period. This corresponds closely with the 90-min equilibration time reported by Bloomer (1965). The albumin-containing dialysate increased the concentration ratios of barbiturate from dialysate to blood, improving the removal rates of quinalbarbitone and pentobarbitone from 17 to 26.2 mg and 26 to 62 mg/hr respectively, though in the latter case the serum barbiturate levels were considerably higher. They were able to show that the haemodialysis/peritoneal dialysis ratio of efficiency for barbiturate removal was of the order of 4 : 1, but that this was increased to a 2 : 1 ratio when 5% albumin was added to the peritoneal dialysate. In a comparison with their own previously reported work (Berman *et al.*, 1956), they showed that for a plasma barbiturate level of a short acter in the region of 3–4 mg%, the removal rate by haemodialysis was 75–110 mg/hr for the first three hours of dialysis, whereas with peritoneal dialysis it was 20 mg/hr, and finally with peritoneal dialysis using an albumin-containing dialysate it was 40 mg/hr. Similar comparison with a long-acting barbiturate with serum levels of 10–15 mg% gave removal rates of 300–400 mg/hr, 92 mg/hr and 140 mg/hr respectively.

An interesting report on a patient poisoned with pentobarbitone (Bloomer, 1965) put into perspective the limited usefulness of alkaline diuresis and peritoneal dialysis in this situation. He determined the distribution of pentobarbitone and its ether extractable metabolites in plasma, peritoneal dialysis fluid and urine, and the elimination of the parent drug and its metabolites by the kidneys and peritoneal dialysis.

Peritoneal dialysis was continued for 29 hours using a total of 16 exchanges involving 32 litres of dialysate. The protein binding of pentobarbitone by *in vitro* dialysis of this patient's plasma was around 55%, whereas the pentobarbitone metabolites were mainly non-protein bound. Mainly pure barbiturate was recovered in the peritoneal dialysis fluid. The pentobarbitone clearance by peritoneal dialysis was calculated at 14 ml/min, representing an elimination rate of pentobarbitone of only 13 mg/hr. Over a 30-hour observation period the plasma barbiturate level was found to decline at 4.5%/hr in spite of the use of forced diuresis and peritoneal dialysis, and the coma duration was not shortened, *i.e.*, it was 45 hr. Brodie *et al.* (1953) had shown that after distribution of an administered pentobarbitone dose in the tissues the plasma level declined at a constant rate of approximately 4%/hr. This carefully prepared report clearly indicated the difficulties in assessing whether a particular form of treatment, in this case peritoneal dialysis, had in any way helped the patient's recovery.

Bloomer's paper was important in another respect as it brought into focus the methods used by others in measuring barbiturates when comparing elimination rates by different techniques. The standard method of barbiturate estimation (Broughton, 1956) measures active drug as well as non-active metabolites (Mark *et al.*, 1963), the latter being water-soluble. Therefore, any apparent increase in the removal rate of barbiturates by dialysis procedures will be misleading unless specific methods for measuring active barbiturate only are used (Bloomer, 1967; Mawer and Lee, 1968) and makes the evaluation of such procedures particularly difficult.

The two largest reported series of cases in which peritoneal dialysis has been used in the management of acute barbiturate intoxication are by Matthew and Lawson (1966) and Hadden *et al.* (1969). In the former report 36 patients, *i.e.*, 4.7% of the total number treated, had peritoneal dialysis and three patients died. Unfortunately, no details are given in this series as to what type of barbiturate poisoning the dialysis was used in, the duration of peritoneal dialysis, the effects on serum barbiturate levels or the total amounts of drug removed. It is not possible, therefore, to comment on whether peritoneal dialysis materially improved the prognosis of individual patients or whether haemodialysis might have been preferable. One of the three deaths reported was inevitable as the patient had a cerebral tumour, but at post-mortem in the other two cases it is noteworthy that both showed changes of bilateral broncho-pneumonia.

In a report on 50 cases of acute barbiturate poisoning, Hadden *et al.* (1969) divided their patients on admission into three therapeutic groups, which were (a) aggressive supportive therapy, (b) mannitol diuresis and (c) peritoneal dialysis. They only considered patients who corresponded to Reed's Grades II to IV depth of coma. No significant differences between the three forms of treatment for quinalbarbitone were found on comparing the mean clearance values. Dialysis and supportive therapy was slightly better than mannitol diuresis for pentobarbitone, and mannitol diuresis was marginally better for mixed quinal- and amylobarbitone poisoning. Irrespective of the treatment group, coma duration was found to be longest in those patients with renal and/or liver disease. It was noteworthy that all three treatments affected the slope of the barbiturate level in the same way, suggesting that aggressive supportive therapy alone was sufficient. In the 16 patients treated with peritoneal dialysis, some important complications of the procedure were noted. There was one incident of bleeding at the trocar site, one of leaking around the catheter site, one of generalised peritonitis, and two of protein loss, electrolyte disequilibrium and localised peritonitis. They concluded that peritoneal dialysis should probably be reserved for those patients with liver and/or renal disease but failed to give any clear indications as to when peritoneal dialysis should be started.

A severe case of poisoning with an intermediate-acting barbiturate, cyclobarbitone, treated with combined haemodialysis, peritoneal dialysis and forced diuresis, was reported by Kennedy et al. (1969). Here, 40% of the total amount of barbiturate removed was eliminated by peritoneal dialysis, although no distinction was made between pure barbiturate and non-active metabolites. They concluded that the amount of barbiturate removed in this case with peritoneal dialysis was significant, and it is of interest to recall that in Bloomer's case (1965) it was mainly pure barbiturate that was removed by peritoneal dialysis.

A number of writers (Maher and Schreiner, 1965; Setter et al., 1966; Kennedy et al., 1969) all consider that peritoneal dialysis should only be used for milder cases of barbiturate poisoning and then only very occasionally. Such recommendations hardly constitute strict criteria for the use of such therapy in acute barbiturate poinsoning and probably reflect on the degree of uncertainty about the efficacy of this form of treatment. In the author's opinion peritoneal dialysis has a very limited role, if any, in the management of this type of case.

The argument that peritoneal dialysis should be reserved for those cases that cannot be safely moved from one unit to another is not convincing. Honey and Jackson (1959), Lee and Ames (1965), Setter et al. (1966) and Linton et al. (1967) have all shown that there is little risk in moving a patient from one place to another provided that adequate ventilation is ensured prior to the patient's removal. Peritoneal dialysis as used in the management of acute renal failure is insufficient when applied to the management of barbiturate intoxication. A much longer equilibration time is required as compared with urea or creatinine, and closely approximates two hr per cycle. Again, to make peritoneal dialysis efficient in this field, the addition of either THAM or 5% albumin would appear to be indicated. This is not only expensive, but fails to significantly reduce the length of peritoneal dialysis. Pulmonary complications are a serious recognised hazard of barbiturate poisoning and these may well be accentuated by peritoneal dialysis. When additional means of drug elimination are required, this indicates a rapid removal technique and there can be no doubt that haemodialysis is more effective than modified peritoneal dialysis.

Cardiovascular complications are common in severe barbiturate intoxications, hypotension ranking first amongst these. Significant protein losses occur during peritoneal dialysis (Berlyne et al., 1964) and can result in hypo-oncotic hypovolaemia in such patients, aggravating existing hypotension and shock. This is quite the converse of the situation often met with in haemodialysis, where the very procedure often enhances the patients' circulatory state (Berman *et al.*, 1964; Pender *et al.*, 1957; Lee and Ames, 1965). As far as the United Kingdom is concerned, no patient is more than a few hours away from a special unit with haemodialysis facilities and, thus, using peritoneal dialysis as a second-best form of eliminative treatment in the very few cases that require it cannot be justified.

HAEMODIALYSIS

The criteria by which a poison may be removed from the human being by haemodialysis have been outlined by Schreiner (1958) and confirmed by Jorgensen and Wieth (1963) and Maher and Schreiner (1967). These are: (1) dialysance or clearance, *i.e.*, that the molecule should be small enough to diffuse through a cellophane membrane at a reasonable speed; (2) distribution, *i.e.*, that a drug is distributed in body water in a freely diffusable or readily dissociable form; (3) time/dose toxic relationship, *i.e.*, that normal mechanisms of elimination (metabolism, conjugation and/or excretion) should be slow compared with haemodialysis; and (4) any additional removal of poison by the dialysis procedure is significant in terms of the patient's recovery.

That the cellophane membrane of a variety of artificial kidneys is not a significant diffusion barrier for barbiturates has been shown in a number of studies on the dialysance of various barbiturates (Henderson and Merrill, 1966; Jorgensen and Wieth, 1963). *In vitro* studies using a four-layered Kiil dialyser (Setter *et al.*, 1964) with blood-flow rates at 400 ml/min have given dialysance values for phenobarbitone of 110 ml/min, amylobarbitone 95 ml/min, pentobarbitone 85 ml/min, quinalbarbitone 65 ml/min. Similar values for a rotating drum kidney and Kolff twin-coil kidney have been shown by Linton *et al.* (1967) for phenobarbitone and butobarbitone.

The number of patients who are going to require haemodialysis treatment is difficult to ascertain. It is generally agreed that something like 5% of all barbiturate poisonings are undoubtedly severe and are likely to require additional intensive eliminative measures such as forced diuresis and haemodialysis, but that the latter treatment will only be required in a small proportion of this group. Many of the series published where haemodialysis has been used in the treatment of acute barbiturate poisoning are selective inasmuch as the patients have been specially referred from other hospitals. However, in one series (Lee and Ames, 1965) a distinction was made between patients admitted directly to the hospital and those referred, and only two patients out of 169 admitted directly to the hospital required haemodialysis. In another series of 1,100 cases (Linton *et al.*, 1967), 100 cases (9%) required forced diuresis therapy, 18 patients (1.6%) required haemodialysis on the basis of criteria established by that group, and 600 of the patients were actually assessed by members of the renal units in that area. In the series as a whole, there were only three deaths and only one death in patients dialysed. This represented a mortality of 0.4% of the patients whose management was controlled by the renal units and an overall mortality rate of 0.28% for the series as a whole. These figures compare very favourably with the average mortality rates of 1% as judged from the general literature. Considering only the serious cases in this series, the mortality rate was 2.7%, compared with an average mortality of about 15% in other series of seriously poisoned patients.

A number of studies have shown quite conclusively (Jorgensen and Wieth, 1963; Setter et al., 1966; Maher and Schreiner, 1967; Linton et al., 1967) that haemodialysis significantly adds to barbiturate removal, as judged by the steeper decline in blood barbiturate levels during dialysis as compared with forced diuresis, and that coma duration is shortened when dialysis is used. There is some divergence of opinion as to which barbiturates are best treated by haemodialysis techniques. From a purely pharmacological standpoint it might seem that the long-acting barbiturates, such as phenobarbitone and barbitone, would be best treated in this way because they are the least protein-bound and mainly distributed in the extracellular fluid compartment and normally the greater part of the ingested dose is excreted renally. However, a number of authors (Lee and Ames, 1965; Setter et al., 1966; Maher and Schreiner, 1967; Matthew and Lawson, 1966) believe, mainly on clinical grounds, that dialysis may more often be successful in the treatment of intoxication with short-acting barbiturates, even though coma duration may not necessarily be shortened. It is particularly important when treating short-acting barbiturate intoxication with haemodialysis that the dialysis procedure goes on long enough. This is because the short-acting barbiturates are distributed in both the extracellular and intracellular fluid compartments and then gradients are established between fat depots and the plasma pool, the movement in the latter case being slower than the movement from the plasma pool to the dialysate. In this context the observation by Setter et al. (1966) is relevant, where in a case of quinalbarbitone poisoning the serum quinal-barbitone was reduced from 7.2 to 2.2 mg% by a 12-hour haemodialysis but at the same time the subcutaneous fat concentration was reduced from 7.2 to only 5.5 mg%.

The first reported cases of barbiturate intoxication treated by haemodialysis were published by Alwall et al. (1952) but it was not until the publication by Berman et al. (1956) that an attempt was made to define the criteria for haemodialysis in this situation. Their recommendations were based on the results of eight cases of severe barbiturate intoxication treated by a Kolff twin-coil haemodialyser, all of whom survived. They suggested that potentially fatal ingested doses and blood levels were 5 g and 8 mg% for phenobarbitone, whilst barbitone was considered less toxic. For short-acting and intermediate-acting drugs, such as pentobarbitone, amylobarbitone and quinalbarbitone, the corresponding amounts were put at 3 g and 3.5 mg%. They were at pains, however, to point out that the clinical evaluation of the total situation should always outweigh any potentially fatal dose or blood level that might be chosen. This view was endorsed by Lubash et al. (1962), who advised that rational evaluations should be made on the basis of physical findings alone and without reference to blood levels of the intoxicating agent. A plea was also made that every effort should be made to reduce the time that elapses between ingestion of drugs and treatment by haemodialysis where required, and this was later re-emphasized by Setter et al. (1966).

Although it had been previously suggested that protein binding of barbiturates might be very important (Sunshine and Leonards, 1954), they were unable to demonstrate any important differences in the in vitro dialysis of pentobarbitone in the plasma as compared with dialysis of the same drug in a saline solution. In three of their cases of poisoning with long-acting barbiturates it was concluded unequivocally that the life of one patient was saved and the coma period markedly shortened in another. They also clearly stated that the presence of severe vascular disease was no contra-indication to haemodialysis. They also drew attention to other important considerations when using haemodialysis, such as the depletion of tissue reserves as the blood levels are lowered and concentration gradients are established, the continued metabolic inactivation of barbiturates during dialysis and, lastly, the ancillary benefits of dialysis, such as stabilization of blood pressure and the improvement in the appearance of arterial blood (Pender et al., 1957; Lubash et al., 1962).

In 1962, Balme et al. reviewed the literature to date on cases of acute barbiturate poisoning treated by haemodialysis. A study of the details in the table printed in that paper reveals some interesting points. Firstly, the percentage of the ingested dose removed by haemodialysis varied considerably, from as little as 3% to as much as 43%, and in most instances no distinction was made between active barbiturate and non-active metabolites. In only four cases, all of whom had taken long-acting barbiturates, was it considered that coma duration had been shortened by haemodialysis. Next, a very considerable variation was noted in the timing of haemodialysis after the onset of coma, varying from as short as 10 hr to as long as 120 hr after the onset of coma. The duration of haemodialysis itself varied from as little as $3\frac{1}{2}$ hr to as long as 8 hr. Finally, a glance at the initial and final blood levels must raise serious doubts as to the part played by haemodialysis in many of the reported cases. This paper clearly pointed out the need for some definite criteria regarding the use of haemodialysis.

In 1964, Linton et al. published their initial observations on haemodialysis in barbiturate poisoning, which were further expanded in another publication in 1967. They dialysed a total number of 18 patients, all of whom were in Reed's Grade IV coma category. Fourteen of these patients were on respirators and there was one death in the group. Haemodialysis time ranged from $4\frac{1}{2}$ to 14 hr and the amount of barbiturate removed ranged from 0.6 to 9.3 g. The percentage of the ingested dose removed ranged from 47% for phenobarbitone to 37% for butobarbitone and 16% and 36% respectively for pentobarbitone and amylobarbitone. They attempted to re-define clearly the criteria for haemodialysis in acute barbiturate poisoning and felt that amongst these, blood barbiturate levels were a reasonable guide to the severity of poisoning. It is of interest that one of the authors, Linton (1967), felt in retrospect that possibly four of the cases who did not require ventilation might not really have needed haemodialysis.

In 1965, Lee and Ames reported their findings on 15 patients, later extended to 19 (Greer and Lee, 1967), with severe barbiturate poisoning requiring haemodialysis, all of whom survived, and corresponded with Reed's Grade IV coma category. This group of patients were of particular interest since no less than nine of them had had cardiac arrests prior to haemodialysis therapy and the vast majority of these patients had been moved from a hospital at considerable distance to the treatment hospital after the initial cardiac arrest. Further, no other cardiac abnormality, such as arrhythmia, was noted during the haemodialysis procedure. All these patients, with the exception of one, were hypotensive prior to haemodialysis and yet in all instances there was a remarkable improvement in the cardiovascular status during treatment (Berman et al., 1956; Pender et al., 1957). These findings are contrary to the opinion expressed by Henderson and Merrill (1966) that haemodialysis itself imposes extra stresses upon the patient. An attempt was again made to define haemodialysis criteria and some emphasis was placed upon serum barbiturate levels. Henderson and Merrill (1966) also gave the same relative merit to blood barbiturate levels in determining whether or not haemodialysis was required.

The relevance of blood barbiturate levels in indicating the need for haemodialysis was severely criticised by Matthew and Lawson (1966). They correctly re-emphasised that serum levels cannot be taken out of context of the overall clinical picture. In their large series of patients they found 83 cases had serum barbiturate levels above the potentially lethal levels that had been postulated by previous authors. Yet in only 27 of these cases were active eliminative measures required. The other 56 patients were satisfactorily managed with basic supportive therapy alone. Conversely, 13 other patients in their series required active therapy for the elimination of barbiturate when the serum barbiturate level was below the ascribed potentially lethal level. It is clear that serum levels alone cannot form an absolute criterion for haemodialysis. Yet most authorities would agree that such levels can be a useful guide in conjunction with the clinical picture. Low serum levels may be more significant in the elderly or the very young, whilst on the other hand high levels may be less significant in patients who have developed tolerance to barbiturate through long-term administration.

The largest series of patients requiring haemodialysis in acute barbiturate intoxication was published by Setter et al. (1966), where 56 out of a total of 163 cases needed haemodialysis. They made some interesting observations on the relationship of serum barbiturate levels to the grading of coma. In 20 cases of phenobarbitone poisoning with serum levels ranging from 1.9 to 29 mg%, they found that Grade I to II coma corresponded with levels of less than 7 mg% with one exception, whereas Grade III to IV coma occurred in all patients with levels greater than 11 mg%, again with one exception. Grade III to IV coma was found in all cases of amylo- and butobarbitone poisoning if the serum levels exceeded 5 mg%, and the same applied to mixtures of quinalbarbitone and pentobarbitone when the serum levels exceeded 3 mg%. Furthermore, coma duration was only related to the serum level of phenobarbitone, pentobarbitone and quinalbarbitone if the patients were seen within 18 hr of ingestion of the drug. Unlike Wright and Raeburn (1969), they observed that the coma duration of both short- and long-acting barbiturates was the same at 42 hr, provided that the patient was seen within 18 hr of ingestion, an observation with which the author would agree. In this series the mean duration of haemodialysis was 9½ hr and in seven cases repeated haemodialyses were required. The serum half-life of all barbiturates was reduced by haemodialysis from 30 to 14 hr for short-acting barbiturates and from 17 to 7 hr for phenobarbitone. Coma duration was shortened by haemodialysis and they felt that this treatment was more often required for poisoning with short-acting barbiturates, an impression confirmed in a later publication (Maher and Schreiner, 1968). Although 17 of the patients treated with haemodialysis died, none of the deaths occurred during haemodialysis or could be attributed to haemodialysis but were rather the consequence of the many complications that can befall a straight severe barbiturate intoxication. Also, many of the patients in this series were referred late to the special centre.

In one patient (Setter et al., 1966), they were able to compare the relative values of haemodialysis, peritoneal dialysis and forced diuresis. They found that the barbiturate clearance through the kidneys was 3–4 ml/min; with ordinary peritoneal dialysis, 4 ml/min; with peritoneal dialysis with 5% albumin, up to 6 ml/min; with THAM in the dialysate, 8 ml/min; and, finally, with haemodialysis, 30 ml/min. An important practical point in Setter et al.'s series in 1966 was that haemodialysis was continued for 12 hr unless the patient improved to Grade I coma or awakened beforehand. This point was emphasised by Linton et al. in 1967 and the author would add the observation by Lubash et al. (1962) that haemodialysis be continued until bowel sounds are restored, this having particular reference to the narcotized gut syndrome (Jorgensen and Wieth, 1963).

A report of particular interest was that by Jorgensen and Wieth in 1963, who treated a group of eight patients referred to their Renal Unit because of renal insufficiency complicating acute barbiturate intoxication. The creatinine clearances in these patients ranged from 0.3 to 19 ml/min, with the exception of one case that had a clearance in excess of 60 ml. All patients were treated with a Skeggs-Leonards dialyser and haemodialysis lasted from four to seven hr. They compared the spontaneous rate of elimination with that of haemodialysis by comparison of the half-life in the plasma, and showed that the barbiturate removal rate was increased from 10 to 60 times by dialysis. By applying their calculations to the results of other workers (Alwall et al., 1952; Kyle et al., 1953; Berman et al., 1956; Schreiner, 1958; Balme et al., 1962) they were able to show similar improved rates of removal. In patients with phenobarbitone poisoning the plasma half-life by spontaneous removal with normal renal function was 95.5 hr, whereas during renal insufficiency this became 117 hr but was reduced by haemodialysis to 9.4 hr. With aprobarbitone, similar figures were 37, 105 and 8.1 hr respectively. When comparing the half-life during renal insufficiency with that during haemodialysis, the efficiency ratios were for phenobarbitone, aprobarbitone and barbitone: 12.5, 13 and 44.5 hr respectively.

Three cases of very severe barbiturate poisoning treated by haemodialysis were described by Kennedy *et al.* (1969). The three drugs that had been ingested were phenobarbitone, butobarbitone and cyclobarbitone, and the authors were in no doubt that haemodialysis had been life-saving in each instance. This report further emphasised the contention that removal of a patient to a unit where haemodialysis facilities are available far outweighs the disadvantages of any hazards of transfer. Modifying their former criteria for haemodialysis, they suggested that when the blood level for a long-acting barbiturate is in excess of 20 mg% or for a short-acting barbiturate in excess of 7 mg%, then the patient should be transferred where dialysis facilities are available. They also reiterated that relatively small amounts of short-acting barbiturates removed by haemodialysis are indeed significant.

Grave doubts have been expressed in some quarters about the need for haemodialysis, with suggestions that haemodialysis itself might interfere with the normal conservative measures afforded this type of patient. Hadden *et al.* (1969) reported a mortality from cardiac arrest in haemodialysis varying between 12.5% and 35%, which 'prohibits meaningful consideration of haemodialysis as a form of treatment at this time'. The author has failed to confirm these figures and indeed would point to his own series of cases (Lee and Ames, 1965) where haemodialysis was successful in a large number of patients who had previously had a cardiac arrest. Elsewhere it was thought that peritoneal dialysis and haemodialysis might interfere with the nursing care of patients because of the technical demands of dialysis procedures (Henderson and Merrill, 1966). However, many would agree with the view of Setter *et al.* (1966) that professional care is often more abundant and expert during dialysis and that the patient can only benefit from all the extra attention.

With the great improvement in aggressive conservative management of barbiturate poisoning over recent years, it is obvious that an ever-decreasing proportion of the cases will require such active measures as haemodialysis or peritoneal dialysis to increase drug removal. However, there are certain groups of patients where such procedures will immediately suggest themselves. For example, in patients with renal insufficiency who have ingested long-acting barbiturates, which are normally excreted mainly through the kidney, it is obvious that dialysis will eliminate the barbiturate more quickly. The same would apply for patients who have ingested short- or intermediate-acting barbiturates and who have liver disease, where this organ is the main route of detoxication for such agents. Special situations will prevail in those circumstances where elderly patients or the very young have taken barbiturates. Another group of patients to benefit in this situation are those known to have chronic respiratory insufficiency, since the possibility of respiratory complications increases with the length of coma even in normal individuals.

In the paragraphs that follow, a therapeutic regime is suggested which will only lead to the use of haemodialysis therapy if appropriate criteria are fulfilled. In all patients with known barbiturate intoxication, the establishment of good conservative measures is vital. The hallmarks of such care are cardiovascular and respiratory support, thus covering the problems created by hypotension, hypothermia and respiratory depression. If the patient is unconscious and is known to have taken either phenobarbitone or butobarbitone, then a forced alkaline diuresis will promote further excretion of the drug (Bloomer, 1965; Bloomer, 1967; Henderson and Merrill, 1966; Mawer and Lee, 1968). If a patient who has taken a short-acting barbiturate is in Grade III or IV coma with a serum barbiturate level in excess of 4 mg% or a known rising level, and in addition is known to have liver impairment, then this presents a fairly strong indication for haemodialysis. Again, in a patient who has taken a large dose of, say, butobarbitone or phenobarbitone, e.g., above 5 g, and is known or found to have renal insufficiency at the outset, then haemodialysis may be considered at an earlier time than might otherwise be the case.

Special indications for haemodialysis unrelated to serum levels but dictated entirely by the clinical state, will be found in the very old and the very young. In those situations where forced alkaline diuresis would be appropriate but is contra-indicated by pre-existing cardiac or renal disease, then, of course, haemodialysis is considered sooner, provided again that the clinical situation demands it. As mentioned earlier, in patients who are known to have severe respiratory insufficiency, haemodialysis will usually be considered sooner if the relevant clinical and biochemical conditions prevail. For reasons detailed earlier, it would seem that haemodialysis would always be the treatment of choice in such situations, rather than peritoneal dialysis.

Some of the poor results of haemodialysis in the management of acute barbiturate intoxication (Alwall, 1967; Setter et al., 1966) are probably due to the late referral of patients to special units. This in turn must result from a lack of clear-cut indications as to when to refer a patient for haemodialysis. In the author's opinion there is no room for a middle of the road course with peritoneal dialysis. Either the energetic conservative management will prevail, i.e., inclusive of forced alkaline diuresis measures, or a rapid elimination procedure is required and this can only be supplied by haemodialysis. The fact that a patient is known to have taken a short-acting barbiturate, which is known to be partly protein-bound, in no way contra-indicates the use of haemodialysis, since it has been shown that significant amounts of such drugs can be removed by this method (Berman et al., 1956; Lee and Ames, 1965; Linton et al., 1967; Maher and Schreiner, 1968). It is a fact that with short-acting barbiturates the actual length of coma duration may not be significantly reduced but, nevertheless, a large proportion of the intoxicating agent can be removed from the organism, which can only be beneficial.

Complications accompanying haemodialysis therapy in acute barbiturate poisoning patients are very rare (see Table 1). In two series of cases (Lee and Ames, 1965; Linton et al., 1967) no complications were reported accompanying the actual procedure, and in both series some cases required more than two haemodialyses. Although

TABLE 1

Mortality rates in some of the larger series of barbiturate poisoning cases treated by dialysis

Authors	No. of cases	Comments	Mortality No.	%
Haemodialysis				
Alwall (1963)	15	Grade III-IV coma; mainly late referrals	3	20
Balme *et al.* (1962)	16	Review of cases in literature up to that time	0	0
Henderson and Merrill (1966)	5	1 case grade II, 4 grade IV coma	2	40
Jorgensen and Wieth (1963)	8	All cases of barbiturate poisoning complicated by renal insufficiency	2	25
Lee and Ames (1965) Greer and Lee (1967)	19	All Grade III-IV coma. 9 cardiac arrests prior to haemodialysis	0	0
Linton *et al.* (1967)	18	All 'severe' or Grade IV coma	1	55
Lubash *et al.* (1962)	21	Grade III-IV coma. Difficult to be sure if all barbiturate poisoning cases	7	33
Setter *et al.* (1966)	56	Includes many very late referrals. Like series Maher and Schreiner (1968) of 77 cases but cannot determine survival rate	17	30.4
Total:	158*		32	20.2
Peritoneal dialysis				
Berman and Vogelsang (1964)	4	? Grade coma. Mainly technical exercise	0	0
Bloomer (1966)	1	Grade IV coma	0	0
Hadden *et al.* (1969)	16	Grade II-IV cases. Many complications	0	0
Henderson and Merrill (1966)	3	2 Grade IV coma	0	0
Matthew and Lawson (1966)	36	Probably Grade III-IV coma. Cannot determine complications	3	8.3
Maxwell *et al.* (1959)	1	? necessity in this case	0	0
Total:	61		3	4.9

* Total experience now said to be over 300 (Maher and Schreiner, 1968)

17 patients died in one series (Setter *et al.*, 1966) it would not appear that any of these deaths could be attributed to haemodialysis. Two out of the eight cases described by Jorgensen and Wieth (1963) died, and one of these from a sub-dural haematoma, where it was queried whether the heparinization during haemodialysis might have been a contributing factor. Both of these patients were aged over 70. Lubash *et al.* (1962) described how four patients went into a decerebrate-type posture during haemodialysis, which they attributed to rapid lowering of the blood barbiturate levels with concomitant electro-motor alteration. Such observations have not been reported by any other workers. Although there were appreciable mortality rates in the series reported by Alwall and Lubash, none of the deaths would seem to be attributable to haemodialysis, but rather in each instance to very late referral of severely ill patients.

Once haemodialysis has been decided upon, it is most important that dialysis is continued long enough. It is clear from a review of the literature that in nearly all series some patients were under-dialysed and thus required a second dialysis. Just as it has been emphasised that the clinical condition is of paramount importance when deciding whether to use haemodialysis or not, equally it should be clinical factors that determine when dialysis finishes, rather than any attention to serum barbiturate levels. The vast majority of patients who require haemodialysis will have absent bowel sounds at the onset of treatment, i.e., a narcotized gut. As a result of increased circulation during dialysis and a lessening depth of coma, further barbiturate may be absorbed from the gut, resulting in a secondary rise in the serum barbiturate level. Thus, in such situations, by prolonging haemodialysis, more drug will be eliminated from the body and the chances of a second haemodialysis being required are lessened. On these grounds, therefore, haemodialysis should be continued until the patient has approached at least Grade I coma category and bowel sounds have been restored or haemodialysis has been maintained for at least eight hours (Jorgensen and Wieth, 1963; Lubash et al., 1962; Lee and Ames, 1965; Setter et al., 1966; Linton et al., 1967).

It is concluded that peritoneal dialysis has a very limited role to play in the management of acute barbiturate poisoning but haemodialysis does have a definite place in a few very select cases. The criteria have been outlined, and if these are used, in conjunction with energetic conservative management, then only those patients who require this treatment will be so treated. Furthermore, unnecessary haemodialysis will be avoided and haemodialysis carried out too late as an afterthought will likewise be precluded.

REFERENCES

ALWALL, N., LINDGREN, P. and LUNDERQUIST, P. (1952), On the artificial kidney: XX. Treatment of severe phenobarbitone poisoning in rabbits by means of forced polyuria, exchange ultrafiltration and dialysis and a preliminary report on dialytic treatment of barbiturate poisoning in patients. Acta med. scand., 143, 299.

ALWALL, N. (1963), Therapeutic and Diagnostic Problems in Severe Renal Failure, Chapter 10. Lund, Berlin.

BAKER, A. B. (1969), Early treatment of the patient unconscious from drug overdose. Med. J. Aust., 1, 497.

BALME, R. H., LLOYD-THOMAS, H. G. and SHEAD, G. V. (1962), Severe barbiturate poisoning treated by haemodialysis. Brit. med. J., 1, 231.

BERLYNE, G. M., HEWITT, V., JONES, J. H., NILWARANGKUR, S. and RALSTON, A. J. (1964), Protein loss in peritoneal dialysis. In: Proceedings European Dialysis and Transplant Association, 1, 177. E.D.T.A., Newcastle-upon-Tyne.

BERLYNE, G. M., LEE, H. A., RALSTON, A. J. and WOOLCOCK, J. A. (1966), Pulmonary complications of peritoneal dialysis. Lancet, I, 75.

BERMAN, L. B., JEGHERS, H. J., SCHREINER, G. E. and PALLOTTA, A. J. (1956), Haemodialysis: an effective therapy for acute barbiturate poisoning. J. Amer. med. Ass., 161, 820.

BERMAN, L. B. and VOGELSANG, P. (1964), Removal rates for barbiturates using two types of peritoneal dialysis. New Engl. J. Med., 270, 77.

BLOOMER, H. A. (1965), Limited usefulness of alkaline diuresis and peritoneal dialysis in pento-barbitone intoxication. *New Engl. J. Med.*, 272, 1309.

BLOOMER, H. A. (1967), Correspondence: Forced diuresis in barbiturate poisoning. *Lancet*, II, 986.

BOEN, S. T. (1961), Kinetics of peritoneal dialysis: a comparison with the artificial kidney. *Medicine (Baltimore)*, 40, 243.

BRODIE, B. B., BURNS, J. J., MARK, L. C., LIEF, E. B. and PAPPER, E. M. (1953), Fate of pentobarbital in man and dog and method for its estimation in biological material. *J. Pharmacol. exp. Ther.*, 109, 26.

BROUGHTON, P. M. G. (1956), Rapid ultra-violet spectrophotometric method for detection, estimation and identification of barbiturates in biological material. *Biochem. J.*, 63, 207.

BUNKER, R. N. V. D. (1959), Correspondence: Artificial kidney in acute poisoning. *Brit. med. J.*, 2, 1402.

BURNS, R. O., HENDERSON, L. W., HAGER, E. B. and MERRILL, J. R. (1962), Peritoneal dialysis, clinical experience. *New Engl. J. Med.*, 267, 1060.

FERGUSON, M. J. and GRACE, W. J. (1961), The conservative management of barbiturate intoxication: experience with 95 unconscious patients. *Ann. intern. Med.*, 54, 726.

GREER, S. and LEE, H. A. (1967), Subsequent progress of potentially lethal attempted suicides. *Acta psychiat. Scand.*, 43, 361.

HADDEN, J., JOHNSON, K., SMITH, S., PRICE, L. and GIARDINA, E. (1969), Acute barbiturate intoxication. *J. Amer. med. Ass.*, 209, 893.

HENDERSON, L. W. and MERRILL, J. P. (1966), Treatment of barbiturate intoxication. *Ann. intern. Med.*, 64, 876.

HONEY, G. E. and JACKSON, R. C. (1959), Artificial respiration and an artificial kidney for severe barbiturate poisoning. *Brit. med. J.*, 2, 1134.

JORGENSEN, H. E. and WIETH, J. O. (1963), Dialysable poisons. Haemodialysis in the treatment of acute poisoning. *Lancet*, I, 81.

KENNEDY, A. C., BRIGGS, J. D., YOUNG, N., LINDSAY, R. M., LUKE, R. G. and CAMPBELL, D. (1969), Successful treatment of three cases of very severe barbiturate poisoning. *Lancet*, I, 995.

KNOCHEL, J. P., CLAYTON, L. E., SMITH, W. L. and BARRY, K. G. (1963), Intraperitoneal THAM: an effective method to enhance phenobarbital removal during peritoneal dialysis. *Clin. Res.*, 11, 246.

KOPPANYI, T. and LINEGAR, C. R. (1942), Cross-circulation as a method in the study of drug fixation and poisoning. *Science*, 96, 562.

KYLE, L. H., JEGHERS, H., WALSH, W. P., DOOLAN, P. D., WISHINSKY, H. and PALLOTTA, A. (1953), The application of haemodialysis to the treatment of barbiturate poisoning. *J. clin. Invest.*, 32, 364.

LANCET (1967), Editorial: Barbiturate poisoning. I, 200.

LEE, H. A., ANDERSON, J. and BROOKS, P. E. (1964), Comparative efficiency of Kolff twin coil, minicoil and peritoneal dialysis. In: *Proceedings European Dialysis and Transplant Association*, 1, 185. E.D.T.A., Newcastle-upon-Tyne.

LEE, H. A. and AMES, A. C. (1965), Haemodialysis in severe barbiturate poisoning. *Brit. med. J.*, 1, 1217.

LINTON, A. L., LUKE, R. G., SPEIRS, I. and KENNEDY, A. C. (1964), Forced diuresis and haemodialysis in severe barbiturate intoxication. *Lancet*, 1, 1008.

LINTON, A. L., LUKE, R. G., BRIGGS, J. D. and KENNEDY, A. C. (1967), Haemodialysis in the treatment of severe barbiturate intoxication. In: *Proceedings European Dialysis and Transplant Association*, 293. Excerpta Medica, Amsterdam.

LUBASH, G. D., FERRARI, M. J., SCHERR, L. and RUBIN, A. L. (1962), Sedative overdosage and the role of haemodialysis. *Arch. intern. Med.*, 110, 120.

MAHER, J. F. and SCHREINER, G. E. (1965), The clinical dialysis of poisons. In: *Transactions American Society Artificial Internal Organs*, 11, 349.

MAHER, J. F. and SCHREINER, G. E. (1968), The dialysis of poisons and drugs. In: *Transactions American Society Artificial Internal Organs*, 14, 440.

MAHER, J. F. and SCHREINER, G. E. (1968), An evaluation of the effectiveness of dialysis for sedative and analgesic poisoning. In: *Proceedings European Dialysis and Transplant A ssociation*, 246. Excerpta Medica, Amsterdam.

MARK, L. C. (1963), Metabolism of barbiturates in man. *Clin. Pharmacol. Ther.*, 4, 504.

MATTHEW, H. (1969), Correspondence on: Early treatment of the patient unconscious from drug overdose. *Med. J. Aust.*, 1, 752.

MATTHEW, H. and LAWSON, A. A. H. (1966), Acute barbiturate poisoning: a review of 2 years' experience. *Quart. J. Med. (N.S.)*, 35, 539.

MAWER, G. E. and LEE, H. A. (1968), Value of forced diuresis in acute barbiturate poisoning. *Brit. med. J.*, 2, 790.

MAXWELL, M. H., ROCKNEY, R. E., KLEEMAN, C. R. and TWISS, M. R. (1959), Peritoneal dialysis. Technique and applications. *J. Amer. med. Ass.*, 170, 917.

MERRILL, J. P. (1967), Discussion. In: *Proceedings European Dialysis and Transplant Association*, 4, 306. Excerpta Medica, Amsterdam.

MYSCHETZKY, A. and LASSEN, N. A. (1963), Urea induced osmotic diuresis and alkalinization of urine in acute barbiturate intoxication. *J. Amer. med. Ass.*, 185, 936.

NAHAS, G. G., GIROUX, J. J., GJESSING, J., VEROSKY, M. and MARK, L. C. (1964), The use of THAM in peritoneal dialysis. In: *Transactions American Society Artificial Internal Organs*, 10, 345.

PALLOTTA, A., BUCHER, G., KYLE, L. and KOPPANYI, T. (1952), The artificial kidney as a method in the study of drug fixation and poisoning. *J. Pharmacol. exp. Ther.*, 106, 409.

PENDER, J. C., BEEBE, R. T., GARRETT, J. J. and KILEY, J. E. (1957), Emergency treatment of barbiturate intoxication with haemodialysis. *Ann. intern. Med.*, 46, 997.

REED, C. E., DRIGGS, M. F. and FOOTE, C. C. (1952), Acute barbiturate intoxication: a study of 300 cases based on a physiologic system of classification of the severity of the intoxication. *Ann. intern. Med.*, 37, 290.

RICHARDS, R. K. and TAYLOR, J. D. (1956), Some factors influencing distribution, metabolism and action of barbiturates: a review. *Anaesthesiology*, 17. 414.

SCHREINER, G. E. (1958), The role of haemodialysis (artificial kidney) in acute poisoning. *Arch. intern. Med.*, 102, 896.

SETTER, J. G., MAHER, J. F. and SCHREINER, G. E. (1966), Barbiturate intoxication: Evaluation of therapy including dialysis in a large series selectively referred because of severity. *Arch. intern. Med.*, 117, 224.

SUNSHINE, I. and LEONARDS, J. R. (1954), Use of artificial kidney for removal of barbiturates in dogs. *Proc. Soc. exp. Biol. Med. N.Y.*, 86, 638.

WRIGHT, N. and RAEBURN, J. A. (1969), Correspondence: Management of unconscious patients. *Brit. med. J.*, 3, 656.

14. the use of ion exchange resins and charcoal in acute barbiturate poisoning

H. Yatzidis

The limitations and dangers of forced diuresis, peritoneal dialysis, haemodialysis, and exchange transfusion in the treatment of acute barbiturate poisoning have directed attention towards other methods of endeavouring to eliminate barbiturate from the body. The use of ion exchange resins or charcoal offers promise in this direction.

ION EXCHANGE RESINS

For many years, ion exchange resins have been used in the treatment of hyperkalaemia, by exchanging either sodium (Resonium A) or calcium (Ca – Zeocarb) for potassium in the intestinal tract. Strongly basic anion exchange resins which act over a wide pH range and readily exchange their chloride or bicarbonate ions for larger or more complex ions are now available (Hurst *et al.*, 1963).

Edwards (1964) tested *in vitro* most of the ion exchange resins in the treatment of acute barbiturate overdosage and found that their efficiency in descending order was as follows: cholestyramine (Merck, Sharp and Dohme), De–Acidite FF, E and H (Permutit), and IRA-400 (Amberlite). The efficiency of a resin appears to increase in proportion to the molecular weight and the complexity of the side chain of the barbiturate, so different barbiturates have varying affinities. In studies on rats, Edwards (1964) also showed that oral administration of cholestyramine reduced the harmful effects of quinalbarbitone overdosage. He concluded that the oral use of ion exchange resins might be useful in the early treatment of drug poisoning, particularly with drugs which are strongly protein-bound and hence poorly dialysable. These compounds are excreted mainly by the liver, and he postulated that they might be absorbed by resins *in vivo* during enterohepatic circulation.

Schreiner (1958) was the first to use ion exchange resins to remove barbiturate from the blood, employing a haemoperfusion procedure in a 37-year-old woman 10 hours after the ingestion of 2.4 g pentobarbitone. Exposure of the patient's blood to a lactate-loaded anion exchange resin column for two 15-minute periods, however, did not result in the removal of a significant amount of pentobarbitone. Pallote and Koppanyi (1960) investigated the treatment of barbiturate poisoning in dogs by pumping the blood through an anion exchange resin column. They were able to remove barbiturate but simultaneously produced serious electrolyte abnormalities. This complication was overcome by Nealon et al. (1966), using a mixture of anion exchange resins in the chloride, bicarbonate, and lactate cycles (Amberlite IRA 900) with satisfactory removal of phenobarbitone from poisoned dogs. A haemoperfusion system of a new resin (Amberlite XAD-2) has been designed by Rosenbaum and Argyres (1969) and effectively applied to treat dogs poisoned by phenobarbitone. Rosenbaum and Mandanas (1967) also succeeded in removing phenobarbitone from intoxicated dogs, using an ion exchange resin in combination with peritoneal dialysis by recirculating fluid through a column of anion exchange resin of chloride and bicarbonate cycle (Amberlite IRA 900).

Apart from the single clinical application by Schreiner (1958) the method of haemoperfusion through ion exchange resins has been studied exclusively in experimental barbiturate poisoning in animals. Maher and Schreiner (1968) concluded that this method was only of limited therapeutic value because of the modest recoveries of the drug and also the significant haemolysis which occurred. We, however, considered it to hold sufficient promise to warrant further evaluation.

ACTIVATED CHARCOAL

Systematic studies of charcoal as a means of treating poisonings were carried out early in the twentieth century. Joachimoglu (1916; 1920; 1923) and Andersen (1946; 1947; 1948) carefully studied the adsorptive power of different activated charcoal-powder preparations; they also investigated the influence on adsorption of the pH of the medium and of gastric and intestinal secretions. Holt and Holz (1963) reviewed the literature on the detoxicant property of activated charcoal. Oral treatment with charcoal has been shown to benefit patients poisoned with many substances and other toxic agents are known to be strongly adsorbed by activated charcoal. These include aconite, antipyrene, barbiturates, mercury, morphine, nicotine, opium, phenol, quinine, salicylate, strychnine and sulphonamides. Oral treatment with activated charcoal is therefore of some value because of its effectiveness in a wide range of poisons whether given early or later in treatment. Some poisonous substances remain for a long time in the gastro-intestinal tract and others are known to be secreted in gastric or intestinal juice; they may be adsorbed by charcoal and prevented from reabsorption.

Intensive investigations in our department between 1961 and 1964 have demonstrated that activated charcoal can absorb in vitro from both plasma and gastro-intestinal juices considerable amounts of urea, creatinine, uric acid, phenols, indican, guanidines and organic acids as well as barbiturates, salicylate, and glutethimide.

After this preliminary research charcoal was used orally and in haemoperfusion for the treatment of chronic renal insufficiency (Yatzidis, 1964a; 1964b) and subsequently we established its value in the management of certain poisonings. (Yatzidis *et al.*, 1965; Dunea and Kolff, 1965; Yatzidis, 1966; Hagstam *et al.*, 1966a; DeMyttenaere *et al.*, 1967).

HAEMOPERFUSION THROUGH A CHARCOAL COLUMN

The study included six patients with severe barbiturate overdosage. The type of barbiturate and the amount taken included 22 g of barbitone; an indefinite quantity of phenobarbitone; 4 g of phenobarbitone together with 0.5 g of levopromazine; 17.5 g of phenobarbitone, approximately 10 g of cyclobarbitone and 13.5 g of butobarbitone. The patients were admitted deeply unconscious with plasma levels of the ingested barbiturate respectively 50.0, 14.8, 12.0, 34.0, 4.8 and 5.6 mg per 100 ml.

Fluid and electrolyte balance was strictly controlled using 5% or 20% glucose, M/6 sodium lactate and 0.9% sodium chloride. Lobeline and cropropamide were administered intramuscularly as respiratory stimulants at two-hourly intervals during the period of unconsciousness. Chloramphenicol 1 g daily was given intramuscularly. Endotracheal intubation was performed in all patients during the first 24 hours after admission and was followed in two cases by tracheostomy in order to maintain adequate respiration. Each patient's blood was perfused on one or more occasions through a cylinder measuring 20 by 6 cm and loosely packed with 200 g activated charcoal (Fig. 1). The charcoal was in granular form (Merck, No. 9624) of 0.5 to 0.75 mm particle size. It had been previously placed for 30 min in a mixture of 1 part alcohol and 9 parts chloroform containing cellulose acetate 0.5 g/l and dried at room temperature. The apparatus was sterilized by heating at 120°C for two hours. The blood is perfused through the charcoal in the column in an anti-gravity direction either by arterial pressure alone or by the pump attached if a flow rate of over 150 ml/min cannot be maintained. More technical information has been given elsewhere (Yatzidis, 1964b).

The details of the haemoperfusions, the clinical course and the laboratory data for each of the six patients are shown in Table 1.

Perfusion of blood through charcoal led in all cases to rapid and satisfactory removal of barbiturate from the blood, the plasma level falling after each perfusion. A considerable decrease of the plasma barbiturate was finally observed by repeated perfusions in a reasonably short time, while the amount of barbiturate excreted in the urine in this period was insignificant.

It would appear that at the start, provided a flow of at least 250 ml/min can be maintained, almost all the barbiturate in the plasma can be removed during one passage through the column. This finding is in accord with many experimental observations (Dunea and Kolff 1965; Hagstam *et al.*, 1966a; Dedrick *et al.*, 1967; DeMyttenaere *et al.*, 1967; De Myttenaere, 1968). However, efficiency is gradually reduced as

TABLE 1

Clinical and biochemical findings in six cases of severe barbiturate poisoning treated by repeated haemoperfusions through a charcoal column of 200 g in a 200–300 ml blood-flow rate per min. Both the mercuric (Zaar and Cornwall, 1961; Curry, 1964) and the ultraviolet spectrophotometric method (Goldbaum, 1952) were used for the plasma and urine barbiturate measurements.

Patient: G.M. ♀ 22 — barbitone, ingested 22.0 g

Hours since ingestion	9	16	17	22	26	31	35	48	72	96
Number of haemoperfusions		1	2	3		4	5			
Duration of haemoperfusion (min)		8	25	70		60	60			
Plasma barbiturate level (mg/l): Before haemoperfusion. Arterial blood from the proximal tubing	500	500	420	500	384	348	200	220	120	30
5 min after the beginning of haemoperf. Blood from the distal tubing		26	5							
30 min after stopping the haemoperf. Blood from proximal tubing			232	448		312	164			
Respiration	shallow	improved	normal	"	"	"	"	"		
Blood pressure (mm Hg)	90/70								100/70	
Temperature (°C)	36								38	
Cyanosis	+	+	–	–	–	–	–	–	–	–
Tendon reflexes	–	–	–	–	–	+	+	+	+	+
Reaction to stimuli	–	–	–	–	–	–	–	+	+	+
Duration of coma (hrs)									70	
Result: (a) Total excreted urine (l) and (b) barbiturate (g) during coma period									(a) 11.00 (b) 2.23 recovered	

Patient: I.V. ♀ 47 — phenobarbitone, indefinite

Hours since ingestion	6	12	19	21	32	56
Number of haemoperfusions		1				
Duration of haemoperfusion (min)		30				
Plasma barbiturate level (mg/l): Before haemoperfusion. Arterial blood from the proximal tubing	148	126	120	120	98	56
5 min after the beginning of haemoperf. Blood from the distal tubing		6				
30 min after stopping the haemoperf. Blood from proximal tubing			69			
Respiration	shallow	improved	normal	"	"	"
Blood pressure (mm Hg)	100/80					
Temperature (°C)	36					
Cyanosis	–	–	–	–	–	–
Tendon reflexes	–	–	–	+	+	+
Reaction to stimuli	–	–	+	+	+	+
Duration of coma (hrs)			20			
Result: (a) Total excreted urine (l) and (b) barbiturate (g) during coma period			(a) 8.00 (b) 1.50 bronchopneumonia recovered			

Patient	Drug							Respiration	B.P.	Temp.					(a)/(b)	Notes
P.X. ♂ 57	pheno-barbitone 4.0	3			120			shallow	110/70	36	−	−	−			abscess on the region of coccyx
		6	1	60	100	17	65	improved			−	−	−			
		8			92			normal			−	−	−			
		10	2	60	86	49	73	"			+	+	−			
	levomo-promagine 0.5	12			69			"		38	+	+	−	18	(a) 6.00	recovered
		16	3	60	53	15	37	"			+	+	−		(b) 0.25	
		24			34						+	+	−			
G.M. ♂ 23	pheno-barbitone 17.5	14	1	20	340	45	227	shallow	100/80	38	−	−	+			bullae on the occular conjunctivae
		17	2	16	255	15	189	"			−	−	+			
		19	3	48	231		150	"			−	−	−			
		23	4	45	172		156	"	col. lapsus		−	−	−			
		28	5	57	170		134	apnea			−	−	+		(a) 10.00	
		33	6	45	132		109	"			−	−	+		(b) 1.80	
		36			150			"			−	−	+	38		died
		38			123						−	−	−			
N.L. ♂ 26	cyclo-barbitone 10.0?	26	1	20	48		39	shallow		37	−	−	−			recovered
		28			41			normal			+	+	−			
M.V. ♀ 50	buta-barbitone 13.5	13	1	9	56	3	25	shallow	100/80	37	−	−	+			broncho-pneumonia, thrombo-phlebitis of the leg,
		16	2	10	31	2	20	"		38	−	−	+			
		18	3	60	39		6	improved			−	−	−			
		22	4	60	29			"			−	−	−			
		25			18			"			−	−	−			
		28			21			"			+	−	−			
		33			21			"			+	−	−			
		60			16			normal			+	+	−	60	(a) 11.00	recovered
		84			12			"			+	+	−		(b) 0.25	
		108			6						+	+	−			

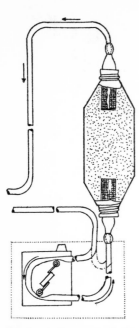

Fig. 1. A diagram indicating the charcoal artificial kidney. The apparatus is sterilized at 120°C for two hours. The blood is perfused through charcoal column in antigravity direction by the arterial pressure alone or with a pump attached to the proximal tubing if a flow rate over 150 ml per minute is desired. More technical information has been described elsewhere (Yatzidis, 1964*b*).

the saturation point of the charcoal in the column is reached. On the other hand, the adsorptive power of charcoal varies, according to Freundlich's isotherm principle, and is proportionate to the concentration of the substance in the liquid phase (Hassler, 1963). We have previously demonstrated that this principle is also true for substances in plasma, but the greater the protein binding of a substance the smaller is the amount adsorbed by the charcoal (Figs. 2 and 3).

There is linear augmentation of the adsorptive power with increase of the concentration. With the exception of barbitone, which is only slightly protein-bound, the adsorptive power of the charcoal was only about half as effective in plasma as in water (Yatzidis and Tsaparas, 1969) (Figs. 2 and 3). Consequently, the efficiency of the charcoal kidney can be expressed as the amount of the substance adsorbed by 200 g charcoal for a given plasma concentration (Yatzidis, 1964*b*; Yatzidis and Tsaparas, 1969). This was calculated for different barbiturates to be approximately 0.5 to 2.5 g for a plasma concentration ranging from 7.5 to 30.0 mg/100 ml plasma. In order to obtain a high removal rate of barbiturate we preferred to use frequent short haemoperfusions, rather than less frequent but more prolonged perfusions, to the point of saturation of the charcoal available.

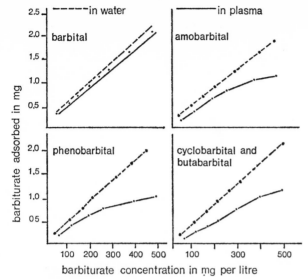

Fig. 2. Fluctuations of adsorptive power of 100 mg charcoal after five minutes contact with 5 ml different concentration of barbiturates in water and plasma. There is a linear augmentation of the adsorptive power with increase of the concentration. With the exception of barbitone, which is only slightly protein-bound, the absorptive power of the charcoal was only about half as effective in plasma as in water (from Yatzidis and Tsaparas, 1969).

COMPLICATIONS

There were no technical difficulties with haemoperfusion in this small number of patients, apart from three occasions when thrombosis occurred in the apparatus and once when the equipment accidentally broke. Heparin in a dose of 2.5 mg/kg body weight appears sufficient to prevent coagulation during a 60-minute perfusion. No bleeding occurred even in two patients in whom five and six consecutive perfusions were carried out in one day. Haemolysis did not occur. A decrease of the arterial pressure was noted at the start of the procedure, but was easily corrected by intravenous infusion of a solution containing 50 mg/l phenylnephrine hydrochloride.

In three cases there was a fall in the platelet count and also the plasma fibrinogen fell to 40–80% of pre-perfusion levels, but these were regained within 48 hours. In subsequent patients these complications were avoided by pretreatment of the activated charcoal with cellulose acetate. Hagstam *et al.* (1966*a*; 1966*b*) demonstrated, using untreated charcoal in perfused rabbits, that deposition of microscopic particles in the internal organs and particularly the lung, spleen, liver and kidney occurred whether they killed the animals immediately or months after the perfusion. Treatment of charcoal with cellulose acetate coats every granule with a very thin permeable layer of cellulose, obviating any damage to or destruction of platelets and also any detachment of charcoal particles by the perfusing blood. Despite the presence of the cellulose acetate, the adsorptive power of the charcoal is scarcely impaired. Using high-speed

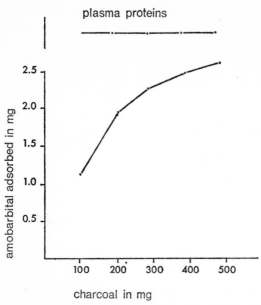

Fig. 3. Adsorption of amobarbital (the barbiturate most bound to plasma protein) by 100–500 mg charcoal after 5 minutes contact with 5 ml of 500 mg amobarbital per litre in plasma. The adsorption augments progressively and 400 mg of charcoal are sufficient to adsorb the total quantity of amobarbital (95%–100%). In the above conditions the charcoal adsorbs the fraction of amobarbital bound to the proteins by a dissociation process, because the concentration of proteins remains constant in the plasma samples (from Yatzidis and Tsaparas, 1969).

centrifugation, we have confirmed that the rinsing fluid from a 200 g column of treated charcoal, following perfusion in a closed circulation for 30 minutes with a flow rate of 200 to 300 ml/min, remains free of microscopic charcoal particles (Yatzidis, 1966; Yatzidis and Tsaparas, 1969).

RESULTS

Clinical improvement during the haemoperfusion was impressive. Respiration improved and cyanosis decreased or even disappeared. Temporary appearance of the tendon reflexes and of the light reflex was invariably noted in all patients, and on some occasions the patient responded to painful stimuli. The only patient who died had ingested 17.5 g of phenobarbitone. He died 38 hours after the ingestion of the drug, despite decrease in the level of plasma barbiturate from 34.0 to 12.3 mg/100 ml in 24 hours. Post-mortem examination showed slight oedema of the brain and small haemorrhagic foci on the intestinal and bladder walls. The remaining five patients recovered completely after periods of coma of 70, 20, 18, 28 and 60 hours, despite the considerable amount of barbiturate ingested and the high level of plasma barbiturate before treatment. These surviving patients remain well two to four years later.

Our clinical results are in agreement with the experimental observations of Hagstam *et al.* (1966*a*, 1966*b*), who used haemoperfusion through charcoal in phenobarbitone-poisoned rabbits. They reported a decrease in the depth of coma during the course of treatment in all of the perfused animals. The grossly abnormal electroencephalogram before perfusion showed a gradual return to normal during treatment. The mean duration of coma in treated animals was 13 hours, while in the control group of animals it was 42 hours.

Haemoperfusion through charcoal is a simple and useful method for the treatment of severe barbiturate poisoning. Its effectiveness on the protein-bound fraction of barbiturates as well as on some other poorly or nondialysable toxic substances of endogenous and exogenous origin is important and merits further consideration (Yatzidis, 1966; DeMyttenaere *et al.*, 1967; DeMyttenaere, 1968; Yatzidis *et al.*, 1969).

REFERENCES

ANDERSEN, A. H. (1946), Experimental studies on the pharmacology of activated charcoal. I. Adsorption power of charcoal from aqueous solutions. *Acta pharmacol. (Kbh.)*, 2, 69.
ANDERSEN, A. H. (1947), Experimental studies on the pharmacology of activated charcoal. II. The effect of pH on the adsorption by charcoal from aqueous solutions. *Acta pharmacol. (Kbh.)*, 3, 199.
ANDERSEN, A. H. (1948), Experimental studies on the pharmacology of activated charcoal. III. Adsorption from gastro-intestinal contents. *Acta pharmacol. (Kbh.)*, 4, 275.
CURRY, A. S. (1964), Rapid quantitative barbiturate estimation. *Brit. med. J.*, 1, 354.
DEDRICK, R. L., VANTOCH, P., GOMBOS, E. A. and MOORE, R. (1967), Kinetics of activated carbon kidney. *Trans. Amer. Soc. artif. intern. Org.*, 13, 236.
DEMYTTENAERE, M. H., MAHER, J. E. and SCHREINER, G. (1967), Hemoperfusion through a charcoal column for glutethimide poisoning. *Trans. Amer. Soc. artif. intern. Org.*, 13, 190.
DEMYTTENAERE, M. H. (1968), Haemoperfusion through a charcoal column for treatment of poisoning. In: D. N. S. KERR, D. FRIES and R. W. ELLIOTT (Ed) *Proceedings of the 5th Conference of the European Dialysis and Transplant Association,* 320. Excerpta Medica, Amsterdam.
DUNEA, G. and KOLFF, W. J. (1965), Clinical experience with the Yatzidis' charcoal artificial kidney. *Trans. Amer. Soc. artif. intern. Org.*, 11, 178.
EDWARDS, K. D. G. (1964), Methods of extrarenal removal of drugs, including the use of dialysis and ion exchange resins in barbiturate poisoning. *Bull. postgrad. Comm. Med. Univ. Sydney*, 20, 89.
GOLDBAUM, L. R. (1952), Determination of barbiturates. Ultraviolet spectrophotometric method with differentiation of several barbiturates. *Anal. Chem.*, 24, 1604.
HAGSTAM, K. E., LARSSON, L. E. and THYSELL, H. (1966*a*), Experimental studies on charcoal haemoperfusion in phenobarbital intoxication and uraemia, including histopathologic findings. *Acta med. scand.*, 180, 593.
HAGSTAM, K. E., LARSSON, L. E. and THYSELL, H. (1966*b*), Charcoal deposition in internal organs haemoperfusion with the Yatzidis' technique in rabbits. *European Dialysis Transplant Ass. Proc*, 3, 352.
HASSLER, J. W. (1963), *Activated Carbon.* Chemical Publ Co., New York.
HOLT, L. M. and HOLZ, P. H. (1963), The black bottle. *J. Pediat.*, 62, 306.
HURST, P. E., MORRISON, R. B., TIMONER, J., METCALFE-GIBSON, A. and WRONG, O. (1963), The effect of oral anion exchange resins on fecal anions. Comparison with calcium salts and aluminium hydroxide. *Clin. Sci.*, 24, 187.
JOACHIMOGLU, G. (1916), Ueber die Adsportionsvermögen der Tierkohle und seine Bestimmung. *Biochem Z.*, 77, 1.
JOACHIMOGLU, G. (1920), Die theoretische Grundlagen der Kohlentherapie. *Chem. Zeitg.*, 44, 780.
JOACHIMOGLU, G. (1923), Adsorptions – und Entgiftungsvermögen einiger Kohlen. *Biochem. Z.*, 134, 493.
MAHER, J. F. and SCHREINER, G. E. (1968), The dialysis of poisons and drugs. *Trans. Amer. Soc. artif. intern. Org.*, 14, 440.

232   H. YATZIDIS

NEALON, T. F., SHEA, W. and FLEEGLER, E. (1966), An extracorporeal device for treatment of barbiturate poisoning. *J. Amer. med. Ass.*, 197, 158.

PALLOTE, A. J. and KOPPANYI, T. (1960), The use of ion exchange resins in the treatment of phenobarbital intoxication in dogs. *J. Pharmacol exp. Ther.*, 128, 318.

ROSENBAUM, J. L. and ARGYRES, S. N. (1969), Resin hemoperfusion to treat barbiturate intoxication in dogs. Paper read at 4th International Congress of Nephrology, Stockholm. (Abstract), p. 421.

ROSENBAUM, J. L. and MANDANAS, R. (1967), Treatment of phenobarbital intoxication in dogs with an anion-recirculation peritoneal dialysis technique. *Trans. Amer. Soc. artif. intern., Org.*, 13, 183.

SCHREINER, G. E. (1958), The role of hemodialysis (artificial kidney) in acute poisoning. *Arch. intern. Med.*, 102, 896.

YATZIDIS, H. (1964a), Recherches sur l'épuration extrarénale à l'aide du charbon actif. *Nephron*, I, 310.

YATZIDIS, H. (1964b), A convenient haemoperfusion microapparatus over charcoal for the treatment of endogenous and exogenous intoxications. Its use as an effective artificial kidney. *European Dialysis Transplant Ass. Proc.*, 1, 83.

YATZIDIS, H. (1966), Further experience with the charcoal artificial kidney. Paper read at 3rd International Congress of Nephrology, Washington. (Abstract), p. 299.

YATZIDIS, H., OREOPOULOS, D., TRIANTAFILLIDIS, D., STAVROULAKI, A., VOUDICLARI, S., TSAPARAS, N. and GAVRAS, C. (1965), Treatment of severe barbiturate poisoning. *Lancet*, 2, 216.

YATZIDIS, H., PSIMENOS, G. and MAYOPOULOU-SYMVOULIDIS, D. (1969), Nondialysable toxic factor in uraemic blood effectively removed by the activated charcoal. *Experientia*, 25, 1144.

YATZIDIS, H. and TSAPARAS, N. (1969), The action of certain factors upon the adsorptive power of charcoal (in Greek). *Bull. Soc. Med. Athens*, 1, 28.

ZAAR, B. and GRONWALL, A. (1961), A micromethod for determination of barbiturates in serum as mercuric complexes. *Scand. J. clin. lab. Invest.*, 13, 225.

15. an assessment of diuresis and dialysis for treating acute barbiturate poisoning

H. A. Bloomer and R. K. Maddock, Jr.

The current enthusiasm for treating serious sedative intoxication with diuresis, peritoneal dialysis, and extracorporeal hemodialysis is founded on the belief that removal of the active agent will reduce the probability of death resulting directly from an extremely high drug concentration or indirectly from the complications of prolonged coma. Despite the fact that this belief is seldom challenged, there are no clear-cut morbidity or mortality statistics to support an aggressive approach, and it is possible that there never will be. At our present stage of development in treating barbiturate overdosage most authorities would agree that any form of treatment which appreciably shortens coma is beneficial, provided that the therapy is of low risk to the patient. It is accepted that, in competent hands, the various types of forced diuresis and of dialysis have low morbidity. The critical issue, therefore, is whether a specific treatment, applied to the removal of a specific intoxicant, actually does remove enough sedative compound to justify the effort.

The biochemical, physiological, and pharmacological principles that determine the effectiveness of a drug removal procedure have been presented in detail by Schreiner (1958). The drug must be accessible, *i.e.* able to pass biological or artificial membranes, and be favorably distributed between plasma water and the other body compartments; the rate of drug removal must add significantly to the endogenous mechanisms for degrading and excreting the agent. Most publications advocating diuresis or dialysis have demonstrated that sedatives can be removed, but have failed to relate the rate of removal to endogenous disposition. Unless this relationship is known it is impossible to select appropriate therapy.

In this chapter we shall explore some of the factors that influence the removal of drugs, particularly the barbiturates, by diuresis and by dialysis. In particular, some problems inherent in the design of studies which attempt to relate removal to endogenous disposition will be analyzed, since some of these difficulties have led to erroneous data or conclusions. Last of all, we shall attempt to define the limitations of selected methods of treatment in hastening recovery from barbiturate coma.

THE ANALYSIS OF DRUGS IN BIOLOGICAL FLUIDS

In order to estimate the rate of plasma disappearance of a specific chemical agent, the rate of its urinary excretion, or its removal into dialysis fluid it is essential that the analytic technique used is both specific and precise. It is critical to know that the data obtained in an experiment relate to the parent sedative compound, and not its metabolites. With the exception of barbital, most of which is rapidly excreted without alteration in the urine (Giotti and Maynert, 1951), all of the commonly used barbiturates undergo significant degradation in the liver. Although various pathways of barbiturate metabolism have been described, the predominant metabolites are formed simply by oxidation of substituents in position 5 of the barbituric acid ring (Mark, 1963). The resulting compounds are relatively polar alcohols, ketones, phenols or carboxylic acids which are poorly bound to plasma proteins and are excreted rapidly in the urine in the free state or as conjugates of glucuronic acid (Bloomer, 1965; Sharpless, 1965). Despite the fact that they still possess the intact barbituric acid ring, they are no longer sedative agents (Schonle et al., 1933; Butler, 1956). Unfortunately, the spectrophotometric techniques that have traditionally been used in investigations of barbiturate disposition depend merely on the presence of the barbiturate ring structure, so that these metabolites, when present in high concentration, contribute appreciably to the measurement of 'barbiturate' in biological fluids (Bloomer, 1965).

When analyses involve only plasma samples, this source of error is small. Because metabolites have low affinity for plasma proteins and are excreted rapidly by the kidneys, their concentrations in plasma are low. Even when relatively polar organic solvents such as chloroform or ethylene dichloride are used to extract the drug from plasma for analysis, metabolite contribution to estimation of total 'barbiturate' is negligible.

When urine is being analyzed the error is much greater because the metabolites are present in high concentration. This is particularly true when the short- to intermediate-acting barbiturates such as pentobarbital, secobarbital and amobarbital are being examined. When no effort is made to increase urinary volume less than 1% of these agents is excreted unchanged in the urine, although as much as 80% of the administered dose can be recovered in the form of various ring-structured degradation products (Schonle et al., 1933; Maynert, 1952; Maynert and Dawson, 1952; Titus and Weiss, 1955; Waddell, 1962). Even during diuresis the concentration of these compounds is many times greater than that of the parent barbiturate. This is shown by the data in Table 1, obtained during mannitol diuresis in a patient intoxicated by pentobarbital (Bloomer, 1965). In this study, the pentobarbital was extracted from urine with a non-polar solvent combination, petroleum ether and isoamyl alcohol, as described by Brodie et al. (1953). Following this, the remaining metabolites were extracted with ethyl ether. Both extracts were analyzed by ultraviolet spectrophotometry. As shown in Table 1, the concentration of metabolites was many times greater than that of the parent pentobarbital, even at high rates of urine flow. When more

TABLE 1

Urinary concentrations of pentobarbital and its metabolites

urine volume (ml/min)	pentobarbital mg/100 ml)	ether-extractable metabolites (mg/100 ml)
3.8	2.9	24.6
4.7	2.5	25.2
5.8	2.9	20.7
9.2	2.5	15.5
7.5	2.5	20.0
5.8	2.5	23.0

polar organic solvents such as chloroform are used to extract urine, appreciable quantities of metabolites will accompany the parent drug and produce erroneously high estimates of urinary 'barbiturate' concentration.

Most studies of the effect of diuresis on barbiturate excretion have used an ultraviolet spectrophotometric technique following extraction of plasma and urine with chloroform (Goldbaum, 1952). In order to estimate the magnitude of the error involved, we have analyzed by three techniques a urine sample obtained from a patient with pentobarbital coma: gas chromatography; ultraviolet spectrophotometry following extraction with petroleum ether-isoamyl alcohol; ultraviolet spectrophotometry following chloroform extraction (Bloomer, 1967). Gas chromatography has the advantage of separating and measuring only the parent drug, whatever the method of extraction, and is sufficiently precise (Bloomer, 1966; Bloomer et al., 1970).

The data are presented in Table 2. The results demonstrate that one can overestimate the concentration of pentobarbital in urine, and therefore its renal clearance, by two and one-half times, depending on the method of chemical analysis, and form an erroneous conclusion about the efficiency of renal drug removal.

TABLE 2

'Pentobarbital' concentrations in urine (mg/100 ml)*

gas chromatography	ether-alcohol	chloroform
0.64	0.77	1.61
0.63	0.84	1.59
0.59	0.81	1.59
0.63	0.84	1.58
Mean 0.6	0.8	1.6

* reprinted by permission of *Lancet*, II, 986, 1967.

The original data presented in this chapter were obtained using analytic techniques specific for the parent sedative compounds. The majority of analyses were performed using gas-liquid chromatography (Bloomer, 1966; Maddock and Bloomer, 1967). In a few instances, analyses were performed by ultraviolet spectrophotometry after extraction of pentobarbital from plasma and urine with petroleum ether-isoamyl alcohol (Brodie *et al.*, 1953), or after phenobarbital extraction with benzene (Waddell and Butler, 1957). All data are suffiiciently precise to permit realistic conclusions about the effectiveness of the various drug removal techniques.

DESIGN OF DRUG REMOVAL STUDIES

Two methods have been used to quantitate the effectiveness of drug removal procedures: first, a comparison of the rate of fall in plasma concentration of drug during diuresis or dialysis with that observed when no measures are employed to increase excretion (Lassen, 1960; Myschetzky and Lassen, 1963; Jørgensen and Wieth, 1963; Hadden *et al.*, 1969); second, a comparison of the total quantity of drug removed per unit time with the rate of disposal by endogenous mechanisms (Bloomer, 1965; Bloomer, 1966; Maddock and Bloomer, 1967). Of these methods, the first is preferable since each patient serves as his own control, provided that the patient is observed for a sufficient time prior to treatment so that an accurate measurement of the spontaneous disposal of the intoxicant can be obtained. Unfortunately, when confronted with an instance of severe coma, it is seldom possible to withhold treatment for very long. Using the second approach, measurements of drug removal are usually made in patients with severe intoxication during active treatment, while estimates of endogenous disposition are made in other patients, frequently less severely intoxicated, receiving only supportive care. Although the removal of sedatives by diuresis or dialysis can be measured precisely by proper analytic techniques, many difficulties are encountered in measuring endogenous disposition, as described below. In spite of the problems inherent in both types of studies, the results obtained and the conclusions reached agree remarkably well.

ESTIMATION OF ENDOGENOUS DISPOSITION

The disappearance of barbiturate compounds from the plasma of intoxicated patients is linear when plotted on semi-logarithmic axes, as in Fig. 1, indicating that total disposal of drug by the various hepatic and renal mechanisms occurs at a constant rate. Since linearity persists over a wide range of plasma concentrations, there is no indication that the endogenous mechanisms involved in the metabolic degradation and excretion of barbiturates ever become saturated or overwhelmed. Provided that gastrointestinal absorption of the drug is complete, that distribution among the various body compartments has reached equilibrium, and that the absolute quantity of drug in the body is known, the rate of plasma disappearance can be used to estimate the absolute quantity of drug degraded and excreted per unit of time. These conditions are not always met in the intoxicated patient.

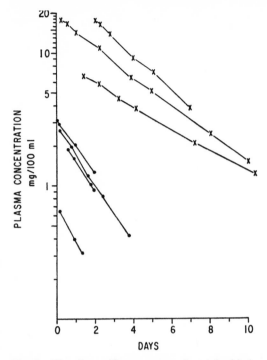

Fig. 1. The plasma disappearance of pentobarbital or secobarbital (•) and phenobarbital (x). The average rate of disappearance for the short-acting barbiturates is 2.2 % hr, while that of phenobarbital is 1.0 % hr. The drugs were ingested at time zero.

GASTROINTESTINAL ABSORPTION

In human subjects given hypnotic doses of barbiturates, absorptions of pentobarbital and secobarbital are complete in two hours, while phenobarbital reaches peak levels in six to twelve hours (Fazekas *et al.*, 1956). However, patients who ingest much higher doses frequently develop paralytic ileus, and may continue to absorb drug for several days (Lassen, 1960). Such an instance, one with a fatal outcome, is shown in Figure 2. The patient was a 21-year-old man who ingested a large quantity of phenobarbital and was admitted in a deeply comatose state with no reflexes or bowel sounds. Shortly after hospitalization, hemodialysis was begun and continued for 14 hours, during which the plasma concentration of phenobarbital fell from 21.4 mg/100 ml to 15.9 mg/100 ml, and bowel sounds returned. However, in the 24 hours following hemodialysis, the plasma level climbed rapidly to 24.9 mg/100 ml, and the patient expired. There is little doubt that phenobarbital absorption continued for 36 hours after ingestion, perhaps augmented by restoration of bowel activity during hemo-

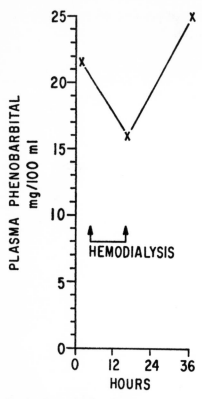

Fig. 2. Late rise in plasma concentration of phenobarbital, presumably resulting from delayed gastrointestinal absorption. The drug was ingested at time zero.

dialysis. If gastrointestinal absorption of a drug continues during study, as may occur in the intoxicated patient, the disappearance rate from plasma will underestimate the actual rate of metabolism and excretion.

Erratic gastrointestinal absorption is particularly troublesome when the offending agent is a sedative of poor water solubility such as glutethimide. Reports have emphasized that the plasma concentration may continue to rise for many hours after ingestion and that significant amounts of unabsorbed glutethimide may be found in the gastrointestinal tract, days after ingestion (Schreiner *et al.*, 1958). Slow gastrointestinal absorption probably accounts for the marked variability in plasma glutethimide disappearance noted (Maher and Schreiner 1961; Maher *et al.*, 1962), and may well be responsible for the prolonged coma produced by this compound.

DISTRIBUTION

Following absorption or intravenous administration, the barbiturates are distributed to all tissues and body fluids. Distribution is rapid, reaching equilibrium in two to three hours (Brodie *et al.*, 1953; Butler, 1952). It has been stated that distribution occurs more or less throughout total body water (Butler, 1952; Wright, 1955). However, this is an oversimplification, since distribution is a dynamic process which is influenced by drug solubility in lipid as well as aqueous media, by binding to plasma and tissue proteins, and by concentration in those organs, liver and kidney, which accomplish drug removal. Some of the physicochemical factors which influence the distribution of the long-acting barbiturate, phenobarbital, and the short-acting agent, pentobarbital, are presented in Table 3.

TABLE 3

Properties of barbiturates

	Binding to plasma protein	Concentration in fat*
Phenobarbital	0.43	0.6
Pentobarbital	0.56	1.1

* mg per kg fat/mg per kg of whole plasma. To calculate the distribution of unbound drug between fat and plasma water, the fat/plasma ratio should be divided by the fraction of diffusible drug (1-fraction bound to plasma protein).

From inspection of these data, it is apparent that any agreement between the actual volume of body water and a virtual space of drug distribution calculated by (quantity ingested/plasma level) is fortuitous. In the case of phenobarbital, the concentration in fat tissue is about the same as in plasma water ($0.6/1-0.43 = 1.05$), while pentobarbital is concentrated in fat ($1.1/1-0.56 = 2.50$). Although the virtual space of distribution of phenobarbital is 70 to 75% of body weight, only slightly greater than plasma water (Wright, 1955; Butler, 1952), the distribution space of pentobarbital must be distinctly greater. In fact, when one calculates from the meager data that have been published (Brodie *et al.*, 1953), the virtual space of distribution of pentobarbital is two or three times the volume of total body water.

These considerations point out the errors that may arise when attempting to calculate the actual quantity of a drug degraded and excreted by endogenous mechanisms in a given time interval. Not only the rate of plasma disappearance, but also the absolute quantity of drug in the body must be known. If the apparent space of distribution is known, the body content of drug can be calculated by plasma concentration times space of distribution (Wright, 1955). Body content of drug and the per cent decrease in plasma concentration can then be used to calculate the actual disposal of drug, so that it can be compared to drug removed by diuresis or dialysis.

Calculations which assume the volume of distribution to be that of total body water are reasonably valid for phenobarbital, but much less secure when pentobarbital is being studied (Bloomer, 1966). However, underestimating the space of drug distribution gives a falsely low estimate of the total body content of drug and of endogenous drug disposal. Such an error tends to exaggerate the contribution of drug removal procedures to total drug disposal. Consequently, the actual efficiency of diuresis or dialysis for removing pentobarbital and other short-acting barbiturates must be considerably less than the maximum estimated by this type of calculation.

A high degree of protein binding and a high solubility in fat tissue, in addition to complicating the interpretation of experiments attempting to evaluate drug removal procedures, markedly impair the efficacy of these treatments by reducing the concentration of diffusible drug in plasma water relative to the total body content. An extremely unfavorable distribution occurs in the case of the nonbarbiturate sedative, glutethimide. Highly bound to plasma protein (70% of plasma level) and extremely fat-soluble (10 to 13 times concentration in whole plasma), only a very small percentage of the ingested dose is present in blood in a diffusible form available for renal excretion or dialytic removal (Maher and Schreiner, 1961). Similar properties are possessed by the ultrashort-acting thiobarbiturates which, fortunately, are seldom used for self-inflicted drug coma.

Despite the variability of the various barbiturates in their patterns of distribution, once equilibrium among body tissues and fluid compartments has been reached the decline in plasma level is proportional to the overall disposition of drug. The rate of barbiturate degradation and excretion is slow in relation to the redistribution of drug among the various tissues and body fluids, so that a fall in plasma level will not result in disequilibrium of drug between plasma water, on the one hand, and drug bound to plasma or tissue protein, or present in adipose tissue, on the other hand. Even when the plasma level has been lowered abruptly by hemodialysis, there is no 'rebound' in plasma concentration after the procedure, as would be expected if drug redistribution were not rapid (Jørgensen, 1963).

COMPARISON OF SELECTED METHODS OF TREATMENT

DIURESIS

Both short- and long-acting barbiturate compounds, as well as other sedative agents, are excreted to some extent in the urine, even at low rates of flow. The major factors which influence the absolute rate of excretion are the filtered load of drug, determined by the plasma concentration and the degree of binding to plasma proteins, and the extent of tubular reabsorption determined by the volume of tubular fluid and its acidity or alkalinity.

The degree of binding to plasma proteins, chiefly albumin, of commonly used sedatives is given in Table 4. Renal excretion of phenobarbital, pentobarbital, secobarbital and glutethimide is strikingly reduced by the fact that the concentrations of these drugs in glomerular filtrate are only 30 to 60% of the concentrations in whole plasma.

TABLE 4

Physicochemical properties of common sedatives.

	Binding to plasma protein	pKa
Barbital	0	7.9
Phenobarbital	0.43	7.2
Pentobarbital	0.56	8.1
Secobarbital	0.70	8.1
Meprobamate	0.21	neutral
Glutethimide	0.71	neutral

At low rates of urine flow the renal clearance of these agents is only 1–2 ml/min, indicating that about 99% of filtered drug is reabsorbed during its passage through the renal tubule. It has been repeatedly demonstrated that an increased urine volume accomplished by water diuresis or the administration of diuretic agents depresses tubular reabsorption and increases urinary excretion of these sedatives (Lassen, 1960; Myschetzky and Lassen, 1963; Maddock and Bloomer, 1967; Setter *et al.*, 1964; Linton *et al.*, 1967). Diuresis, by increasing the volume of fluid present in the various segments of the nephron, reduces passive back-diffusion by lowering the concentration gradient for drug between tubular fluid and blood.

The influence of plasma protein binding and of urine flow rate on drug clearance is shown in Figs. 3 and 4. In both plots, renal excretion of drug increases with urine flow. However, as shown in Fig. 3, the plasma clearance of meprobamate only 20% bound to plasma protein is distinctly higher at all rates of urine flow than that of either pentobarbital or glutethimide, which are more highly bound to plasma protein. When renal excretion is plotted as the clearance of filtrable drug, UV/F, Fig. 4, this difference disappears, indicating that the degree of tubular reabsorption of the various chemical agents is roughly the same at any rate of urine flow.

In addition to these factors, alkalinization of the urine has a definite additive effect on those weak organic acids, such as phenobarbital or salicylate, whose pKa is less than 8.0, the upper limit of urinary pH (Bloomer, 1966; Kelley *et al.*, 1966; Weiner *et al.*, 1959). These drugs exist in tubular fluid both as the undissociated acid, which is highly lipid-soluble, and as the water-soluble salt. The proportion of total barbiturate present as acid or salt depends on the pH of tubular fluid. The acid moiety diffuses readily through cell membranes while the ionic form does not. Alkalinity of tubular fluid, which increases ionization, depresses tubular reabsorption and increases excretion by trapping barbiturate as its sodium salt in tubular fluid. Predictably, alkalinity of the urine has little effect on the excretion of barbital, pentobarbital, or secobarbital (Giotti and Maynert, 1951; Bloomer, 1966), each of which has a higher pKa (Table 4), or on the excretion of neutral drugs such as meprobamate or glutethimide. This phenomenon is examined in Figs. 5, 6 and 7.

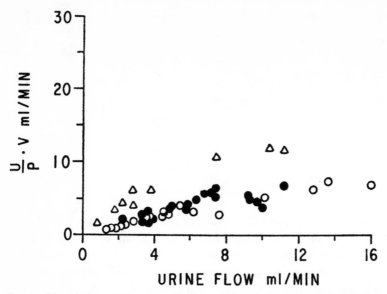

Fig. 3. The relation between rate of urinary flow and the clearance from whole plasma of pento-barbital (•), glutethimide (o) and meprobamate (Δ). Clearances were calculated from: (U/P) V, where U and P are drug concentrations in urine and plasma, and V the rate of urine flow.

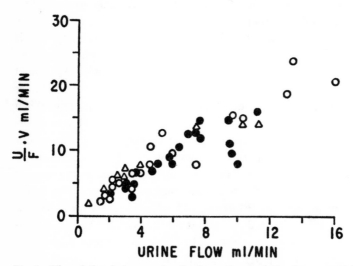

Fig. 4. The relation between rate of urinary flow and the clearance of filtrable pentobarbital (•), glutethimide (o) and meprobamate (Δ). Clearances were calculated from: (U/F) V, where U and F are drug concentrations in urine and plasma filtrate, and V the rate of urine flow.

Fig. 5 shows the theoretic ratio of concentration in urine to concentration in plasma filtrate at each urinary pH for a weak organic acid of pKa 8.1, as well as data obtained from patients intoxicated by pentobarbital and secobarbital. Increasing the urinary pH to its maximum even at low urine flows does not concentrate either of these short-

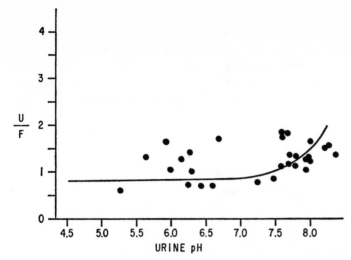

Fig. 5. The effect of pH on the concentration of short-acting barbiturates in urine. The curve portrays the theoretic ratio of concentration in urine to concentration in plasma filtrate, U/F, at each urinary pH for an organic acid of pKa 8.1. The data points are ratios observed in patients intoxicated by pentobarbital and secobarbital. (Reprinted from *J. Lab. clin. Med.*, 67, 898–905, 1966, by permission of C. V. Mosby.)

acting barbiturates in urine. On the other hand, Fig. 6 shows that a urine pH above 7.5 does actually concentrate phenobarbital in urine as much as fourfold.

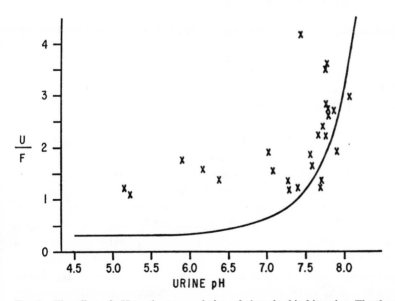

Fig. 6. The effect of pH on the accumulation of phenobarbital in urine. The theoretic ratios for an organic acid of pKa 7.2 are shown by the curve and the ratios measured in patients by the data points. (Reprinted from *J. Lab. clin. Med.*, 67, 898–905, 1966, by permission of C. V. Mosby.)

This enhancement of phenobarbital excretion by alkalinization of the urine is also apparent from the clearance data shown in Fig. 7. In these studies only data obtained from urines of pH 7.5 or greater are shown, and differences in excretion due solely to protein binding have been adjusted by using the clearance of filtrable barbiturate, UV/F. At each level of urine flow up to at least 6 or 7 ml/min the clearance of filtrable phenobarbital clearly exceeds that of either pentobarbital or secobarbital.

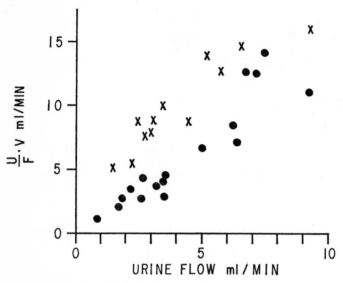

Fig. 7.   The relation between rate of urinary flow and the clearance of pentobarbital or secobarbital (•) and phenobarbital (X). All data points were obtained from urines of pH 7.5 or greater. (Reprinted from *J. Lab. clin. Med.* 67: 898–905, 1966, by permission of C. V. Mosby.)

The method by which increased urine flow and pH are achieved does not seem to matter. At any level of flow and pH, the excretion of a barbiturate is about the same whether the subject is undergoing water diuresis, or has been given an osmotic diuretic like urea or mannitol or a pharmacologic agent such as furosemide (Linton *et al.*, 1967). Similarly, the effect of alkalinity is the same whether produced by the administration of bicarbonate or by inhibition of renal carbonic anhydrase. Both the osmotically active alkaline buffer, tris (hydroxymethyl) aminomethane, and the carbonic anhydrase inhibitor, acetazolamide, have been advocated for treatment of phenobarbital intoxication (Kelley *et al.*, 1966; Balagot *et al.*, 1961). Although either agent might be convenient in a given situation, neither possesses special properties which make it a superior form of treatment.

Granted, then, that increased urine flow promotes excretion of various barbiturates and that alkalinization of the urine produces an additive effect for certain long-acting drugs such as phenobarbital, how effective a therapeutic maneuver is diuresis? It has been established that alkaline diuresis will approximately double the rate of elimination of long-acting barbiturates and will shorten coma, whereas diuresis with or without alkalinization will increase the disposal of short-acting agents by only 15 or 20% (Bloomer, 1965; 1966; Lassen, 1960).

Using the rate of plasma barbiturate disappearance, Lassen found that alkaline diuresis increased the elimination rate of barbital, aprobarbital, phenobarbital and diallyl barbituric acid by 30 to 180% over that observed in untreated control patients (Lassen, 1960; Myschetzky and Lassen, 1963). Lassen calculated the effect of increased elimination on the period of unconsciousness and predicted that coma would be shortened by 30 to 70%. Unfortunately, no observations were made on patients intoxicated by short-acting drugs.

Support for Lassen's data can be obtained by a different approach (Bloomer, 1966). The plasma disappearance of phenobarbital under non-diuretic conditions is about 1% per hour. Provided that intestinal absorption and tissue distribution are complete, a 70 kg patient who ingests 5000 mg of this drug will achieve a plasma level of about 10 mg per 100 ml and will eliminate approximately 50 mg/hr by hepatic degradation and renal excretion. At low urinary pH and flow rate, most of phenobarbital disposal will occur by hepatic metabolism. The clearance of filtrable phenobarbital at a urine flow of 1 ml/min and urinary pH less than 7.5 is about 2 ml/min. At a plasma concentration of 10 mg per 100 ml, only 6 or 7 mg would be excreted per hour. About 43 or 44 mg would be degraded by hepatic metabolism in the same period.

At a urine pH greater than 7.5 and a urine flow between 5 and 10 ml/min, the clearance of filtrable phenobarbital is about 15 ml/min, as shown in Fig. 7. At the same plasma level, urinary drug excretion will increase to 51 mg/hr, and total disposal will double.

This method of calculation is less secure for the short-acting barbiturates, whose apparent volume of distribution is greater than that of phenobarbital. Nevertheless, when similar assumptions and calculations are made it becomes obvious that diuresis is much less effective for treating a comparable degree of intoxication by pentobarbital or secobarbital. Assuming a body distribution similar to phenobarbital, a 70 kg subject who ingests 2000 mg of pentobarbital will achieve a plasma concentration of about 4 mg per 100 ml. Pentobarbital is metabolized at a more rapid rate, about 2.2% per hour. In spite of the lower plasma level, total drug disposal will be approximately 44 mg per hour, of which only 2 mg is excreted in the urine at low rates of urine flow. During diuresis, the clearance of filtrable pentobarbital reaches 10 or 12 ml/min, an absolute excretion of about 12 mg/hr. Renal excretion of drug has risen 10 mg/hr, an increase in disposal of only 20 or 25%. As pointed out earlier in this chapter, this method of calculation provides a maximum estimate of the effectiveness of treatment, so that the actual increase in disposal is well below 20%.

Since the effect of diuresis on the total disposal of short-acting barbiturates is minimal, the advisability of applying this form of treatment must be questioned. In fact, one might predict that diuresis would have no measurable effect either on the rate of plasma disappearance of drug or on the duration of coma. Although the data are scanty, a recent study suggests that this is so (Hadden, 1969).

PERITONEAL DIALYSIS

The fraction of plasma barbiturate not bound to plasma proteins readily diffuses into peritoneal fluid. Both the parent barbiturate and its metabolites are removed by peritoneal dialysis (Bloomer, 1965). The absolute rate of sedative removal depends on the degree of plasma protein binding.

In Fig. 8, the accumulation of various sedatives in peritoneal fluid is shown. During 90 minutes of equilibration, glutethimide (about 70% bound to plasma protein) has reached a concentration in peritoneal dialysate only 20% of that in whole plasma, while meprobamate (only 20% protein bound) has reached 60% of its plasma level. Pentobarbital and phenobarbital, which have intermediate degrees of binding, fall between these extremes.

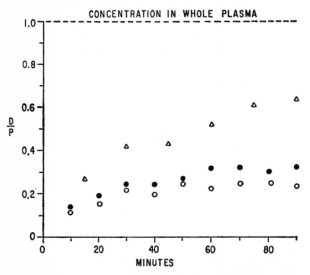

Fig. 8. The accumulation of drugs in peritoneal fluid, plotted as the ratio of concentration in dialysate to concentration in whole plasma D/P. Pentobarbital accumulation is shown by (•), that of glutethimide by (o) and meprobamate by (Δ). Instillation of dialysate was completed at time zero.

When the peritoneal concentrations of these drugs are plotted against their concentrations in plasma filtrate as in Fig. 9, each of these drugs accumulate at about the same rate, comparable to that of the highly diffusible substance, urea. Diffusion equilibrium is not achieved by 90 minutes. During the equilibration period usually allowed during peritoneal dialysis, 45 to 60 minutes, drug concentration in peritoneal fluid has reached about two-thirds of the concentration of diffusible drug in plasma.

Using these observations, it is simple to calculate the rate of barbiturate removal by standard peritoneal dialysis. A patient with a plasma phenobarbital concentration of 10 mg per 100 ml has a diffusible concentration of 6 mg per 100 ml. During 60 minutes of equilibration, the concentration of phenobarbital in peritoneal dialysate will reach

4 mg per 100 ml, or 80 mg per 2-liter exchange. Each 2-liter exchange will remove 80 mg of phenobarbital in the 90 minutes required for its completion, so that about 53 mg will be removed each hour. According to the calculations used in the preceding section, such a patient will eliminate approximately 50 mg/hr by hepatic metabolism and renal excretion. Therefore, standard peritoneal dialysis will double total disposal of phenobarbital and has about the same effectiveness as a brisk alkaline diuresis.

The patient with a comparable degree of pentobarbital intoxication at a plasma level of 4 mg per 100 ml, will achieve a dialysate concentration of only 1.2 mg per 100 ml after 60 minutes of equilibration. Peritoneal dialysis will remove 24 mg of pentobarbital per 90-minute exchange, or 16 mg/hr. Since hepatic and renal mechanisms remove about 44 mg during the same period, overall disposal is increased by about 35%. These calculations overestimate the effectiveness of therapy, so that the actual contribution of peritoneal dialysis to total riddance of drug is somewhat less. Although slightly more efficient in drug removal than diuresis, standard peritoneal dialysis can have little effect on the rate of decline in plasma concentration or on duration of coma, a conclusion which recently has gained support (Hadden *et al.*, 1969).

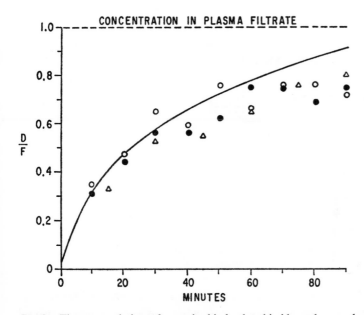

Fig. 9. The accumulation of pentobarbital, glutethimide and meprobamate in peritoneal fluid, plotted as the ratio of concentration in dialysate to concentration in plasma filtrate, D/F. Peritoneal accumulation of urea is shown by the curve.

Two clever maneuvers have been used to increase peritoneal removal of barbiturates: addition of albumin to dialysate; and alkalinization of dialysate. Berman and Vogelsang (1964) used 5% albumin solution for dialysis and noted that the peritoneal concentrations of secobarbital, pentobarbital, and phenobarbital after 60 minutes of equilibration were approximately twice as high as the concentrations reached in protein-free dialysate. This augmented peritoneal accumulation is shown in Fig. 10, for glutethimide, a drug highly bound to plasma protein. During the two peritoneal exchanges shown in this graph the plasma level dropped from 5.1 mg per 100 ml to 4.5 mg per 100 ml, and the concentration in plasma filtrate changed little. After 60 minutes of equilibration, glutethimide concentration in dialysate containing 5% albumin was over twice that found in ordinary dialysate. Therefore, adding 5% albumin to each peritoneal exchange will double the rate of peritoneal removal for those drugs with significant binding to plasma proteins. Increasing the albumin concentration in dialysate above that in plasma will not produce a further increase in peritoneal removal.

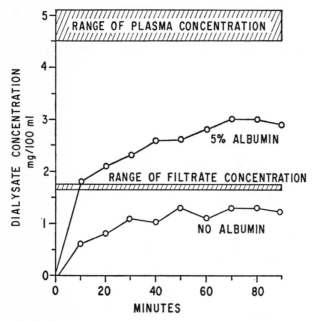

Fig. 10.   The accumulation of glutethimide in ordinary peritoneal dialysis solution, the lower curve, and in dialysate containing 5% human albumin (the upper curve).

Knochel *et al.* (1964) and Knochel and Barry (1965) have buffered peritoneal dialysate with tris (hydroxymethyl) aminomethane to enhance dialysis of phenobarbital and secobarbital from dogs. By maintaining the pH of peritoneal fluid at 8.2 or greater, above the pKa of either drug and a full pH unit higher than that of ordinary dialysate at the end of equilibration, considerable trapping of water-soluble barbiturate anions was achieved. The rates of peritoneal removal were strikingly increased. We have encountered no reports applying this promising technique to human subjects.

HEMODIALYSIS

Extracorporeal hemodialysis with the artificial kidney is the most effective method for removing barbiturates from the body. As with diuresis and peritoneal dialysis, absolute removal depends directly on the concentration of diffusible drug in plasma, which is determined by the degree of binding to plasma protein and by the partition of drug among the various tissues and fluid compartments. The highly bound and lipid-soluble short-acting barbiturates are removed at much lower rates than are the long-acting drugs. Nevertheless, a standard artificial kidney with a dialysis membrane surface area of two square meters will remove even the short-acting barbiturates at rates at least two or three times those accomplished by diuresis or peritoneal dialysis, and is even more efficient when a long-acting agent is involved (Jørgensen and Wieth, 1963; Maddock and Bloomer, 1968).

The influence of protein binding is shown in Fig. 11. Three drugs with different affinities for albumin were dialyzed *in vitro* from a reservoir of plasma, using the disposable coil kidney. Clearances for these drugs and for 14-C-urea were obtained simultaneously. The clearance of meprobamate, which is only 20% bound to plasma protein, was higher than that of either pentobarbital or glutethimide, but much lower than the urea clearance. Similar results have been obtained by Setter *et al.* (1964).

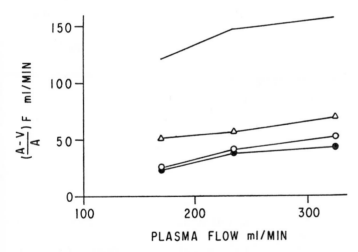

Fig. 11. The clearance of pentobarbital (•), glutethimide (o) and meprobamate (Δ) from plasma *in vitro* by the disposable-coil artificial kidney. The clearance at each plasma flow was calculated from: (A-V/A) F, where A and V are the concentrations of drug at the inlet and outlet of the dialyzer respectively and F is the plasma flow through the coil. Concentrations of drugs in the bath were negligible. Urea clearances obtained simultaneously are shown in the upper curve.

They studied the dialyzability of phenobarbital, amobarbital, pentobarbital, and secobarbital, and found that the rates of removal varied inversely with the degree of protein binding. Phenobarbital, least bound to albumin, was removed at a rate about 50% higher than that of secobarbital, the agent most highly bound.

Note also from Fig. 11 that there is little increase in the rate of clearance for either urea or the sedatives at plasma flow rates over 200 ml/min, a fact also pointed out by Setter and his coworkers (Setter et al., 1964). As blood flow through the artificial kidney is increased, extraction of urea or drugs falls rapidly. At higher rates of blood flow, this fall in extraction more or less balances the increase in delivery of drug to the dialyzer, so that the clearance rate changes little. Therefore, during hemodialysis of an intoxicated patient there is little to be gained in striving for blood flow rates over 200 ml/min.

The effectiveness of the artificial kidney in removing long-acting barbiturates from an intoxicated patient has been well documented. Jørgensen and Wieth (1963) found that the plasma levels of barbital, amobarbital, and phenobarbital decline two to five times more rapidly during hemodialysis than during osmotic diuresis. These investigators published no data on the removal of short-acting barbiturates.

Similar results are obtained by comparing the removal of a barbiturate by the artificial kidney with its rate of endogenous metabolism (Maddock and Bloomer, 1968). At a blood flow rate of 200 ml per min, the dialysance* of phenobarbital is about 75 ml/min and that of pentobarbital is about 65 ml/min when the disposable coil kidney is used (Setter et al., 1964). At these clearance rates, the artificial kidney will remove about 450 mg of phenobarbital per hour from a patient whose plasma level is 10 mg per 100 ml, and about 155 mg/hr of pentobarbital from a patient with intoxication of comparable severity at a plasma level of 4 mg per 100 ml. Endogenous mechanisms would dispose of 50 mg of phenobarbital and about 44 mg of pentobarbital during the same period. Therefore, hemodialysis removes phenobarbital nine times as rapidly as does spontaneous metabolism and removes pentobarbital over three times as rapidly. When compared with diuresis and peritoneal dialysis, extracorporeal hemodialysis increases the total disposal of both drugs between three and five times.

---

* Dialysance, (A-V/A-B)F in ml/min, is frequently used in hemodialysis literature to express the removal rate of a drug by the artificial kidney. It differs from artificial kidney clearance, (A-V/A)F in ml/min, only in that (B), the concentration of that drug in the bath, is taken into consideration. In theory, dialysance has the advantage of factoring absolute drug removal, (A-V)F, by the actual concentration gradient across the dialysis membrane, (A-B). In practice, using dialysance has two major disadvantages. First, since drug concentration in dialysate, (B), is very low, considerable analytic error may be introduced. Second, published dialysance data cannot be converted directly to absolute drug removal per unit time unless the concentration gradient, (A-B), is given. On the other hand, absolute drug removal can be calculated from clearance figures by multiplying: clearance times plasma concentration.

When bath concentration of drug, (B), is negligible, dialysance equals clearance. This assumption is made in the above calculations. The error introduced is to overestimate actual removal by the artificial kidney by a small amount.

CONCLUSIONS

Forced diuresis, peritoneal dialysis, and extracorporeal hemodialysis are widely used for treating patients with barbiturate intoxication. The efficiencies of these therapeutic maneuvers differ, depending mainly on the physicochemical properties of the barbiturate preparation being treated. The following table (Table 5) summarizes the maximum effectiveness of each procedure for treating patients with comparable degrees of intoxication by phenobarbital, a representative long-acting barbiturate, and pentobarbital, a short-acting agent.

TABLE 5

	Total disposal (mg/hr)	Increase in disposal
Phenobarbital (10 mg/100 ml)		
Spontaneous disposal	50	—
a) plus alkaline diuresis	94	+ 85%
b) plus peritoneal dialysis	103	+106%
c) plus hemodialysis	500	+900%
Pentobarbital (4 mg/100 ml)		
Spontaneous disposal	44	—
a) plus diuresis	54	+ 23%
b) plus peritoneal dialysis	60	+ 36%
c) plus hemodialysis	200	+350%

Our current practice is to treat mild to moderately severe cases of long- or short-acting barbiturate intoxication by conservative methods alone, to employ alkaline diuresis in the occasional case of moderately severe coma produced by long-acting barbiturates, and to reserve hemodialysis for severe intoxication by either type of agent. Admittedly, it may be justifiable to use diuresis or peritoneal dialysis to treat severe barbiturate intoxication when extracorporeal hemodialysis is not available. However, the responsible physician should be aware of the distinct limitations of these maneuvers, especially when short-acting barbiturates are involved.

REFERENCES

BALAGOT, R. C., TSUJI, H. and SADOVE, M. S. (1961), Use of osmotic diuretic – THAM – in treatment of barbiturate poisoning: Alkalinizing action of drug and its ability to increase elimination of electrolytes in urine appears to facilitate clearance of barbiturates. *J. Amer. med. Ass.*, 178, 1000.

BERMAN, L. B. and VOGELSANG, P. (1964), Removal rates for barbiturates using two types of peritoneal dialysis. *New Engl. J. Med.*, 270, 77.

BLOOMER, H. A. (1965), Limited usefulness of alkaline diuresis and peritoneal dialysis in pentobarbital intoxication. *New Engl. J. Med,*. 272, 1309.

BLOOMER, H. A. (1966), A critical evaluation of diuresis in the treatment of barbiturate intoxication. *J. Lab. clin. Med.*, 67, 898.

BLOOMER, H. A. (1967), Forced diuresis in barbiturate poisoning. Letter to the editor in *Lancet*, II, 986.

BLOOMER, H. A., MADDOCK, R. K., JR., SHEEHE, J. B. and ADAMS, E. J. (1970), The rapid diagnosis of sedative intoxication by gas chromatography. *Ann. intern. Med.*, 72, 223.

BRODIE, B. B., BURNS, J. J., MARK, L. C., LIEF, E. B. and PAPPER, E. M. (1953), Fate of pentobarbital in man and dog and method for its estimation in biological material. *J. Pharmacol. exp. Ther.*, 109, 26.

BUTLER, T. C. (1952), Quantitative studies on the metabolic fate of mephobarbital (N-methyl phenobarbital). *J. Pharmacol. exp. Ther.*, 106, 235.

BUTLER, T. C. (1956), The metabolic hydroxylation of phenobarbital. *J. Pharmacol. exp. Ther.*, 116, 326.

FAZEKAS, J. F., GOLDBAUM, L. R., KOPPANYI, T. and SHEA, J. G. (1956), Study on the effect of overdoses of pentylenetetrazol and barbiturate combinations in human volunteers. *Amer. J. med. Sci.*,231, 531.

GIOTTI, H. and MAYNERT, E. W. (1951), The renal clearance of barbital and the mechanism of its reabsorption. *J. Pharmacol. exp. Ther.*, 101, 296.

GOLDBAUM, L. R. (1952), Determination of barbiturates: ultraviolet spectrophotometric method with differentiation of several barbiturates. *Analyt. Chem.*, 24, 1604.

HADDEN, J., JOHNSON, K., SMITH, S., PRICE, L. and GIARDINA, E. (1969), Acute barbiturate intoxication: Concepts of management. *J. Amer. med. Ass.*, 209, 893.

JØRGENSEN, H. E. and WIETH, J. O. (1963), Dialysable poisons: haemodialysis in the treatment of acute poisoning. *Lancet*, I, 81.

KELLEY, W. N., RICHARDSON, A. P., JR., MASON, M. F. and RECTOR, F. C., JR. (1966), Acetazolamide in phenobarbital intoxication. *Arch. intern. Med.*, 117, 64.

KNOCHEL, J. P. and BARRY, K. G. (1965), THAM dialysis: An experimental method to study diffusion of certain weak acids in vivo: II. Secobarbital. *J. Lab. clin. Med.*, 65, 361.

KNOCHEL, J. P., CLAYTON, L. E., SMITH, W. L. and BARRY, K. G. (1964), Intraperitoneal THAM: An effective method to enhance phenobarbital removal during peritoneal dialysis. *J. Lab. clin. Med.*, 64, 257.

LASSEN, N. A. (1960), Treatment of severe acute barbiturate poisoning by forced diuresis and alkalinisation of the urine. *Lancet*, II, 338.

LINTON, A. L., LUKE, R. G. and BRIGGS, J. D. (1967), Methods of forced diuresis and its application in barbiturate poisoning. *Lancet*, II, 377.

MADDOCK, R. K., JR. and BLOOMER, H. A. (1967), Gas chromatography of meprobamate. *Clin. Chem.*, 13, 333.

MADDOCK, R. K., JR. and BLOOMER, H. A. (1967), Meprobamate overdosage: evaluation of its severity and methods of treatment. *J. Amer. med. Ass.*, 201, 999.

MADDOCK, R. K. and BLOOMER, H. A. (1968), Limitations of diuresis and dialysis as treatments for sedative intoxication. *Clin. Res.*, 16, 166.

MAHER, J. F. and SCHREINER, G. E. (1961), Acute glutethimide poisoning: II. The use of hemodialysis. *Trans. Amer. Soc. artif. int. Org.*, 7, 100.

MAHER, J. F., SCHREINER, G. E. and WESTERVELT, F. B., JR. (1962), Acute glutethimide intoxication: I. Clinical experience (twenty-two patients) compared to acute barbiturate intoxication (sixty-three patients). *Amer. J. Med.*, 33, 70.

MARK, L. C. (1963), Metabolism of barbiturates in man. *Clin. Pharmacol. Ther.*, 4, 504.

MAYNERT, E. W. (1952), The distribution and fate of dialkylbarbiturates. *Fed. Proc.*, 11, 625.

MAYNERT, E. W. and DAWSON, J. M. (1952), Ethyl (3-hydroxy-1-methylbutyl) barbituric acids as metabolites of pentobarbital. *J. biol. Chem.*, 195, 389.

MYSCHETZKY, A. and LASSEN, N. A. (1963), Urea-induced, osmotic diuresis and alkalization of urine in acute barbiturate intoxication. *J. Amer. med. Ass.*, 185, 936.

SHARPLESS, S. K. (1965), Hypnotics and sedatives: 1. The barbiturates. In: L. S. Goodman and A. S. Gilman (Ed) *The Pharmacological Basis of Therapeutics*, 3rd ed., 120. Macmillan, New York.

SCHREINER, G. E. (1958), The role of hemodialysis (artificial kidney) in acute poisoning. *Arch. intern. Med.*, 102, 896.

SCHREINER, G. E., BERMAN, L. B., KOVACH, R. and BLOOMER, H. A. (1968), Acute glutethimide (doriden) poisoning: the use of bemegride (megimide) and hemodialysis. *Arch. intern. Med.*, 101, 899.

SETTER, J. G., FREEMAN, R. B., MAHER, J. F. and SCHREINER, G. E. (1964), Factors influencing the dialysis of barbiturates. *Trans. Amer. Soc. artif. int. Org.* 10, 340.

SHONLE, H. A., KELTCH, A. K., KEMPF, G. F. and SWANSON, E. E. (1933), Question of elimination of barbituric acid derivatives in urine with special reference to iso-amyl ethyl barbituric acid (sodium amytal) and 1-methyl-butyl ethyl barbituric acid (pentobarbital sodium). *J. Pharmacol. exp. Ther.*, 49, 393.

TITUS, E. and WEISS, H. (1955), Use of biologically prepared radioactive indicators in metabolic studies: metabolism of pentobarbital. *J. biol. Chem.*, 214, 807.

WADDELL, W. J. (1962), The metabolic conversion of secobarbital to 5-allyl-5-(3-hydroxy-1-methyl-butyl) barbituric acid. *Fed. Proc.*, 21, 182.

WADDELL, W. J. and BUTLER, T. C. (1957), The distribution and excretion of phenobarbital. *J. clin. Invest.*, 36, 1217.

WEINER, I. M., WASHINGTON, J. A. and MUDGE, G. H. (1959), Studies on the renal excretion of salicylate in the dog. *Bull. Johns Hopk. Hosp.*, 105, 284.

WRIGHT, J. T. (1955), The value of barbiturate estimations in the diagnosis and treatment of barbiturate intoxication. *Quart. J. Med.*, 24, 95.

16. acute barbiturate poisoning in children

A. K. Done

Definitive comparisons of acute barbiturate poisoning in children and in adults are not available. Consequently, even though animal data suggest that immaturity may be associated at least with quantitative differences in response to barbiturates, it is difficult to document age-dependent differences in the course of intoxication in human beings. Thus, much of what follows is necessarily speculative or based upon empirical observations.

Generally speaking, barbiturate poisoning in children resembles that in adults and is treated similarly. Consequently, the reader should refer to other chapters for general discussions of pathology, symptomatology, diagnosis and treatment. Emphasis here will be on known or suspected differences between children and adults in the course of acute barbiturate poisoning. Aspects of development or immaturity which may be pertinent to barbiturate poisoning are listed in Table 1. In some instances, clinical observations support the suggestion of an influence; the other factors should at least be suspected of being influential. It need hardly be emphasized that further investigation of these factors is needed. Also it is obvious that whatever influence is exerted by them would be expected to be greater in the younger the child. Beyond about four or five years of age, or perhaps even earlier, one would expect the response to be essentially identical to that seen in adults.

CIRCUMSTANCES OF OCCURRENCE

Barbiturate poisoning in pre-school children is usually accidental, resulting from the ingestion of drug which has been left within reach. Although barbiturates do not rank high among substances accidentally ingested by children, there are appreciable numbers of fatalities every year. In the United States, for example, barbiturates usually account for 1 % or less of accidental ingestions among toddlers, but rank sixth as the cause of fatal accidental poisoning; among drugs, they are exceeded only by salicylates as a cause of fatal accidental poisoning in children.

TABLE 1

Potential factors differentiating childhood from adult barbiturate poisoning.

Circumstances of occurrence
  Usually accidental
  Usually 'pure' poisoning

Severity of poisoning
  ? Coma with lower levels
    Receptor sensitivity
    Distribution differences

  ? Prolonged
    Slower detoxification and/or excretion
    Tolerance less likely

Complications
  Respiratory obstruction more likely
  Acid-base-electrolyte disturbances more common
  ? Cerebral edema more common
  ? Pneumonia more common

Treatment problems
  Special attention to airway
  Induced diuresis less effective and more dangerous
  Dialysis more difficult
  ? Exaggerated response to analeptics

Among older school-age children and adolescents, most cases result from the wilful ingestion or injection of barbiturate. Wilful abuse of barbiturates for their mind-altering effects is common in this age group; results include both addiction and accidental overdosage. There are, of course, occasional *bona fide* suicide attempts by seriously disturbed children, especially adolescents, which carry the same import as similar acts on the part of adults (see Chapter 18). More commonly, however, intentional barbiturate poisoning among young children represents a rather special psychological circumstance which should be recognized for what it is; otherwise it is impossible to interpret the significance of the incident properly and to provide guidance accordingly. In my experience, the majority of children who become intentionally poisoned under the age of about 15 years, and certainly the very young child (under the age of about 12 or 13 years, and sometimes as young as 7 or 8 years of age), do not have serious psychopathology, but rather are reacting either to fantasy or intolerable environmental factors. In this age group, the individual usually does not consciously seek death in the sense of oblivion, permanency, or even departure. Rather, they envisage a temporary situation, a 'long sleep' during which they can observe the regret of family and acquaintances. Many actually give no real thought to the consequences, but are escaping an intolerable situation such as a family argument, avoiding a confrontation with parents regarding school grades, and the like. Indeed, our studies of children under these circumstances have revealed that they do not at all equate the drug effect with the same type of 'death' that they associate with disease, accidental injury, or old age. The practical implications are that in such cases the parents can usually be reassured that their child does not have a devastating mental illness, that he did not truly wish to die, and that he is not a prime candidate for future suicide attempts providing that the precipitating factor is dealt with adequately. The latter usually requires only relatively minor environmental manipulations, counseling, and understanding on the part of parents and friends. It should be emphasized, how-ever, that difficulties in distinguishing between the situation just described and one which denotes serious psychopathology make it mandatory that psychiatric evaluation be undertaken in all cases.

Whatever the reason for the poisoning, children are more likely to have 'pure' bar-biturate intoxication rather than a mixture of various intoxications. In this institution, for example, less than 20% of children with barbiturate poisoning ingested additional materials; by contrast more than two-thirds of the adult cases were mixed poisoning in which at least one other substance was involved, and in nearly half there were two or more additional substances ingested. Most frequently, the adults took their barbitu-rates in conjunction with alcohol, tranquilizers, opiates, anticonvulsants or non-bar-biturate sedatives.

SEVERITY OF POISONING

Surprisingly, it is not really known whether barbiturate poisoning tends to be more or less severe in children than in adults. It is my empirical observation that, all other factors being equal, young toddlers have a disproportionately high rate of morbidity and mortality, but to my knowledge this has never been documented. Moreover, if the observation is valid, there are insufficient data to determine whether the difference is dependent upon immaturity *per se* or simply reflects a greater likelihood that a child will ingest a potentially dangerous dose.

Several studies (Done, 1964; Done, 1966a; Yeary *et al.*, 1966; Fouts and Hart, 1965) have shown that infant experimental animals have an increased susceptibility to the toxic effects of barbiturates. A similarly enhanced toxicity of morphine in the newborn rat is attributable to the achievement of higher brain levels of the drug relative to the levels in plasma (Kupferberg and Way, 1963). It would be logical to assume that a similar factor may be operative in the case of barbiturates. However, infant animals die with lower brain concentrations of pentobarbital than do adult animals (Bianchine and Ferguson, 1967). These and other findings (Kato *et al.*, 1964, and Kalser *et al.*, 1969) suggest that receptor sensitivity to barbiturate is actually enhanced by imma-turity, and that the increased response during immaturity is not necessarily related to greater overall penetration of the drug into the brain because of immaturity of the 'blood-brain barrier'. Other studies (Domek *et al.*, 1960) have demonstrated onto-genetic differences in the distribution of barbiturate among various areas of the brain, and it may be this phenomenon which is important.

Whether the enhancement of barbiturate toxicity in immature animals is attributable to differences in distribution within the brain, permeability of the 'blood-brain barrier', greater sensitivity or affinity of receptor sites, or other factors, we can only speculate as to whether similar characteristics are shared by the human infant or the young child. In my own experience, when severity of barbiturate poisoning has belied relatively low blood levels it has usually been in young children. However, as is noted below, it is difficult to determine with certainty whether this is directly attributable to increased sensitivity or related to a predisposition to certain complications. An illustrative case which appears to demonstrate exceptional sensitivity during early childhood follows:

Case 1. This ten-month-old girl ingested an unknown number of 100-mg secobarbital capsules and became comatose, apparently within minutes. The child was immediately rushed to the hospital where she was found to be flaccid, unresponsive even to painful stimuli. The deep tendon reflexes were diminished, but present; corneal and gag reflexes were absent, and the pupils were somewhat constricted and were responsive to light. Respiration was adequate initially and the blood pressure and temperature were normal. The blood barbiturate level obtained at about one hour post-ingestion was 2.5 mg/100 ml (secobarbital). Shortly after admission, respiration became shallow and infrequent and it was necessary to assist breathing using a mask and bag. After about an hour, respiration became difficult and so endotracheal intubation was performed. During intubation all spontaneous respirations ceased and the heart-rate dropped to 20 beats per minute. She was quickly given positive pressure respiratory assistance through the tube, and her condition improved. After stabilization, gastric lavage was performed using normal saline. Artificial respiration was required for about two hours after which adequate spontaneous breathing was sustained. After about 5 hours it was possible to remove the endotracheal tube. She remained unresponsive except to deep painful stimuli for about 9 hours, after which she gradually became more responsive. At 12 hours she awakened, but was markedly ataxic. By the following day, however, ataxia had disappeared and the child was discharged in normal condition.

Considerable data reviewed elsewhere (Done, 1964) suggest that the immature of many species, perhaps including the human, may have relatively inefficient processes for the detoxification and/or excretion of various substances. Indeed, all of the phase I (reduction and oxidation) processes which have been studied in experimental animals have been found to be relatively inactive during infancy. This appears also to be true with regard specifically to barbiturates (Fouts and Hart, 1965; Kato *et al.*, 1964; Kalser *et al.*, 1969; Catz and Yaffe, 1967) which have greatly prolonged effects in infant animals. The status of the immature human is unknown, but the probability is that at least during early infancy detoxification and/or excretion of barbiturates is deficient; the transition to adult levels of activity then is a gradual one and it is not possible at this point to state at what age the processes can be expected to be fully mature.

Again, data cannot be found to indicate whether children at poisoning-prone ages tend to inactivate or eliminate barbiturates at a slower rate than do adults, thereby experiencing prolongation of the features of poisoning. We are badly in need of studies of serial blood levels of barbiturate in children who have been accidentally poisoned at various ages. The expectation that the course of barbiturate poisoning may be prolonged in childhood comes not only from animal experiments, but also from the theoretical consideration that children are less likely to have had previous experience with barbiturate. Such exposure, at least in experimental animals, may be reflected in an increased rate of metabolism of the drug (Pantuck *et al.*, 1968).

It is this author's experience, again empirical, that the most prolonged cases of barbiturate intoxication seem to occur in children, but this point would require documentation of a larger number of cases than would be available to any one individual. At least among patients having coma of grade IV severity, classified according to Reed *et al.* (1952) it has been my experience that a disproportionate percentage of the individuals who remain comatose for several, rather than two or three, days are young children. With lesser degrees of coma a real difference in duration has not been discernible. The following representative case seems to illustrate both prolonged barbiturate effects and enhanced sensitivity to relatively low levels of barbiturate:

Case 2. This two-year-old boy ingested twelve 32 mg phenobarbital tablets and within a few minutes became irritable and was noted to be staggering and falling frequently. He was seen at the hospital within about 45 minutes. Initially, he was sleeping, but could be aroused to respond to verbal commands. Shortly, however, he became completely unresponsive and within one and a half hours of ingestion he had suffered two respiratory arrests from which he was successfully resuscitated by positive pressure applied through an endotracheal tube. Gastric lavage was then performed as soon as his condition had stabilized. The blood barbiturate at the time of admission was 3.9 mg/100 ml (phenobarbital). At that time, physical findings included flaccidity, sluggish deep tendon reflexes, dilated reactive pupils and normal blood pressure. The barbiturate level, repeated at 6 hours and again at 20 hours, had not changed! The level of consciousness improved very gradually, and the patient did not awaken until the third day, at which time he was irritable, groggy, and grossly ataxic. These findings improved, but the patient was still ataxic on the sixth day. He was discharged on the seventh day, at which time he was essentially normal.

COMPLICATIONS

The complications of barbiturate poisoning are similar in children and in adults and will not be enumerated here. There are, however, certain complications which seem to occur with increased frequency in childhood. Again, however, complete documentation is wanting.

In my experience the complication which is both most characteristic of, and poses the greatest danger to, children with barbiturate poisoning is respiratory obstruction. The sudden and unexpected occurrence of respiratory obstruction not infrequently converts what should be relatively inconsequential poisoning into a life-threatening situation in young children. The most likely explanation for this predisposition of young children is the small caliber of the respiratory passages, especially relative to the respiratory needs of the child. This not-infrequent (among children) occurrence is illustrated by the following representative case in which a nearly-fatal outcome was dictated almost solely by the occurrence of respiratory obstruction:

Case 3. This four-year-old boy with a seizure disorder had been receiving diphenylhydantoin, 200 mg, and phenobarbital, 32 mg, twice daily for several months. In the day of admission he was found by his mother to be extremely lethargic, whereupon she found that approximately 39 of the phenobarbital tablets were missing. He was taken to another hospital where vomiting was induced by ipecac. He was referred here within 3 hours following ingestion, at which time the blood barbiturate level was 4 mg/100 ml (phenobarbital). It was not known what transpired during the transfer, but when the boy arrived here he was lying on his back, apneic and moderately cyanotic. Upon turning the patient on his side, placing an oral airway momentarily, and with artificial respiration, he awakened within a few minutes and was able to stand and look about, although still somewhat obtunded. He had no further difficulty and was discharged the following day in normal condition.

As in other pathological conditions, barbiturate poisoning is more likely to be associated with acid-base and electrolyte disturbances in children than in adults because of the greater turnover of water and electrolytes, the relatively higher metabolic activity, and immature homeostatic capacities. In point of fact, however, acid-base or electrolyte disturbances are not common in barbiturate poisoning except in patients whose coma is exceptionally long or where acid-base disturbances are initiated by respiratory problems. Respiratory arrest or prolonged respiratory insufficiency can, of course, be associated with severe acidosis, which requires energetic intervention. In the majority of cases, however, acid-base-electrolyte problems can be prevented or corrected by ensuring adequate ventilation and fluid and electrolyte intake.

Less well established than the foregoing is the possibly greater tendency of children to develop cerebral edema or pneumonia than the adult. It has seemed to me that children are especially prone to develop these complications, and such would certainly be expected by analogy with other clinical situations. Thus, we commonly institute treatment for the prevention or correction of cerebral edema (osmotics and steroids) in children who have periods of significant hypoxia. We also undertake energetic measures to prevent the development of hypostatic pneumonia, including the use of intermittent positive pressure augmentation of respiration, frequent turning, and meticulous tracheobronchial toilet.

TREATMENT PROBLEM

The therapeutic approach used by the author is described elsewhere (Done, 1966*b*; and Done, 1969) and does not differ substantially from that described for adults in Chapter 11. It is important, however, that the approach to treatment take cognizance of the above factors as well as others which have specific pertinence to the treatment of children.

In view of the occurrence of unexpected respiratory obstruction or disproportionate depression in young children even with relatively minor degrees of intoxication, it is important that they are observed for the first few hours, almost regardless of the magnitude of the blood barbiturate level. It is our practice either to admit to the hospital or at least to retain in the emergency ward any child who has ingested barbiturate and shows any degree of depression of conscious level; since most such difficulty occurs within the first two or three hours, a period of observation of four hours should suffice if one is satisfied that the conscious level is not becoming more depressed. This also provides sufficient time to ascertain whether further barbiturate absorption is occurring. If respiratory obstruction occurs, we favor endotracheal intubation, preferably with a cuffed tube to prevent aspiration. Only rarely have we felt it necessary to resort to tracheotomy, even when prolonged (three or four days) intubation is required. In patients whose respiration can only be maintained marginally because of such factors as extensive pneumonia, it is occasionally important to perform tracheotomy not only for maintenance of a patent airway but also to lessen the respiratory dead-space. It should be remembered that the latter may be proportionately far more important to the small child than to the larger individual.

Induced diuresis, whether osmotic, alkaline or simple water diuresis, tends to be less effective and more dangerous in young children than in adults. This is because the child, at least during infancy, has a limited ability to excrete either a water or an osmotic load and has a limited ability to excrete an alkaline urine during stress. Consequently, the administration of water, osmotic agents or alkali in amounts sufficient to produce the desired result is fraught with the danger of circulatory overload in young children. In children with phenobarbital poisoning, we endeavor to alkalinize the urine, but do not persist with such efforts if the urine does not alkalinize readily. We have not employed osmotic diuretics extensively in children and feel that until more data are available such procedures either should be approached cautiously or not used at all in children. Although dialysis is fraught with some special difficulties in young children (see below) our tendency is to resort to those procedures rather than forced diuresis in children who have potentially lethal levels of barbiturate. However, it has been the observation that the vast majority even of children with barbiturate poisoning will recover with supportive care alone and that efforts to hasten the elimination of barbiturate are rarely indicated.

The problems with dialysis in children relate mainly to the small size of the individual. Extracorporeal hemodialysis should be approached with even more caution and reluctance in children than in adults because of the difficulties of avoiding dangerous shifts of extracellular fluid volume. If a dialysis team is available which has had extensive experience with small children, this difficulty is to some extent obviated. However, the limits within which the fluid fluctuations of the artificial kidney can be regulated are sometimes as large as the total extracellular fluid volume of the small child. The dangers are considerably less with peritoneal dialysis, but the efficiency is far less. The complications of peritoneal dialysis are essentially the same in children as in adults except, perhaps, for a greater tendency for herniation of omentum or other structures through the incision unless a very small one is used. In very small infants whose barbiturate levels must be reduced rapidly in order to preserve life, we consider exchange transfusion to be the procedure of choice.

I agree with those who feel that analeptic drugs rarely, if ever, are worthwhile in the treatment of barbiturate poisoning even in adults (Done, 1969). Children, beyond the newborn period, have a lower seizure threshold than do adults. Although there are no definitive data it is logical to suppose that they may, therefore, have an exaggerated response to analeptic drugs. My experience with the use of analeptic drugs in barbiturate poisoning has confirmed this supposition, and has caused even greater reluctance to employ such drugs in the treatment of children.

REFERENCES

BIANCHINE, J. R. and FERGUSON, F. C., JR. (1967), Acute toxicity and lethal brain concentration of pentobarbital in young and adult albino rats. *Proc. Soc. exper. Biol. (N.Y.)*, 124, 1077.

CATZ, C. and YAFFE, S. J. (1967), Strain and age variations in hexobarbital response. *J. Pharmacol. exp. Ther.*, 155, 152.

DOMEK, N. S., BARLOW, C. F. and ROTH, L. J. (1960), An ontogenetic study of phenobarbital-C^{14} in cat brain. *J. Pharmacol. exp. Ther.*, 130, 285.

DONE, A. K. (1964), Developmental pharmacology. *Clin. Pharmacol. Ther.*, 5, 432.

DONE, A. K. (1966a), Perinatal pharmacology. *Ann. Rev. Pharmacol.*, 6, 189.

DONE, A. K. (1966b), Intoxications of the nervous system. In: V. C. Kelley (Ed), Brennemann-Kelley. *Practice of Paediatrics*, Vol. 4, 1–52. Prior, Hagerstown, Md.

DONE, A. K. (1969), Pharmacologic principles in the treatment of poisoning. *Pharmacol. for Phycns*, 3, 1.

FOUTS, J. R. and HART, L. G. (1965), Hepatic drug metabolism during the perinatal period. *Ann. N.Y. Acad. Sci.*, 123, 245.

KALSER, S. C., FORBES, E. and KUNIG, R. (1969). Relation of brain sensitivity and hepatic metabolism of hexobarbitone to dose-response relations in infant and young rats. *J. Pharm. Pharmacol.*, 21, 109.

KATO, R., VASSANELLI, P., FRONTINO, G. and CHIESARA, E. (1964), Variation in the activity of liver microsomal drug-metabolizing enzymes in rats in relation to the age. *Biochem. Pharmacol.*, 13, 1037.

KUPFERBERG, H. J. and WAY, E. L. (1963), Pharmacologic basis for the increased sensitivy of the newborn rat to morphine. *J. Pharmacol. exp. Ther.*, 141, 105.

PANTUCK, E., CONNEY, A. H. and KUNTZMAN, R. (1968), Effect of phenobarbital on the metabolism of pentobarbital and meperidine in fetal rabbits and rats. *Biochem. Pharmacol.*, 17, 1441.

REED, C. E., DRIGGS, M. F. and FOOTE, C. C. (1952), Acute barbiturate intoxication. A study of 300 cases based on a physiologic system of classification of the severity of the intoxication. *Ann. intern. Med.*, 37, 290.

YEARY, R. A., BENISH, R. A. and FINKELSTEIN, M. (1966), Acute toxicity of drugs in newborn animals. *J. Pediat.*, 69, 663.

17. barbiturate automatism

R. C. B. Aitken

'For the great enemy of the truth is very often not the lie – deliberate, contrived and dishonest – but the myth, persistent, persuasive and unrealistic.'

John Fitzgerald Kennedy (1962)

The term *automatism* was 'borrowed' in 1934 by Richards, a lecturer in Forensic Medicine at Aberdeen, to explain three cases of poisoning by barbiturates. Each patient on recovering consciousness claimed to remember taking only one or, at the most, two doses, though obviously more must have been taken. Richards suggested that 'the knowledge of the need for another tablet persists, while the memory is so affected by the drug that the patient does not realize that he has already satisfied the need, and automatically repeats the dose at intervals'. Clearly, Richards attributed the amnesia to clouding of consciousness due to sedation.

The phenomenon of drug automatism continues to be widely quoted (Lieberman, 1963; Backett, 1965; Goodman and Gilman, 1965; Leading Article, 1965; Meyler, 1966; Berger, 1967; McCarthy, 1967; Today's Drugs, 1968). The concept is entrenched firmly in the minds of the medical profession and general public. It provides a credible explanation of drug overdose which is socially acceptable; and it allows verdicts of accidental death to be recorded in cases of poisoning, which otherwise would have been classified as suicide.

In 1960, Long reviewed the evidence on barbiturate automatism as a cause of death. He defined automatism as 'any action performed without the doer's intention or knowledge', and then reported that he could find nothing in the literature which proved the existence of barbiturate automatism as a clinical entity. This was also the view of Litman and his colleagues in 1963.

Long traced how this explanation for some cases of barbiturate poisoning was quoted from one source to another, but without the addition of new evidence on which to substantiate it. He quoted cynically from an apparently authoritative editorial in the *New England Journal of Medicine* in 1957: 'Undoubtedly, an occasional poisoning from automatism has occurred.' Long's opinion was that 'to affirm the soundness of Richards' conclusions on the meagre evidence of his three cases is an appeal to credulity which ought not to be attempted in an intelligent society.'

It is difficult to conceive how an adult could swallow sufficient barbiturate by accident rather than intention, unless there was a particular kind of purposive behaviour caused by clouded consciousness. It is always intrinsic in the accounts of the phenomenon that serial consumption takes place as a result of pharmacological action producing amnesia. Yet in other kinds of clouded consciousness either drowsiness inhibits sensory and motor function uniformly, or it produces a delirious state with some of the following features:

- Impaired grasp of activity in the environment
- Liability to perceptual disturbance
- Restless unconstructive behaviour
- Vagueness of thought
- Incoherence of speech
- Fluctuating disorientation
- Patchy and diffuse amnesia

Despite the lack of these ever being mentioned in descriptions of the phenomenon, the patient with drug automatism is considered to have been capable of sufficient purposive behaviour to have acquired and repeatedly ingested small doses of drugs. The feasibility of such an explanation must be open to considerable doubt.

That the amnesia on recovery could be a psychogenic defence used at the time of recall has not been considered with sufficient care. If ingestion were due to accident, there should be no reason for a psychogenic defence mechanism to be necessary and these patients should be relatively free of the psychopathology found in other self-poisoners.

In order to investigate this, Aitken and Proudfoot (1969) assessed 994 admissions of poisoned patients, 295 of which were due to barbiturates. They could find only two patients who had amnesia for ingestion, yet who accepted that more drug must have been consumed than could be remembered. In both cases, there was evidence of pre-existing psychopathology and circumstances to conclude that amnesia at the time of recall on recovery was credible as a psychological mechanism. Apart from drowsiness, none of the other features commonly found in pathological clouding of consciousness were noted; the amnesia was quite specific and crucial only to the acts of overdose.

One patient was a nurse with an anxious, histrionic personality; she was often dependent on barbiturates, and had taken an overdose before. Prior to admission, semi-comatose due to barbitutate poisoning, she was distressed by grief following the death of a male patient whom she nursed. She had heard of the entity of barbiturate automatism; clearly admission of deliberate self-poisoning would have threatened her self-esteem among colleagues in particular.

The other patient also had been admitted previously, after barbiturate poisoning following desertion by his wife. While unconscious then he sustained a burn which resulted in chronic osteomyelitis. Subsequent to this he had not worked and had lived alone in lodgings. There was other evidence of inadequate, depressive and sociopathic traits in his personality. On this occasion he was only drowsy at admission and later claimed that he could not remember taking more than his usual dose of pentobarbitone, despite evidence that he must have done so. On the previous day he had returned to his lodgings from a stay with his sister's family and was overcome by loneliness. His distress was attributed to chronic physical ill-health with inter-personal problems due to dissatisfaction with his dependency needs. Clearly there was reason to deduce abnormality of mental state prior to ingestion.

Aitken and Proudfoot (1969) also looked at the group of patients (31 admissions in 29 patients) who simply denied the act of self-poisoning despite evidence to the contrary. In comparison with the other patients who admitted ingestion the denial sample was older and more of them had been more deeply unconscious due to barbiturates. The distribution of their psychiatric diagnoses did not differ from those who admitted the act. More of them had attempted suicide before. The same proportion had been treated previously as in-patients at psychiatric hospitals and required transfer there on this occasion. As a group, they too had ample evidence of pre-existing psychopathology.

Scandinavian observers reported a high incidence of automatism in cases of poisoning, the explanation for which may lie partly in their definition of the term. Ettlinger and Flordh (1955) considered that 28 % of 500 cases of attempted suicide were due to 'serial consumption' of drugs, applying this when the patient 'showed amnesia for his actions and even for his intentions'. Jansson (1961; 1962) found that no less than 25 % of 488 cases of attempted suicide by various drugs were due to automatism. Jansson defined automatism as 'poisoning, where the person involved gradually has consumed an overdose of hypnotics in order to get to sleep without any intention to commit suicide'.

This definition did not demand that these patients necessarily had amnesia, either at the time of ingestion or on recovery, only that the assessment of motive was not suicide. The act of self-poisoning could well have been an appeal for help, rather than a dangerous disturbance of behaviour resulting purely by accident from barbiturate action. Indeed, Kessel (1965) preferred the diagnosis to be called self-poisoning rather than attempted suicide. Not only is self-poisoning an accurate description, but it does not require retrospective assessment of motive. To call the majority of cases 'attempted suicide' is both clinically inapplicable and misleading. The fact that by Jansson's definition the patients did not intend suicide did not make their behaviour *automatism*. Moreover, Jansson found the same incidence of repetition of overdose in those cases thought to be due to automatism and those classified as serious attempts at suicide, so they were not free of psychopathology.

In England and Wales in 1964, 506 deaths were certified by doctors, or after coroners' inquests, as due to *accidental* barbiturate poisoning; these deaths accounted for 25 % of all those coded as due to barbiturate poisoning (Registrar General). In the same year in the United States, 478 died similarly (McCarthy, 1967). In both groups 99 % of the patients were over the age of 15 years.

In Scotland, the number of deaths due to *accidental* poisoning has fallen from a peak in 1962; but the proportion by barbiturates has increased steadily (Fig. 1). Hence in

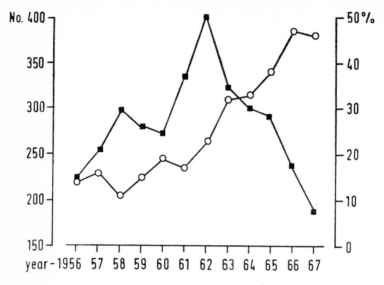

Fig. 1. Comparison of deaths due to accidental poisoning with proportion due to barbiturate poisoning in Scotland; ■ = number of accidental deaths, o = percentage due to barbiturates.

recent years the total number of deaths due to *accidental* barbiturate poisoning has remained fairly constant. The number of admissions to hospital in Edinburgh between 1962 and 1967 for self-poisoning by barbiturates has also remained fairly constant, though the number by other drugs has increased considerably (Aitken *et al.*, 1969). While the unreliability of mortality statistics regarding cause and motive is notorious, the relative constancy of suicide rates is remarkable (Stengel, 1964). The fluctuations in the number and cause of *accidental* deaths from ingested poison in adults seems as likely to reflect an artefact of certification as a reality of behaviour.

The lack of evidence to support disturbed behaviour due only to clouding of consciousness at the time of ingestion, and the abundant evidence of pre-existing psychopathology, seem to render automatism untenable as an explanation for barbiturate poisoning. This is in agreement with the Hill Report (1968) which concluded 'that the majority of the deaths in adults (due to poisoning) are the result of deliberate self-administration'.

Self-poisoning should always be regarded as a plea for help, and this applies as much to patients who claim amnesia for ingestion as to those who admit the act. A diagnosis of barbiturate automatism, like that of hysteria, suggests that the underlying psychopathology need not be explored further, the term being sufficient explanation for the behaviour. As this does not seem to be so, it is concluded that the use of the term contributes nothing to the clinical management or accuracy of mortality statistics. Hence the term 'drug automatism' should be abandoned and the concept discarded as a cause of barbiturate poisoning.

ACKNOWLEDGMENT

The author is indebted to Dr. A. T. Proudfoot for his contribution to this paper, the ideas for which developed initially in a joint publication.

REFERENCES

AITKEN, R. C. B. and PROUDFOOT, A. T. (1969), Barbiturate automatism – myth or malady? *Postgrad. med. J.*, 45, 612.
AITKEN, R. C. B., BUGLASS, D. and KREITMAN, N. (1969), The changing pattern of attempted suicide in Edinburgh, 1962–67. *Brit. J. prev. soc. Med.*, 23, 111.
Annual Reports of the Registrar General for Scotland for 1956–1967. HMSO, Edinburgh.
BACKETT, E. M. (1965), *Domestic Accidents*. WHO. Public Health Papers, No. 26, 99.
BERGER, F. M. (1967), Drugs and suicide in the United States, *Clin. Pharmacol. Ther.*, 8, 219.
Editorial. (1957), Sedative-hypnotic drugs. The barbiturates. *New Engl. J. Med.*, 256, 77.
ETTLINGER, R. W. and FLORDH, P. (1955), Attempted Suicide. *Acta psychiat. scand.*, Supp ., 103, 17.
GOODMAN, L. S. and GILMAN, A. (1965), *The pharmacological Basis of Therapeutics*, p. 123. Macmillan, New York.
HILL REPORT (1968), *Hospital Treatment of Acute Poisoning*, p. 8. HMSO, London.
JANSSON, B. (1961), Drug automatism as a cause of pseudo-suicide, *Postgrad. Med.*, 30, A 34.
JANSSON, B. (1962), A catamnestic study of 476 attempted suicides, with special regard to the prognosis for cases of drug automatism. *Acta psychiat. scand.*, 38, 183.
KESSEL, N. (1965), Self-poisoning. *Brit. med. J.*, 2, 1265, 1336.
Leading Article (1965), Dependence on barbiturates and other sedative drugs. *J. Amer. med. Ass.*, 193, 673.
LIEBERMAN, A. (1963), The case of the barbed barbiturate. *J. Indiana med. Ass.*, 56, 1426.
LITMAN, R. E., CURPHEY, T., SHNEIDMAN, E. S., FARBEROW, N. L. and TABACHNICK, N. (1963), Investigations of equivocal suicides. *J. Amer. med. Ass.*, 184, 924.
LONG, R. H. (1960), Barbiturates, automatism and suicide. *Postgrad. Med.*, 28, A 56.
McCARTHY, M. A. (1967), Selected types of poisoning as causes of accidental death: United States, 1964. *United States Public Health Report*, 82, 1025.
MEYLER, L. (1966), *Side Effects of Drugs*. Vol. V, p. 38, Excerpta Medica, Amsterdam.
Registrar General's Statistical Review of England and Wales for the year 1964 (1966), HMSO, London.
RICHARDS, R. (1934), A symptom of poisoning by hypnotics of the barbituric acid group. *Brit. med. J.*, 1, 331.
STENGEL, E. (1964), *Suicide and Attempted Suicide*, p. 18. Penguin, Harmondsworth.
Today's Drugs (1968), Hypnotics. *Brit. med. J.*, 2, 409.

18. psychiatric aspects of acute barbiturate poisoning

N. Kessel

The tasks of the psychiatrist on behalf of a patient with barbiturate poisoning are:
1. to discover and deal with any psychological consequences of the poisoning, whether accidental or deliberate, and
2. to explore the psychological and social circumstances leading to the act and examine the recovered patient so as to carry out the appropriate psychological and social treatment.

The first of these functions is not commonly required because it is unusual for barbiturate poisoning to have psychological sequelae. The second is by far the more important and is always necessary if the poisoning has not been accidental. Since accidental barbiturate poisoning in adults is exceedingly rare and since the determination of whether the poisoning was deliberate or not is usually made during the course of the psychiatric history-taking, the best course in practice is to carry out the psychological enquiry for every patient.

This chapter, which is concerned only with adult patients, is divided into four parts. The first deals with the psychological sequelae of barbiturate poisoning whether accidental or deliberate. The second (for which I have drawn on previous papers) reviews briefly our knowledge of the psychological and social features of patients who deliberately poison themselves, and of their motivation. In the third part this knowledge is used to discuss the clinical approach to such patients. Lastly, the arrangements which need to be made to permit the functioning of a proper psychiatric service are described.

The term psychiatrist refers throughout to the doctor who carries out the psychological history-taking and clinical examination and makes the appropriate decisions. Where a service for poisoned patients is properly organized this doctor will be a trained psychiatrist and will have the assistance of a social worker. In many places, however, the evaluation will have to be made by a doctor without special training in psychiatry. He will need to acquire the knowledge and skills here described. This is not especially difficult, given the will to do so. In the same way a trained social worker can with experience carry out the social work functions described even without the special skills of psychiatric social work.

PART ONE

PSYCHOLOGICAL CONSEQUENCES OF BARBITURATE POISONING

Usually there are none. During the phase of recovery of full consciousness, or shortly after, withdrawal symptoms may occur. These, in the time order in which they happen, are: (1) acute tremulousness, sometimes accompanied by brief, disorganized, visual hallucinations and some disorientation; (2) fits; and (3) delirium tremens.

Not all these features need occur in the same patient, though they all form part of the general excitatory syndrome, a 'rebound' phenomenon of the cerebral cells escaping from the influence of sedation. Fits are met with more commonly than the others. They are clinically the same as grand mal attacks and, in the absence of a history of epilepsy, of any recent symptoms suggesting cerebral involvement or of a head-injury in association with the poisoning, they are not of much importance and do not warrant extensive neurological investigation.

Fits do not usually occur in the recovery phase unless the patient has been taking barbiturates for a fairly considerable time, months if not years. In animal experiments (Jaffe and Sharpless, 1965), two weeks of barbiturate intoxication were necessary before spontaneous fits followed withdrawal. The clinical significance of a fit during the recovery phase, then, is to draw attention to the probability of chronic intoxication and hence of the possibility of barbiturate dependence. However, the same sequence of withdrawal symptoms follows withdrawal of alcohol from regular excessive drinkers, and as deliberate self-poisoning is common among alcoholics this is the first possibility that should spring to mind. Tremulousness and delirium are commoner in alcohol withdrawal than in barbiturate withdrawal.

The general excitatory syndrome, whether it arises from barbiturate withdrawal or alcohol withdrawal, can be abolished or prevented with chlorpromazine. Once the condition is established large doses are necessary, up to a gram a day. If restlessness or fear is uncontrollable, the dose may be supplemented by intramuscular injection of chlorpromazine 75 mg, not more often than two-hourly. In the writer's experience, chlordiazepoxide cannot be as well relied upon, although it has its exponents (Glatt *et al.*, 1965).

If the patient is known to be an alcoholic, chlorpromazine, 150 mg three times per day, should be given prophylactically by mouth as soon as the patient is sufficiently conscious, and continued for one week. If tremulousness develops the dose should at once be increased.

Status epilepticus requires treatment with further doses of barbiturates intravenously, notwithstanding the fact that the patient is recovering from barbiturate poisoning.

One other feature of the recovery from barbiturate poisoning deserves mention. Because of the very rapid development of some tolerance to barbiturates the patient may, during the recovery phase, reach consciousness still with a level of barbiturate in the body that would have been sufficient to render him unconscious during the absorption phase. The clinical psychological examination may therefore be carried out when there is still a significant blood level of barbiturate. It has been suggested (Haider and Oswald, 1970) that the residual barbiturate produces, by its sedative action, a state of unnatural calm which acts to conceal some of the psychological depression or anxiety present. Certainly the psychiatrist must resist any attempt to have him decide about the patient before he is satisfied that full consciousness has been restored, but if he is so satisfied we have not found that patients failed to reveal significant psychological abnormalities.

PART TWO

PSYCHOLOGICAL AND SOCIAL CHARACTERISTICS OF SELF-POISONERS

The principal function of the psychiatrist is to elicit the circumstances of the act and the mental state of the patient and to render the appropriate treatment. In order that this should be understood it is necessary to give some general account of the people who take overdoses. This description is limited to those who survive their acts, since we have no special interest in suicides. Mostly these characteristics apply whatever the ingestant chosen but where there are special features about those who take barbiturates these are stated. Much of the information was obtained from a detailed study over a number of years of patients at the Edinburgh Poisoning Treatment Centre, by the author (Kessel, 1965; Kessel, 1966; Kessel and McCulloch, 1966; Kessel et al., 1963). Later accounts from this and other centres have confirmed the findings.

A. Social factors
These are extensively treated in Chapter 19. Here I have singled out only those characteristics which influence diagnosis and treatment.

Sex and Age. Female rates outnumbered male by a ratio of approximately three to two in Edinburgh in 1962. By 1967 the sex ratio had approximated nearer to unity (Aitken et al., 1969). The earlier difference in sex rates was almost entirely attributable to people below the age of 50 and the recent change has been because of an increase in young male rates. Self-poisoning in its current proportions is still of unstable epidemicity and shifts in its demographic characteristics may be expected for some time yet.

For both sexes now the great preponderance of cases occur among people below the age of 35. Although for self-poisoners in general there are high rates among teenagers, doctors do not so readily prescribe barbiturates to these youngsters, and thus their rates for barbiturate poisoning are somewhat lower. Conversely, relatively more people over the age of 55 chose this method.

Marital state, marital relationships and other personal relationships. A very high proportion, male 30% and female 26%, of married patients, had had their marriages unnaturally interrupted by separation and divorce. In a sixth of these instances the break had been recent, within a month, and it probably played a part in causing the self-poisoning act. Generally, however, the separation was of long duration; nearly half the broken marriages had ended five or more years before. Moreover, for the marriages that subsisted, husband and wife, whoever had taken the overdose, usually agreed that marital relations were bad. Frequent hostility characterized 85% of the marriages of male and 68% of those of female patients and the psychiatric social worker graded half the marriages as poor or bad (See Chapter 17). Unfaithfulness, jealousy, gambling and drinking on the part of one or other partner, generally the husband, were the chief causes cited. On the other hand, only a minority of patients, and their spouses, actually wished the marriage would end. When either party did express such a wish the prognosis for the marriage was far from good. It was not always the patient who was responsible for the unfortunate state of the marriage; sometimes it was both parties. Certainly the other partner was not blameless. McCulloch's assessment found only half the spouses normal. The remainder mostly exhibited character disorders, though a proportion of the wives of male patients were psychiatrically ill.

Seventy per cent of the men and 59% of the women who were single, or whose marriages had ended, got on badly with whomever was the principal figure in their life situation. This bad relationship was the dominant theme in the story of nearly every patient, whether the account was given by the patient or by an informant.

More than any other factor these bad personal relationships, within or outwith marriage, provided the setting for the self-poisoning act. Yet in many cases they but set the seal on a life pattern characterized by adverse circumstances – a bad work record, chronic debt and constant changes of home, often the product of separations. Moreover, these life stories seemed to repeat similar stories in the parents' lives and there had been a great amount of parental absence during the childhood of the patients.

This is the background upon which precipitating social factors are superimposed. Table 1 shows the frequency with which certain items occurred and were important in the stories we obtained. Excessive drinking was prominent. Unemployment played its part with men. Money worries were often mentioned, housing problems less commonly. Girls in particular were sometimes driven to the extremity of poisoning themselves by a broken or a breaking love affair.

Living circumstances. Self-poisoning is associated with bad living conditions. High case rates were found to be associated with indices of overcrowding and family dislocation. There was no significant association with living alone. A new housing estate to which people from a bad social area had been moved *en bloc* had high rates. A new housing area to which there had been selective entry of families where the breadwinner had a job on a local industrial development had low rates.

B. Psychological factors
   Diagnosis. The vast majority of patients surviving self-poisoning acts do not have

TABLE 1

Major precipitating factors. Percentages of approximately 165 males and 350 females (except for marital disharmony and forced separation, which are based on 68 married males and 147 married females). More than one factor might be present. Factors occurring in less than 10% of cases have been omitted. They included bereavement, gambling, and sexual problems.

	Percentage of males	Percentage of females
Marital disharmony	68	60
Drinking a problem	51	16
Financial difficulties	44	31
Unemployment	34	18
Kin disharmony	28	30
Isolation	15	
Crime	15	
Housing difficulties	14	19
Difficulties at work	14	
Love affairs going badly		16
Forced separation	12	

the more severe forms of mental disorder. Most patients suffer from depression or from personality abnormalities or from both. Table 2 shows the diagnostic distribution of 515 patients studied between 1962 and 1963, although, as I then wrote, 'the appropriate terms of conventional psychiatric nomenclature – depression, neurosis, personality abnormality, and the like – are ill-suited to describing, differentiating, or even pigeon-holing the patients. We have been forced into unreal decisions whether a patient's manifest unhappiness should be attributed to a depressive illness or regarded as understandable distress at intolerable living circumstances. We have had to distinguish, with what success I cannot judge, between normality and personality disorder.'

TABLE 2

Diagnoses, in percentage

	Males (165)	Females (350
Organic psychiatric illness	5	4
Depression	26	43
Other psychoses	5	5
Other neuroses	5	12
Personality disorder only	32	16
No psychiatric illness	26	20

When these findings were first published eyebrows were raised about the 26% of men and 20% of women with 'no psychiatric illness'. Some argue that to poison oneself is such an abnormal act that everyone who does so must be psychologically ill. We did not accept this, since it made the recognition of psychiatric illness no more than a dependent phenomenon. Instead, we reasoned as follows: the diagnosis of a psychiatric condition must be made from positive features. These are detected either from the history or on clinical examination. If all the information about the patient's mental state at the time of his act, obtained both from him and from an informant, does not indicate any departure from normal, and if clinical examination after physical recovery fails to reveal any significant disorder, then there are no grounds for concluding that the patient is psychiatrically ill. This view will not be acceptable to everyone. There are psychiatrists who assign the soubriquet of abnormality of personality very readily. But even if they would have labelled as suffering from a character disorder some of those whom we have judged to be normal, that disorder was certainly not pronounced. It was not enough in itself to explain their self-poisoning acts. Nor is this unexpected. Distress drives people to self-poisoning acts, and distress is not the exclusive province of the mentally ill. Now, there was in the American Psychiatric Association's diagnostic manual a category: 'Acute situational reaction'; in the current British classification (General Register Office, 1968) this appears in the guise of 'Transient situational disturbance'. Were these patients not suffering from this? Exquisitely they were. It is difficult, however, to make any of these terms bear a psychiatric implication. The important thing, though, is not to split hairs but to emphasize that many self-poisoned patients are not particularly abnormal individuals.

The significance of the finding that so many patients had no psychiatric disorder is that it focuses attention upon the purposes of the act and makes us concentrate upon personal relationships in their social setting.

Those with no psychiatric illness tended to be younger; those with organic illnesses were generally old. Apart from this the relation between diagnosis and age was not close.

Quite commonly patients who were suffering from depression had an underlying character disorder. The combination of depression and psychopathy often occurred. This conjunction seems especially prone to manifest in self-poisoning acts. Personality disorder, either as a principal or as an accessory diagnosis, was recognized in 41% of men and 27% of women patients, and about half of these were classed as psychopaths. A smaller proportion appeared to us to be abnormally immature in their outlook. No other sort of personality abnormality occurred frequently.

Associated diagnostic factors included alcoholism, drug addiction, epilepsy, and subnormality. Fifty-two per cent of men had one or more of these conditions, and the dominant factor was alcoholism. Thirty-nine per cent of the men and 8% of the women were alcoholics, seasoned drinkers, unquestionably addicted, many of them bearing the physical signs of chronic alcoholism. Alcoholism is a major factor predisposing to self-poisoning. So is alcohol itself: 56% of the men and 23% of the women had been drinking just before the act took place, with, one presumes, potentiation of the barbiturate taken.

Intention and motivation. In most countries of the world for which statistics are available there has been an enormous increase in self-poisoning in the last two decades. Detailed figures are available for Edinburgh (Fig. 1) which show that the increase

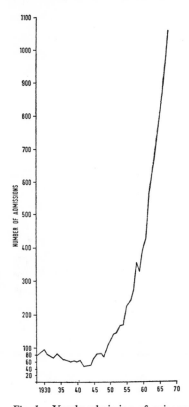

Fig. 1. Yearly admission of poisoned patients to the Royal Infirmary of Edinburgh (1928–1968)

began in the late nineteen-forties and has continued ever since. Similar figures have been published for many different areas in many parts of the world. National data for England and Wales are available from the Hospital In-patient Enquiry (Ministry of Health, 1968) (Table 3).

TABLE 3

Admissions to hospital for treatment of poisoning (England and Wales)

	1957	1958	1959	1960	1961	1962	1963	1964
All poisoning	15,900	17,500	20,200	23,300	27,900	33,600	45,900	50,400
Barbituric acid and derivatives	6,100	6,600	7,500	8,800	10,500	12,100	16,500	16,300

It can be surmised that, for the Edinburgh figures, some of the rise is because of an easier admission policy since the introduction of the National Health Service, but the shape of the curve largely reflects the mounting extent of this behaviour. It is not credible that this great growth represents an increase in the frequency with which citizens of Edinburgh attempt to kill themselves. If that were so it would call out most strenuously for an explanation. There has been no change in our national social condition or psychological status to account for it. Certainly an undesirable phenomenon has become fashionable but the activity is unlikely to be the attempt to kill oneself. Many authors have shown that most of those said to be attempting suicide are not addressing themselves singlemindedly to death. Stengel and Cook (1958) have described their acts as Janus-faced. The semantic justification of the phrase 'attempted suicide' has thus been destroyed. It is time we discarded it, since its meaningless residuum leads to incorrect clinical management.

The rise in number of self-poisoning acts has come about in conjunction with a great increase in the number of powerful preparations employed therapeutically and a contemporaneous increase in prescribing habits. Drugs are readily available to a populace aware both that they are comparatively safe and that their dosage can, with discretion, be regulated by the taker. Both the factual and the fictional taking of overdoses is widely publicized; moreover it is now widely appreciated that it is customary to survive such overdoses. To die is the exception rather than the rule; Stengel (1964) for instance, when describing a much publicized death by poisoning, in a work written for the general public, made it plain that 'the large majority of similar cases of intoxication survive today'. It is common knowledge that one can take a lot of pills, lose consciousness and later return to it none the worse for the experience. Doctors, of course, know this too, but some of them, some psychiatrists in particular, fail to accept the information is general. Instead, they incline to assume a degree of lethal intent in all acts of self-poisoning. By making this assumption they are deceiving rather than enlightening themselves.

The term 'attempted suicide' is now misapplied to acts with a wide variety of intentions (the notion of an attempt must always imply some intention), all of which are expressed in similar types of behaviour, namely acts of self-poisoning or self-injury. Shneidman (1963) explains how it is that we get the term. He draws attention to the four traditionally recognized modes of death: natural death, accident, suicide and homicide. Nomenclature intended for mortality classifications is now applied, with varying degrees of pertinence, to morbid states without fatal issue. So acts against the self that do not end in death come to be labelled as attempted suicide. We would do well, however, to extend Shneidman's concept with a further parallel. When a Manchester United supporter punches a Manchester City supporter on the nose he is charged with assault but not with attempted murder. A clear distinction is drawn between the two sorts of act because it is realized that they have different intentions. We can accept without difficulty that there are harmful acts against someone else which have no lethal intent. But exactly the same applies to acts against the self. They are not all attempted suicide because they do not all have lethal intent and, if we seek a general term to embrace all such acts, then attempted suicide will not do.

To approach patients who have poisoned or injured themselves already convinced that there was some degree of lethal intent in their acts is not only unreasonable; it prevents one ever ascertaining the opposite. The quality of the act itself, the history obtained both from an independent informant and from the patient, and the patient's own statement of his intent at the time, all show that acts of self-poisoning or self-injury can frequently be performed without lethal intent. In the work in Edinburgh we devised an *index of endangering life* by which to characterize each act from the patient's point of view. The index (Fig. 2) used two measures: first, an estimate of the

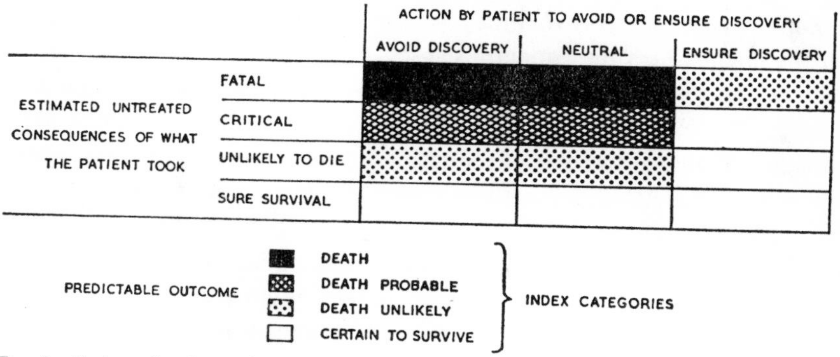

Fig. 2. Index of endangering life

consequence of what the patient had done, had no treatment been available; and second, the steps he took to avoid, or to ensure, discovery. By combining these items we derived four categories of predictable outcome of the act: death, death probable, death unlikely and certain to survive. Only a fifth seemed to have escaped a projected death (Table 4). These figures were for all cases of self-poisoning. But if only barbiturate poisoning were considered, they would not be much different. It is important to note that nearly half the patients did not, from their point of view, jeopardize their lives at all.

TABLE 4

Index of endangering life, in percentage

Predictable outcome of act	Males (170)	Females (352)
Death	19	19
Death probable	11	11
Death unlikely	28	21
Certain to survive	40	49
Unclassified	2	0

The next pieces of evidence are provided by the history, obtained from both the patient and an informant. Sometimes a wish to die, however muddled, was revealed in one or other of these accounts of how the patient was at the time, or just before, the act took place. More often, however, both concurred, independently of each other, that they did not believe there was any such wish. In a substantial proportion of cases the recovered patients expressly denied any intention of dying; they had acted in the belief that they would recover. Patients sometimes conceal their intentions, but this is generally because they feel that they would be censured if the truth were known. They do not do so if they are aware that our sympathy and concern for them will be unaffected by what they tell us. A large group said that they could not remember having formed any intention one way or the other. They had acted in the heat of the moment without forming any objective of what they were trying to do. Once again, it may be argued that the intent which the patient discloses, even if he is doing his best to be truthful, may not be correct. But apart from the act itself and the mental state after physical recovery, these sources of information are our only available evidence about the patient's state of mind at the time of the act; it is unrealistic to reject it because of the possibilities that the relative did not know what was in the patient's mind or that the latter's recollections were subject to retrospective falsification. Evidence should only be discounted when there are factual, not merly speculative, objections.

Shneidman (1963) describes patients' intention in respect of *cessation* of consciousness. Cessation implies that consciousness has ended and cannot be restored. *To die, to sleep. No more.* But consciousness, as Shneidman points out, can also suffer *interruption.* It may be abolished, but temporarily only; some time later consciousness will reassert itself and the activities of life continue. Many people who poison or injure themselves seek only interruption. A desperate situation arises for them, often quite suddenly, though perhaps on a basis of long strain. It may be a violent marital quarrel; it may be being jilted; it may be alcoholic remorse. In the cold and subsequent light of day the event will often appear trivial, but at the time it overwhelms. The patient knows, to the temporary exclusion of everything else from his thinking, that the present is unbearable. He can see no solution to his difficulties. He feels trapped and so he acts irrationally and often impulsively to effect his removal by the readiest means to hand. He may previously have thought about dying, but such acts are rarely the result of planning. 'It just came over me', the patients say, 'I had to get out of it'. And when they are asked, 'For ever?' they reply, unhesitatingly, 'No!'

Sometimes the act itself, by its very shock, brings about a favourable change in the situation. Often the patients, once physically recovered, consciously use the act to effect such a manipulation. But that is not why the tablets were taken. The reason was the urgent and insupportable distress, to obtain relief by withdrawing from the situation. 'I want out,' the Scots say. But it is a temporary withdrawal that is sought. Interruption. *Sleep that knits up the ravell'd sleave of care. . . Balm of hurt minds.* The play is different, but we are still among the tragedies.

Sleeping tablets are taken to give excess of that very function for which they were prescribed. To make certain of interrupting the painful consciousness of distress the patient knowingly takes an overdose. But overdoses can be regulated and this the patient does, even when acting without forethought. His judgement may not be as nice as a physician's, but all the same he exercises it. It was a minority of our patients who took all the tablets that were available. They certainly were not physically prevented from taking them all.

Many patients, admitted to hospitals after having poisoned themselves, were using drugs in just this way. They felt the need to sleep more securely, more deeply, for longer. Doctors are the designers of the fashion of self-poisoning. We have invented and we prescribe dangerous substances, hypnotics and sedatives like sorcerers and these patients are our apprentices. Like their fictional counterpart they frequently endanger their lives, but that is not their intention. They want eventually to wake.

The unifying basis to self-poisoning acts is distress, distress and despair. This may arise from within, from a morbid appreciation that the patient has of himself in the world; such is the person with a depressive illness. Often it is generated from outside, from the intolerable yet insoluble social situation in which he is caught; that is why so many patients cannot be classed as ill. Sometimes it springs from both sources. Nobody takes poison, a little or a lot, to live or to die, unless at that moment he is distressed beyond what he can bear and so desperate that he cannot see a more rational solution. He does not think that no solution exists, but he cannot himself find it. The suicide says, in effect, 'There is no way out,' but people who poison themselves are saying, 'I cannot see a way out.' They find themselves trapped. They are desperate; and their distress drives them to an action that is both stupid and, at the same time, a blow for liberation, to an action that is both senseless and purposeful. We must respect the conjunction of these epithets. Almost always the patients can. Many of them do even as they are taking the tablets.

A married woman of 27 whose husband was threatening to leave her took 50 aspirins: 'I didn't think they'd kill me. I thought they might. I hoped they wouldn't. I thought of my mother and father. I couldn't let them be hurt. I hoped really it would bring John back. If it didn't I might as well die.'

Senseless and purposeful, it is a paradox that we have to accept.

Impulsiveness and premeditation. Two-thirds of all acts were impulsive. Five minutes, sometimes only one minute, before the act took place the idea of taking poison was not in the person's mind. He may have, often he had, thought about doing it in the past. Hours of rumination may have preceded the determination which was formed in a single moment. But in the event, at the event, a feeling of despair arose, often suddenly, from a trivial cause, and was as suddenly acted upon. It was no culmination of a gathering plan. 'Why did you do it?' the patients are asked. 'I don't know; it just came over me,' they reply. And they do not know. It is not that they have forgotten. They are not prevaricating. They never worked it out. They never had a period when they were intending to do it. It just came over them.

A 30-year-old woman, who had long endured an unhappy marriage to an aggressive ne'er-do-well, related how one day they had a protracted quarrel.

There was violence and she collapsed, crying, in an armchair. What was she to do? While she was weeping she remembered that a little while earlier a bottle of sleeping tablets had slipped down the back of the chair and she had never retrieved it. She reached down her hand, found the bottle, and took twenty Seconal capsules.

We could multiply that case over three hundred times with similar impulsive instances. Men and women acted impulsively in equal proportions. Impulsive acts were not related to alcoholism and were no more common among the inebriated than among the others. They had little bearing on the method adopted. Impulsiveness was more common than premeditation at all ages, though its incidence was rather less in women of 55 and over, because of an increase in depressive illness in this group. Patients with formal psychiatric illnesses premeditated self-poisoning more often than did others, but even among them impulsiveness characterized just over half the acts.

Repeating the act. Even with a good psychiatric service, almost a fifth of patients will repeat a self-poisoning act within 12 months. (Most repetitions will occur within four months.) The patients who do so are largely those with personality disorders of an antisocial type and there is a particular risk for alcoholics and those who are drug-dependent. Another group of patients more prone than most to repeat are housewives whose depression springs from intolerable marital circumstances. This latter group, more perhaps than the others, can be helped by the offer of continuing support, whether by psychiatrist or by social worker, at the psychiatric clinic. With regard to alcoholics, it is unfortunately the case that these particular alcoholics, by virtue of their personality disorders, are least likely to be helped by the offer of anti-addictive treatment at an alcoholism clinic. Nevertheless the offer should be made. The subsequent suicide rate of self-poisoned patients is widely agreed to be between 1% and 2% per year, (Ettlinger, 1964; Kessel and McCulloch, 1966; Greer and Lee, 1967). McCulloch *et al.* (1969) have shown, conversely, that 25% of suicides in Edinburgh had had a previous episode of self-poisoning within the preceding ten years. Suicide is particularly frequent among alcoholics who have previously had an episode of self-poisoning. There is no justification whatsoever for the view that if someone has 'attempted suicide' he will not subsequently kill himself.

However, even where the patient had been determined to kill himself, the act seems to exhaust, for the time being, his suicidal potential. This is of practical importance. While the patient is in the general ward during the few days after recovery of consciousness and before transfer to a psychiatric ward it is very seldom that any suicidal precautions need to be taken.

The relation of toxicological severity to psychological severity. The extent of physical damage is no criterion either of the seriousness of psychiatric illness or of the need for psychiatric care. This is a matter of great importance. Too often the decision to make a psychiatric assessment is allowed to depend on whether the patient is physically ill enough to require admission to a bed or a medical ward. When this is the case the psychiatrist is called in but if the patient is dealt with in the accident room of the hospital he may be allowed to go home without any psychological evaluation because consciousness has not been greatly impaired.

Tables 5 and 6 show that neither the index of endangering life (the patient's-eye-view of the overdose) nor the depth of coma on admission (the toxicological criterion) relate to the disposal in terms of psychological treatment required.

TABLE 5

Index of endangering life and disposal in percentage

	Predictable outcome			
	Death	Death probable	Death unlikely	Certain to survive
In-patient psychiatric care (131)	40	23	22	23
Out-patient psychiatric care (190)	30	45	40	39
No further psychiatric care (179)	30	32	38	38

TABLE 6

Depth of coma on admission and recommended psychiatric management of self-poisoning cases in 1968, in percentage (Matthew et al., 1969)

	Level of consciousness			
Disposal	Conscious or drowsy	Unconscious but responsive	Unconscious and unresponsive	All cases %
In-patient care	20	31	28	22
Out-patient care	36	38	34	37
Other	44	31	38	41
Total	100 (N=788)	100 (N=179)	100 (N=32)	100 (N=999)

This must be obvious. A patient who is forcibly prevented from taking more than three or four out of a hundred tablets is likely to be as psychiatrically disturbed as the patient who has swallowed them all. As the Ministry of Health report puts it in its recommendations (1968):

'All cases of deliberate self-poisoning should therefore receive psychological and social evaluation and help. The physical condition resulting from the poisoning is no indication of the extent to which such help is needed . . . . A psychological and social evaluation needs to be made whatever the motive may appear to have been without distinguishing between 'suicidal gesture', 'attempted suicide', and other such formulations.'

PART THREE

CLINICAL EVALUATION AND TREATMENT

We have needed this appreciation of the social and psychological setting in which self-poisoning acts occur, and of their motivation in order to study the clinical approach of the psychiatrist to the patient. The relationship of the psychiatrist's role to that of the physician is a curious one, unique in the calendar of medicine. For although the physician's intervention will have been life preserving and may have been life saving, it yet remains irrelevant to the prevailing illness or the underlying situation that generated the incident. To discharge the patient from hospital care at the point of physical recovery, therefore, without evaluating the psychological situation, is incomplete medicine. Put at its most crude, the mortality rate of poisoned patients from subsequent suicide is likely to be higher than the immediate mortality rate from the barbiturate poisoning itself. However, the aim of psychological intervention is not limited to the prevention of suicide. We have seen that the act occurs in a setting of intolerable distress and it is the duty of the doctor to discover the sources of that distress, whether they lie within the patient or in the social situation, and to try to alleviate them.

The necessary evaluation of every patient therefore consists in:
1. ascertaining the circumstances surrounding the ingestion;
2. assessing the psychological status of the patient at that time;
3. assessing the situation of the patient at that time, the pressures and stresses to which he was then subject;
4. determining the past and the current psychiatric history of the patient;
5. examining the psychological status of the patient after physical recovery.

To obtain this information it is necessary not only to question the patient but also to talk to at least one other person who can give an account of the patient at or about the time of the ingestion, in the immediate past and in the more remote past. The questioning of an informant in this way is standard practice in any psychological evaluation, since no one can give a complete picture of himself:

O, wad some Pow'r the giftie gie us
To see oursels as others see us!

In the particular circumstances of deliberate self-poisoning by barbiturates it is all the more important; the patient may have good reasons either for exaggerating or for concealing the true position. To omit to question an informant is always dangerous. The patient's own denial of suicidal intention, either at the time he took the tablets or at that moment, may be deliberate, so as to facilitate his discharge, thereby enabling him to take a further overdose.

It is advantageous to question the informant as soon as possible after the patient comes to hospital. Then he will be most forthcoming, perhaps because he sees the clinical situation as grave and presumes that any information he can give may assist the patient's chances. By the time the patient has recovered consciousness and is clearly no longer in danger, collusion sometimes occurs between the patient and his relatives to play down the whole situation so as to obtain speedy discharge.

We have found that the best procedure to adopt is for any accompanying relative to be asked to stay so that the doctor or social worker can take a history. If he knows little of the situation, or if the patient is not accompanied, a relative is asked to come, either forthwith, if it is during the daytime, or first thing the following morning if the admission is at night. For convenience it is also requested that any remaining tablets or containers be brought. The patient, however physically fit, does not go home until the relative is seen, unless there are very special circumstances, such as his being already well known to the hospital or the local authority services. Should the patient insist on leaving before the psychological situation has been explored it is proper to detain him against his wishes for a brief period until a relative can be found, in order to be satisfied that there is no suicidal risk. In practice such compulsory powers need seldom be used.

1. The circumstances surrounding the ingestion

The first thing that needs to be established is whether the barbiturates, in the quantity ingested, were deliberately self-administered or taken by accident. (The number of instances where there was deliberate administration by someone else is very small but from time to time this possibility has to be considered.) It frequently happens that the patient says the overdosage was accidental: 'I must have forgotten I'd taken them.' But diligent and persistent enquiry reveals that the poisoning was deliberate, once the patient's fear of criticism and even punitive action by the staff has been allayed. When it is made clear to the patient that the facts are required only to see how he or she can be helped, the true story is readily disclosed and he admits that he perfectly remembers taking all the tablets.

Those who deal with very many cases of barbiturate poisoning know that the so-called barbitutate automatism (e.g., Jansson, 1961; 1962) so beloved of coroners – the view that the patient took a normal dose of sleeping tablets, became confused and took more and so on – happens very rarely in clinical practice.

In any individual instance the conclusion that the tablets were taken accidentally should only be arrived at after very careful enquiry. It should certainly not be formed hurriedly by a casualty officer. Sometimes viewing the overdose as accidental is considered to be a kindness to the patient because it gives him the benefit of the doubt. It is no benefit, however, to a patient, to be discharged with his depression undiscovered and untreated, so that he may repeat the act. The overwhelming majority of overdoses in adults are deliberate.

The next circumstance to be discovered concerns the exact tablets taken and their number and strength. This information will also be required by the physician but, whereas he is only concerned with the quantity ingested, the psychiatrist needs also to know the number left untaken. Moreover, if someone takes a hundred tablets and is discovered by chance shortly after and if another does the same, but announces the event immediately to his family – 'See what I've done' – the physician will be faced by two patients equally intoxicated, but there is a wealth of difference in the interpretation of these acts. The psychological evaluation seeks to discover not only how much of what has been taken but also any steps taken by the patient to avoid or to ensure discovery. It is also necessary, once the patient is conscious, to try to find what he imagined would be the effect of his action. The possibility of more than one kind of tablet or drug having been taken simultaneously should not be overlooked, and frequently, as has been mentioned, barbiturates are taken by men who have already had a certain amount to drink.

2. *The psychological status of the patient at the time of the act*

This can only be determined by inference. The data required are: (a) the reports of those who last saw the patient or talked to him, concerning both his demeanour and his statements at the time, together with (b) a knowledge of how the patient took the tablets and what he did about it, and of course (c) the recovered patient's own account. Under the procedure advocated an informant will have been questioned already so that it is possible, when talking to the patient, to face him with any discrepancies between his account and the informant's. This need not be done in any spirit of criticism. Indeed, especially where there is a marital problem, there can be no assumption that the informant is right and the patient wrong. Nevertheless, circumstances certainly exist where the patient under-reports his depression, out of guilt or shame, or to be discharged so as to do it again. It is necessary then to mention to him that his wife says that he has been very miserable lately and so on: 'Isn't that so? Haven't you been more depressed than you say?' The opposite can also obtain; the patient, once she is sure that she is safe, makes the utmost of her situation in order to manipulate things to her maximum advantage. It may then have to be pointed out to her that her family say that she had seemed quite cheerful right up to the morning of the crisis day. Admission to the ward, having poisoned oneself, can be for instance a powerful weapon in bringing back errant boy-friends. The girls who resort to it are, all the same, very much distressed; in their despair they do something stupid and senseless, and it works. Should we judge them harshly on that score? Perhaps what we most resent is that, though there was probably a negligible risk to life, they are held by their circle of friends to have narrowly escaped death. They have had their drama; to us it only means work. But we can hardly expect our patients to have borne that in mind. The fact that they manipulate afterwards, however, should not lead us to assume that they took the tablets expressly in order to achieve this end.

Statements of intention to take tablets are very important, especially if they have been made just before the act. In our Edinburgh study 34% had communicated their intent; nearly everybody who had premeditated the act had done so. Commonly the warning goes unheeded (Table 7).

TABLE 7

Prior indication of intention, in percentage. This was given in connection with 175 acts (34%). There were no differences between the sexes.

Timing		Appreciation and action	
On the day	46	Not noticed	17
1–7 days before	16	Noticed but ignored	62
8–30 days before	6	Noticed and some action taken	21
More than a month before	32		

3. The situation of the patient at the time

It is important for the psychiatrist to obtain from the same sources a history of the patient's current life situation. If he was seeking to escape from some intolerable fix or some intolerable psychological pain the psychiatrist needs to know of it. He must determine whether that situation still continues. The very act of getting admitted to hospital with barbiturate poisoning often awakens the patient's entourage to his feelings and difficulties and sometimes the situation has taken care of itself without the psychiatrist's intervention. It must be said, however, that bedside reconciliations seldom last.

Here again the psychiatrist attempts to balance the patient's account (probably correct as to the stress on him) with the informant's (more likely to be correct as to fact). At the same time he is able to assess the sensitivity of the spouse or other informant to the patient's emotional needs.

This is probably the most important section of the history-taking.

4. The past and the current psychiatric history of the patient

It must go without saying that the psychiatrist needs to know the patient's history. He must know whether the patient is currently under psychiatric care, from his general practitioner or from a psychiatrist. If the tablets taken were intended for the patient's own use he needs to know why they were prescribed; more precisely, he needs to know the cause of the insomnia. He will also want to know whether other drugs are being prescribed for the mental state and if this is the case he will pass the information on to the physician, since not infrequently more than one type of tablet has been taken in overdosage.

He needs also to discover any past history of psychiatric illness, and in particular whether there have been previous episodes of self-poisoning or self-unjury and, if so, the details. He must also enquire for a history of drug dependence or of alcoholism. Enquiry of the patient's general practitioner is recommended for obtaining this information.

5. The psychological status of the recovered patient

When the patient is sufficiently conscious to permit proper psychological examination (and not before) the psychiatrist takes his history from the patient and conducts his clinical examination. The details of this examination do not differ from those of any psychiatric examination: it seeks to discover any abnormality in the functions of consciousness, cognition, affect, volition and reality testing, and if so what type of abnormality, and also to characterize the personality of the patient. The appropriate questions will be asked (see, *e.g.*, Mayer-Gross *et al.*, 1969) and any necessary psychological tests carried out.

However, the history-taking and the examination have some special features to which the psychiatrist may not be accustomed. In the first place, the patient is not seeking the consultation and may be afraid, ashamed, resentful, or hostile. He will have to be persuaded that it is in his best interests to let the psychiatrist take a hand in his future. In addition, the patient is at a time of crisis. This makes the impact of the psychiatric interview all the greater but it means that both patient and psychiatrist are denied the perspective that time might bring.

Lastly, the patient is usually in in a night-dress, pyjamas or dressing-gown, often not his own, if he is not actually in bed. This is hardly the appropriate clothing or position for a responsible discussion with a psychiatrist. These circumstances operate to increase his belief, not ill-founded, that the psychiatrist has the power to keep him there or, worse, to send him to a mental hospital.

The interview, then, needs to be conducted very gingerly. The psychiatrist will need to demonstrate that he is not in any way judging or criticizing his patient. Though the patient may have, by his own action, led to a great amount of medical work, no hint of this must appear. The reason for the psychiatric assessment is to see if any help can be offered to the patient. Any other approach will not lead to a medically useful conclusion. At present, regretfully, in some hospitals it appears that the only common ground between doctor and poisoned patient (they are often called 'poison patients' in such hospitals) is the wish that the patient should leave as soon as possible. This, though the collusion is covert, is speedily effected.

The psychiatrist must also know that, in very many circumstances, the enquiry and examination in the ward will be all the psychiatry that the patient needs or gets. The interview then must be therapeutic as well as diagnostic. Not only must the psychiatrist recognize the problems and try to seek a solution, but the patient must be led to do likewise. All in all the patient receives a very considerable dose of psychological treatment during his comparatively brief stay in the unit. This, which I have termed stösspsychotherapy – psychological treatment in a single massive dose – administered at a time of crisis, can be very beneficial.

Yet, in other instances, he is sowing the seeds of a more lasting relationship, letting the patient see that he is a helpful person, worth coming to for further treatment to continue to sort out his personal problems.

However, the psychiatrist needs at the initial interview to be more than usually firm. He cannot allow the patient to be discharged if there remains anything more than a slight suicidal risk and he cannot therefore allow the patient to evade examination. 'Acts have consequences,' I used to say to patients, 'and the consequence of your having taken an overdose is that we have to be satisfied you will not do it again if we can possibly prevent it.' The patient has to accept the truth, that his disposal will be decided by the psychiatrist. At the same time he has to know that the psychiatrist will act solely in his interests.

About a quarter of all patients in a poisoning treatment centre need to have a period of in-patient psychiatric care following the episode, and of the remainder a variable proportion, depending partly on local circumstance, will be asked to attend as out-patients. It is known (Matthew *et al.*, 1969) that only about half of these will actually keep their appointment and this fall-out from even a good service reinforces the need to establish the best possible relationship at the initial clinical interview.

Besides the immediate and the on-going psychological treatment of the patient himself it is very often necessary for the psychiatrist or social worker to work with the key relatives. Sometimes it needs to be pointed out very forcibly to insensitive partners just how much unhappiness their behaviour is bringing upon their spouses. Sometimes the boot is on the other foot and the patient's spouse needs help in dealing with the difficult patient with a personality disorder. Often there is a concatenation of social problems which seems overwhelming but them the social worker can help render manageable by getting the patient and his family to tackle them piecemeal. Often they have got into financial difficulty by not knowing their way about the intricate problems of rent, hire purchase, etc. In the subsequent treatment of poisoned patients social casework plays as large a part as psychological treatment.

PART FOUR

The organization of psychiatric services

Any plan for the organization of psychiatric services (including social work) for acutely poisoned patients has to be modified according to local circumstance. However, there are certain principles that must be adhered to if the patients are to receive proper care.

In the first place all poisoned patients must receive psychological and social assessment. Although this widely obtains for patients who are admitted to medical beds, there is still too much discretion placed on junior doctors in accident rooms or casualty departments whether or not to arrange such an evaluation. This is a responsibility they do not relish, nor, usually, have they the necessary data on which to form a judgment. Thus casualty officers should not be asked to form hasty opinions about whether poisoning has been deliberate or accidental, nor should they be encouraged to categorize the acts as 'attempted suicide', 'suicidal gesture', 'suicide bid' or some similar useless term. The reasons why not have already been presented. It is easier for them, and better medicine, to arrange a psychological and social evaluation in every case of self-poisoning. The few instances that are accidental can be sorted out by the psychiatrist when full information is available. The psychiatrist should not be asked to make his assessment before the patient is fully conscious.

Secondly, arrangements have to be made for an informant to be seen and for the patient to stay until this has been done.

Both of these place strains upon an accident room which may not have good facilities for patients to spend some time there – often difficult patients, still mildly intoxicated. Nevertheless, the number of cases of self-poisoning now occurring really demands that accident rooms be equipped with such facilities.

At the same time the psychiatrist must be prepared to come without delay when asked to do so. This point has been made by us for some years now and was recently echoed by Watson (1969). It also features in the Ministry of Health report (1968): 'Arrangements must be made for psychiatrists and social workers to be available every day of the week, whether these personnel are employed by the general hospital or detached for a considerable part of each day from the local psychiatric hospital'. The number of cases occurring renders it impossible to provide this service on an emergency call basis. Those responsible for hospital medical staffing must be prepared to implement this recommendation.

We have also drawn attention to the need for a social worker, who will in fact begin history-taking from an informant even before the patient is well enough to be interviewed.

Most of the logistic difficulties disappear when there is a psychiatric unit in the district general hospital where the accident room is located.

When the patient has to be admitted, there are good reasons from the point of view of toxicological management why all patients should go to a special unit. Psychiatric reasons support this. First, a good working relationship develops between the medical team and the psychiatric team, which is to the patient's benefit. Second, many of these patients, especially during the recovery phase, can be difficult to manage, aggressive, truculent, restless and seeking to leave. Many wards and many ward sisters find this intolerable and by their reaction they exacerbate the situation. A ward which is used to receiving numbers of these patients learns to take them for the most part in its stride. Even so, they do put a strain on the nursing staff and if there is a psychiatric team constantly there they can help morale in this important matter.

The psychological evaluation should be carried out while the patient is in the medical ward and not arranged as a subsequent out-patient psychiatric consultation. If the history-taking from an informant has been done in advance, the discharge of the patient from the acute medical unit need not be delayed by the psychiatric assessment, which can be made as soon as the patient is fit. This speedy service to a poisoning unit must be provided by the psychiatric team. If the patient requires further in-patient psychiatric care it should ideally be under the same team in the psychiatric wards of the same hospital. If this cannot be, and the patient has to be transferred to another psychiatric hospital, that hospital must accept him without delay; an acute poisoning treatment unit cannot function if beds are blocked by patients awaiting transfer.

If out-patient treatment is recommended this, too, should preferably be carried out by the same team, unless the patient is already in the care of another psychiatrist. The need for continuing psychiatric after-care is considerable, both to relieve distress and to prevent repetition. The first four months after discharge are the most important in this respect. The mental health resources of the local authority may also be brought to bear, particularly if the patient is known to the department.

When the patient is discharged a full report of the psychological evaluation and treatment must be sent to his general practitioner. Here there is scope for prevention, for the risk of allowing the patient further access to dangerous tablets, barbiturate or other, must be stressed. The family doctor might take steps to remove any unused stocks currently in the patient's home. Further prescriptions must be for small quantities only. Statements by the patient at any subsequent time, however vague, should be regarded seriously and are indications for further preventive action.

The acute event of barbiturate poisoning, it should be said once more, is an incident in a chronic psychological illness or social problem situation. The full and correct medical management (in the broadest sense) must operate to deal promptly and effectively with the present emergency and then go on to provide an extended service of treatment to deal with the protracted underlying cause. The efficient working together of a therapeutic team, comprising different specialities, to further this end is one of the most satisfying combinations in medicine.

ACKNOWLEDGMENTS

It gives me great pleasure to state my debt to Dr. Henry Matthew, and before him to the late Dr. J. K. Slater, to Mr. Wallace McCulloch and to Sister Parr and before her Sister Macfie and to numerous registrars, all of whom at various times have, by their encouragement, instruction and assistance, taught me so much of the content of this chapter.

REFERENCES

AITKEN, R. C. B., BUGLASS, D., and KREITMAN, N. (1969), The changing pattern of attempted suicide in Edinburgh, 1962–1967. *Brit. J. prev. soc. Med.*, 23, 11.

ETTINGLER, R. W. (1964), Suicides in a group of patients who had previously attempted suicide. *Acta psychiat. scand.*, 40, 363.

General Register Office (1968), A glossary of mental disorders. *Stud. med. popul. Subj.* 22.

GLATT, M. M., GEORGE, H. R., and FRISCH, E. P. (1965), Controlled trial of chlormethiazole in treatment of the alcoholic withdrawal phase. *Brit. med. J.*, 2, 401.

GREER, S. and LEE, H. A. (1967), Subsequent progress of potentially lethal suicides. *Acta psychiat. scand.*, 43, 361.

HAIDER, I, and OSWALD, I. (1970), Late brain recovery processes after drug overdose. *Brit. med. J.*, 2, 318.

JAFFE, J. H. and SHARPLESS, S. K. (1965), The rapid development of physical dependence on barbiturates. *J. pharm. exp. Ther.*, 150, 140.

JANSSON, B. (1961), Drug automatism as a cause of pseudo suicide. *Postgrad. Med.*, 30, A–34.

JANSSON, B. (1962), A catamnestic study of 476 attempted suicides, with special regard to the prognosis for cases of drug automatism. *Acta psychiat. scand.*, 38, 183.

KESSEL, N. (1965), Self-poisoning. *Brit. med. J.*, 2, 1265, 1336.

KESSEL, N. (1966), The respectability of self-poisoning and the fashion of survival. *J. psychosom. Res.*, 10, 29.

KESSEL, N. and McCULLOCH, J. W. (1966), Repeated acts of self-poisoning and self-injury. *Proc. roy. Soc. Med.*, 59, 89.

KESSEL, N., McCULLOCH, J. W., and SIMPSON, E. (1963). Psychiatric service in a centre for the treatment of poisoning. *Brit. med. J.*, 2, 985.

MATTHEW, H., PROUDFOOT, A. T., BROWN, S. S., and AITKEN, R. C. B. (1969), Acute poisoning: organization and work-load of a treatment centre. *Brit. med. J.*, 3, 489.

MAYER-GROSS, W., SLATER, E., and ROTH, M. (1969), Clinical Psychiatry, 3rd ed., Bailliere, Tindall and Cassell, London.

McCULLOCH, J. W., PHILIP, A. E., and CARSTAIRS, G. M. (1967), The ecology of suicidal behaviour. *Brit. J. Psychiat.*, 113, 313.

Ministry of Health (1968), Hospital treatment of acute poisoning. HMSO, London.

SHNEIDMAN, E. S. (1963), Orientations towards death: a vital aspect of the study of lives. In: R. W. White (Ed), *The Study of Lives*. Atherson Press, New York.

STENGEL, E. (1964), Suicide and attempted suicide, Penguin Books, London.

STENGEL, E. and COOK, N. G. (1958), Attempted suicide. Chapman and Hall, London.

WATSON, J. P. (1969), Psychiatric problems in accident departments. *Lancet*, 1, 877.

19. *social aspects of acute barbiturate poisoning*

J. W. McCulloch

SOME SOCIAL ASPECTS

It is necessary to begin this chapter with an apologia, since much of the available data concerning the social, sociological, and psychological aspects of self-poisoning covers *all* drugs. Kessel (1965) has pointed out that, in acts of self-poisoning, people of different ages tend to employ different methods, and that the use of barbiturates appears to increase with increasing age. He explains this trend by pointing out that insomnia is complained of more often as age advances and that, as a result of this, more barbiturates are prescribed for older people. However, since he has also made the point that self-poisoning tends to be an impulsive act, it would perhaps be difficult to make a convincing case to demonstrate that, apart from the factors which determine the 'availability' of a particular drug, there are factors which would distinguish those people who take overdoses of barbiturates from those who use any other type of drug. In essence, it is assumed that the social aspects of acute barbiturate poisoning will not be exclusive to overdosage of that particular family of drugs but will have much wider relevance.

THE DELAY IN SOCIAL RESEARCH

Research into the social aspects of attempted suicide has lagged behind research into the clinical aspects of this kind of behaviour. Stengel and Cooke (1958) pointed out that there was a general reluctance to carry out research into the phenomenon of attempted suicide and suggested that this was due to feelings of sympathy mixed with veiled contempt for unsuccessful undertakings. They advanced many reasons as to why attempted suicide should be studied as a behaviour pattern of its own and they maintained that, far from being a failed attempt at self-destruction, attempted suicide could frequently be seen as a plea for help to overcome difficult life situations or as a bid to influence personal relationships in such a way that life and not death would be the more desirable outcome of the act. They also pointed out that the studies which set out to investigate attempted suicide used the same retrospective techniques as were used in studies of completed suicide, with the result that the problems which beset the patient at the moment of the act of self-poisoning were difficult, if not impossible to understand.

Farberow and Shneidman (1961), on the basis of a statistical study which compared sociological factors involved in attempted and completed suicides, emphasized that it was wrong to combine attempted suicides and suicides, and call them both suicidal, without emphasizing a number of differences which may be extremely important.

Undoubtedly, it was the failure to acknowledge that these may be separate populations, although there may be overlaps, which caused research into this kind of behaviour to be so long delayed. If, as was for so long thought, suicide and attempted suicide were so closely related, it is indeed surprising that so little effort was made to investigate the circumstances which surrounded the attempts which did not succeed. Stengel and Cooke (1958) have described the psychiatric post-mortem investigations that had been carried out as being as frustrating as would be those on persons who had died from a physical illness but whose bodies were not available for dissection.

One of the main reasons for the delay in social investigation into acts of deliberate self-poisoning was the fact that many of the early investigations emanated from mental hospitals and were therefore sponsored almost exclusively by psychiatrists. This may also have accounted for the assumption that the attempted and the completed suicide were alike in all aspects save one – the fact of survival. If one assumes that not all persons who had deliberately poisoned themselves and lived, but only those who were most seriously psychiatrically sick, were admitted to mental hospital, then one can understand why investigations into this very select population showed that they resembled a group of persons whose deliberate self-poisoning had resulted in death.

The law also played its part in masking the size and the nature of the problem of suicidal behaviour, for until 1961 it was an offence to attempt suicide in very many countries, including England and Wales. This undoubtedly led to a good deal of 'covering up' by relatives and family doctors.

Another delaying factor was the view that suicidal behaviour was, *ipso facto*, evidence of mental illness. Because of this, it is likely that many attempts were hidden so that family members who had poisoned themselves would not be shut up in asylums – partly because of the stigma and also because many of them did not appear to be mentally ill on physical recovery from the effects of their action. This latter reason also tended to weight the severity of the illness of patients who were admitted to mental hospital, with the resultant perpetuation of the view that suicide and attempted suicide were the same phenomenon differing only in terms of success or failure. The size of the problem was minimized still further by the belief that there was a direct association between the quantity of drugs taken and the seriousness of the action. Persons who had not ingested a sufficient quantity of drugs to warrant hospitalization for treatment of the physical effects were not considered to be more than 'attention seekers' and were therefore not considered to be in need of psychological treatment either. Even now many patients admitted to general hospitals following acts of self-poisoning are discharged after physical treatment without any psychiatric or social screening. Kessel et al. (1963) pointed out that those who were referred to a psychiatrist by general physicians or surgeons tended to come from three groups of patients: those who patently remained suicidal, those who had seriously endangered their lives, and those with whose disposal the clinicians wanted help.

In the field of psychiatry, Wagner (1864) was perhaps the first person to deviate from the conception that suicidal behaviour could be equated with mental illness, but even he opined that suicide was probably a hundred times more common in mentally diseased than in mentally sound people. Morselli (1881), supported by Masaryk (1881), introduced the idea that suicide could result from 'the difficulties of practical affairs' and was not necessarily symptomatic of mental illness. From these three studies a new dimension appeared – the influence of environmental factors. No statistical studies concerning the influence of social factors resulted, however, until that of Durkheim (1897) when he produced the results of his systematic sociological research into the phenomenon of suicide. He was not concerned to discover the circumstances that lay behind suicide in individual cases, but tended to concentrate on those factors which affected society as a whole. He concluded that the incidence of suicide in any society would be the outcome of inter-related social causes and that suicide was necessarily a collective phenomenon. He studied the relationship of suicide rates to environmental factors; to the effects of race and heredity; to the process of imitation; and to many other factors, including cosmic ones. He came to the conclusion that, in order to understand the problem, one must look to dynamic social factors rather than to isolated individual motives. This conclusion was based on his finding that where social solidarity is strong there is little suicide, and where it is weak there is more. He was able to demonstrate increased rates of suicide during periods of economic stress when social cohesion was low, and decreased rates among societies, especially religious ones, where common beliefs and practices hold their members together. In the compilation of his comparative tables, however, he perhaps placed too much reliance on reported incidence rates at a time when there was a very high possibility of faulty reporting and of 'covering up' for religious and other reasons. His finding that isolation and detachment from the group was conducive to suicide has received much support in many more recent studies but one could argue with some of his findings on many grounds. It is important, however, to remember that almost three-quarters of a century have passed since Durkheim made his magnificent contribution to the study of suicidal behaviour.

The work of Sainsbury and Barraclough (1968) has shown that immigrants, as a group, are more at risk for suicide than the native population, and one must therefore question the 'protection of the cohesive minority' suggested by Durkheim (1897). Methodologically it is a dangerous procedure to relate, for example, decreased rates of suicide in time of war to high social cohesion, since it is virtually impossible to interpret pre-death behaviour in the face of enemy action. It would be impossible, for instance, from the evidence available to distinguish between persons killed in air-raids who wanted to go on living and those who did not or who were indulging in the kind of 'Russian roulette' described by Stengel (1964) by leaving the outcome of an air-raid purely to chance and refusing to take any precautionary action. Nevertheless, Durkheim's work and his systematic approach clearly led the way in the study of the social aspects of suicidal behaviour. Despite all his efforts, investigations in the early part of this century continued to lack method and to ignore the part played by social influences. It was not until 1925 that researchers really sought to investigate the possibility of motive being something other than directed by physical or mental ill-health. Mosdzien (1925) did look for motives in the areas of 'conflict with the law' and 'financial distress'. However, his main hypothesis concerned the relationship between suicide and physical disease and not unnaturally this was the aspect that received most of his attention.

The second quarter of the twentieth century saw the first of the comparative studies between suicide and attempted suicide, and Halbwachs (1930) showed that there were almost twice as many attempts as there were completed suicides. He demonstrated parity of incidence between the sexes for attempted suicide but, for completed suicide, a sex ratio of two males to one female. Despite his findings, Halbwachs, like most of his predecessors, still grouped suicide and attempted suicide under the common heading of suicidal behaviour, with the inference once more that the dividing line between the two groups was simply the difference between success and failure. However, he did take a major step forward when he suggested that 'suicidal behaviour' could be regarded as due on the one hand to nervous disturbance with organic cause, and on the other to a 'disturbance of balance caused by social factors'. He did not suggest that there was any association between these two groups and the two groups of 'success' and 'failure'. The main implication was that both the latter groups lay somewhere along the same continuum with causes common to both, the most frequent being mental illness.

Among the earliest works which investigated attempted suicide exclusively was that of Stelzner (1906) who showed that more than 15% of the patients in her study displayed no psychiatric symptoms but concluded that although no illness was apparent during the post-suicide attempt interview, a cathartic effect must have occurred in the 'violent discharging of the suicidal act'. She did, however, tentatively suggest that in some cases there were motives which, of themselves, appeared to be sufficient explanation of the act. Her finding that patients who, on recovery, displayed no psychiatric symptoms were not mentally ill compares favourably with the much more recent findings reported by Kessel (1965), but he argued rather differently when he said: '... the diagnosis of a psychiatric condition must be made from positive features. These are detected either from the history or on clinical examination. If all the information about the patient's mental state at the time of his act, obtained both from him and from an informant, does not indicate any departure from normal, and if clinical examination after physical recovery fails to reveal any significant disorder, then there are no grounds for concluding that the patient is mentally ill.' Kessel further postulated that distress drove people to poison themselves but that distress was not the exclusive province of the mentally ill.

SOCIAL FACTORS IN ATTEMPTED SUICIDE

One of the first British studies of attempted suicide was that carried out by East (1913) on 1,000 male admissions to Brixton prison following suicidal attempts. He compared this highly selected group with studies of completed suicides. By virtue of the location of his study all females were excluded as were, presumably, persons suffering from the more severe forms of mental illness. It is hardly surprising that in differentiating the groups he concluded that mental disease caused more suicides and alcoholism more attempted suicides. It is of interest that Menninger (1938) referred to alcoholism as 'chronic suicide' while Kessel and Grossman (1961) began their paper with the words 'many alcoholics kill themselves' and went on to demonstrate an extremely high rate of suicide among alcoholic persons admitted to mental hospitals — 75 to 85 times the expected rate for males of the same age in Greater London. The part played by alcohol in suicidal behaviour has been well documented by Zmuc (1968). Although he was reporting a study conducted in Jugoslavia, the author provides some 48 international references on the topic. However, East (1913) observed and documented social factors which he regarded as being important in the causation of suicidal acts. Since this time, many researchers have shown that there are associations between social factors and attempted suicide, and these have been reviewed by McCulloch and Philip (1967). This review looked at the various social factors involved under the several headings of: emotional problems (papers on jealousy, anger, spite, and hate); problems involving close interpersonal relations (comment and writings on such aspects as broken homes, marital disharmony, amatory problems, and bereavement); and problems involving the wider social sphere (problems of finance, crime, loneliness, and alcohol). The authors of this review concluded that, although the factors associated with suicidal behaviour included social ones where these were present, they were frequently multiple and often of long standing. They postulated that the presence of interacting social factors often told more about the patient's personality than about the motivation for the act itself; and they ended with the caution that it is dangerous to accept that there is a causal relationship between social and other factors, frequently referred to as 'precipitants', and suicidal behaviour. They stressed the point that, although patients may be prepared to say 'I did it because . . .', the interpretation of motive and intent may still have to be inferred. It is easier for a person so distressed as to poison himself to produce a motive from a real-life stress situation than have to admit to himself that he did not really know why he had behaved as he had done. Suicidal behaviour is usually impulsive and many persons who behave this way never truly formulate their intention or think carefully about the possible outcome of their act. It becomes imperative, therefore, to know more about the kind of person who indulges in this impulsive behaviour and about the social milieu in which he lives. Imperative because, if research is to have any real value in the study of suicidal behaviour, it must have as its aim prevention. This is particularly important in view of the fact that the trends reported for attempted suicide over the last decade or so have been in a markedly upward direction (Sclare and Hamilton, 1963; Kessel, 1965; Parkin and Stengel, 1965; Bridges and Koller, 1966; Ellis *et al.*, 1966; Kessel and McCulloch, 1966; Evans, 1967; Graham and Hitchins, 1967; Whitlock and Schapira, 1967; Aitken *et al.*, 1969; *Brit. med. J.*, Leader, 1969).

Primary prevention must, of course, be extraordinarily difficult to effect, but secondary prevention, it is hoped, will become much more of a practicable proposition. That is to say, it may be possible to identify persons who, having attempted suicide and recovered, will be more likely than others to repeat this dangerous behaviour, and to ensure that their behaviour is to some extent controlled in so far as it is of a suicidal nature.

THE INFLUENCE OF SOCIETY ON HUMAN BEHAVIOUR

Generally speaking, individuals are controlled by the society (and sub-society) to which they belong. This control begins with the network of training practices and social learning through which they become 'socialized' at an early age and which is normally maintained so that their behaviour as adults is also controlled. According to McDavid and Harari (1968), these sources of control are both external and internal. The external sources include such practices as direct reward and punishment from adults, other authorities and peer groups, and threatened retribution. These agents help to control the child's early social learning by the provision of models to demonstrate appropriate behaviour as well as by rewarding or punishing.

It could be postulated that, on the one hand, if the sources of external control are faulty and/or the models are missing, then internal control will become less complete while, on the other hand, if the model of appropriate behaviour includes behaviour which diverges from the modal behaviour of the society in which the individual lives, there may be a perpetuation of the 'learned' deviant behaviour.

The internal sources arise from the social training which is intended to make the individual accept society's standards as his own. These include 'learned' rewards and values, the wish to behave in socially acceptable ways, and the development of a 'conscience'. Again, if the internalized controls are incomplete or at variance with the concept of a modal personality, impulsive behaviour or a pattern of behaviour may occur which is different from the norm, and often not acceptable.

Durkheim (1897), looking at the society in which an individual lives in order to try to provide explanations for suicidal behaviour, underestimated the possible value of studying, individually as well as collectively, persons who had behaved in this way. For, while society shapes the individual, the individual also helps to shape society.

In addition, as we shall see, an understanding of the society in which individuals live can be achieved by quantifying the data concerning individuals who present with a particular behaviour pattern such as attempted suicide. According to McDavid and Harari (1968), environmental conditions surrounding a particular social system often operate to produce certain uniformities in the conditions of social learning and the kinds of experiences from which individual members of a society learn their values and behavioural habits. The same processes, within a given social system, which are involved in socialization and in the development of personality – training practices, family structure and kinship systems, religious beliefs and practices, moral values, the law, political systems and social desirability – are all mutually interdependent and it appears that they must not be split if we are ever to discover the true motivation for suicidal behaviour.

Within each sub-group of a larger society smaller systems of socialization occur and, while an overall set of practices and values still operates for the majority of its members, particular sub-sections may evolve their own patterns. This is especially true of social class sub-groups. It is also true that within societies and sub-societies it is possible to discern individual behaviour differences, and Fig. 1 shows a conceptual scheme of the relationship between socialization, personality, and behaviour, including suicidal behaviour.

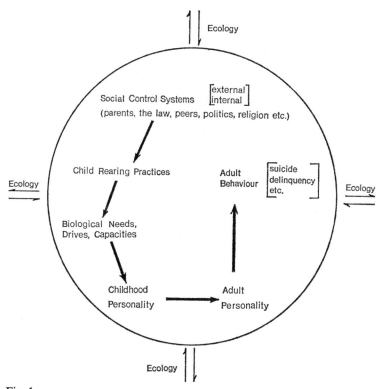

Fig. 1.

The effects of childhood deprivation

Writers as varied in their theoretical outlook as Freud, Jung, and the early behaviourists such as J. B. Watson placed great store on early relationships within the family. Other writers, among whom Bowlby (1940; 1956; 1960 and 1969) is the most noted, have concerned themselves with the effects of maternal deprivation and the emotional problems of early childhood. There are also many works dealing with disturbances in parent/child relationships. These have been well reviewed by Clarke and Clarke (1960) and Casler (1961). The former authors stressed two main types of deprivation. The first is, in nature, socio-economic and cultural and therefore shows wide variations in time and place, and the second includes five distinct forms of deprivation. These are social isolation, cruelty and neglect, institutional upbringing, adverse child-rearing practices, and experiences of separation. Among the factors which they consider relevant in deprivation are the duration and intensity of the experience, previous experience of similar deprivation, the age at occurrence, and other aspects which can be thought of as being influenced by the personality of the child at the time. In their summary they offer four main conclusions. First, there are considerable differences in vulnerability. Second, individuals show varying degrees of recovery even from very severe deprivation. Third, gross deprivation such as prolonged isolation usually has profound psychological effects. Last, they comment on the 'amazing resilience of the young human being to tolerate wide variations in its early experience'.

In the course of prolonged and varied studies of suicidal behaviour in the city of Edinburgh during the period 1958 to 1966, cases were uncovered by the author which appear to go a long way towards demonstrating the effects of cruelty, neglect and adverse child-rearing practices. Later, it will be shown that there is value in quantifying data such as is graphically shown in the two abbreviated case histories that follow, which show that, despite the resilience of some children to adverse early experiences, others are much less fortunate.

The case of Mrs. H. R.

This patient's first of many admissions to the Poisoning Treatment Centre at the Royal Infirmary of Edinburgh was at the age of 20. She was the fifth child in a family of eight. She had taken an overdose of barbiturates while intoxicated. Although at the time of her first admission both her parents were alive and living together and she had spent her entire childhood and adolescence living with them, her history revealed that within the nuclear family there was much evidence of social disorganization. The effects of this on the patient were evidenced in many ways. As a child she frequently played truant and was often kept off school to help with domestic chores, not always because her mother was ill. Interestingly, the patient's own children have truanted and also have had many absences from school because of her frequent domestic and social troubles. Her parents have both been at odds with the law and the patient herself has had many appearances in court for breach of the peace. She has also been placed on probation for endangering the lives of her children while attempting to gas herself. Following this attempt her children were removed to 'a place of safety'. Although Mrs. H. R. was never herself involved in a road accident, one of her children, then aged two, was knocked down and injured by a car some two miles from home.

Since her first admission to the Centre in 1962, Mrs. H. R. has been admitted on 15 other occasions, all of them following acts of self-poisoning or gassing or self-inflicted injury or severe drinking-bouts. Although on some of her admissions this patient was clearly depressed, the underlying diagnosis was that of 'psychopath with habituation to alcohol and drugs'.

Prior to Mrs. H. R.'s first admission, an elder sister had been admitted to the Poisoning Treatment Centre on four occasions following acts of self-poisoning, the last one being fatal.

The case of the White family

Fig. 2 shows the pedigree of a family which demonstrates even more graphically than the case of Mrs. H. R. how a peculiar child-parent relationship can be handed down from generation to generation. The first generation of this remarkable family showed no psychopathology on the female side until the grandmother of our series poisoned herself. In the grandfather's family, however, there was much evidence of social disorganization, alcoholism and mental illness. Indeed, one of his sisters has spent some 65 years in a hospital for the mentally sub-normal. Her admission followed involvement in a road accident in which her mother was killed. The great-grandfather remarried and none of the children of his first marriage had a good or satisfying relationship with their stepmother. The grandfather, who had been treated frequently for alcoholism and alcoholic psychosis, was the first of three generations to be admitted to the Poisoning Treatment Centre of the Royal Infirmary of Edinburgh. The second generation consisted of nine children, one of whom (A) died in infancy. Only one of the remaining eight children has not (to date) been admitted (F). In addition, the spouses of two of the second generation have also indulged in behaviour of a suicidal nature. The daughter of (C) was the first and to date the only member of the third generation to be admitted to the Unit. By the time she was 16 years old she and her mother were both cohabiting in the same house. The mother's cohabitee was also well known as a frequent patient in the Poisoning Treatment Centre. The third generation patient had poisoned herself following a row with her cohabitee, who had also been previously admitted to the Unit following a fracas in prison when he was stabbed by a fellow inmate. In all, the 12 members of this family who have indulged in suicidal behaviour have, between them, done so on more than 40 occasions. The last episode concerning second generation (C) was fatal. Of the first and second generations there have been, in addition to these acts of self-poisoning, many hospitalizations for lengthy periods for alcoholism and mental illness, and imprisonment for acts of crime. It is likely that in indirect help (hospital, prison, cost of rearing children in children's homes, etc.) this family has been a charge on the state to the extent of approximately one hundred and fifty thousand pounds. Since its work record is almost non-existent, it is probable that, direct grants from the Ministry of Social Security and other sources taken into consideration, the cost to the country will have exceeded half a million pounds sterling.

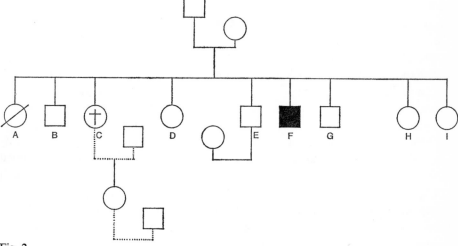

Fig. 2.

PATHOLOGICAL PERSONALITY AND SOCIAL PATHOLOGY

In addition to these two cases there have been many instances of parent and child admissions to the Poisoning Treatment Centre in Edinburgh. In the course of one year approximately 6% of the patients admitted had a close relative who had also attempted suicide or was to do so subsequently. From the records of 118 such relationships it was found that between them there had been at least 218 episodes of suicidal behaviour of which 17 had resulted in death. Clinical diagnoses were only available for 100 of the cases involved and of these 61 were diagnosed as having abnormalities of personality, compared with only 31% found in the study carried out in the same Unit by Kessel (1965). Forty-four of this group were alcoholics or habituated to drugs, compared with only 25% of the Kessel series. As was found in the two cases quoted in detail, a high incidence of 'pathological personality' was found in this group of patients and many of the families concerned displayed severe psycho-social pathology: alcoholism, neglect, brutality, delinquency and crime. In the main these were people who grew up in an environment in which impulses are not merely fantasied but real because they are acted out. Petty crime, prostitution and many other forms of degradation are witnessed as part of daily living. These people have been reared in a world where actions speak louder than words; where impulsiveness is dominant; and where people live from day to day with weak ties to a meaningful past and little investment in the future. To this way of life it is nearly certain that we must now add 'suicidal behaviour'.

These cases and other clinical studies such as that of Kreitman et al. (1969) have pointed to the importance of parent/child relationships in the study of suicidal behaviour and it is felt that they are quite consistent with the sociological model (Fig. 1) discussed earlier. From the many works concerning the emotional development of children which have been reviewed by Clarke and Clarke (1960) and Casler (1961) there is strong evidence to suggest that disturbances in the child/parent relationship have a profound effect on the child.

More specific to the present work, Leese (1969) found that 75% of the adolescents in her study of attempted suicide were diagnosed as having a personality disorder, while 60% of her sample 'had an unnatural or unhealthy background'. Philip and McCulloch (1966) demonstrated very high correlations between the incidence of attempted suicide and the incidence of repeated attempted suicide, overcrowding, children taken into care, contact (as a child) with the Royal Scottish Society for the Prevention of Cruelty to Children, vandalism and juvenile delinquency. These correlates were derived from 'cold' statistical data and the technique used in the analysis was typically sociological. It does not necessarily follow that information so gathered and analysed tells more than that certain areas are characterized more than others by the high incidence of the variables examined. However, McCulloch and Philip (1967) showed that persons who had been admitted to the Poisoning Treatment Centre of the Royal Infirmary of Edinburgh following a suicidal attempt manifested these same variables to a remarkable degree (see Table 1).

TABLE 1

Social indices present in a group of patients admitted consecutively to the Poisoning Treatment Centre of the Royal Infirmary of Edinburgh following attempted suicide*

	Males (n = 36)	Females (n = 59)	Both sexes (n = 95)	Both sexes: Lifetime rates per 1,000 patients	Both sexes: annual city rates per 1,000 persons at risk
Repeated attempted suicide	15	27	42	442.12	0.45
Overcrowding	10	18	28	294.74	106.00
Prosecutions	22	17	39	410.53	39.60
Children in care	9	10	19	200.00	3.38
School absences (not sickness)	24	41	65	684.21	2.07
Referrals for cruelty to children	4	6	10	105.26	6.57

* The rates for this population are incomplete lifetime rates and the annual rates for the city are shown only as a guide. We know of no other comparative data for our indices. We also point out that with the exception of school absences and repeated attempted suicide the indices seldom occurred more than once. The observed rates for each of the indices shown in the table are strikingly high.

Men had more prosecutions than women (Chi square = 9.6375, 1 d/f., p = 0.002). Men and women played truant in approximately equal proportions but there was a tendency for women to have been kept off school for domestic reasons more often than men.

The same authors (Philip and McCulloch, 1967) used the same variables to construct a scale of social pathology and related these to the Personal Illness (PI) and Character Neurosis (CN) scales of the Symptom Sign Inventory (Foulds, 1965, 1967) and the NSQ or Neuroticism Scale Questionnaire of Scheier and Cattell (1961). Using the PI scale it was found that only 12% of their sample of 84 patients could be classified as normal; 56% were identified on the CN scale as being character neurotics and the remaining 32% were found to be personally ill but not character neurotics. They found that the patients who scored highest in 'social pathology' were not more personally ill than those who displayed fewer of the social indices but that they did have more features of character neurosis.

Kessel (1965) stressed the importance of assessing the personal relationships and social backgrounds of persons who had poisoned themselves, as have the majority of the reports listed earlier which were concerned with the fast rising rates for this kind of behaviour. All of these reports have stressed the growing demand on the social services as well as on the medical and psychiatric services. It is somewhat surprising that, until recently, little use has been made of the standardized psychological tests in cases of attempted suicide, despite the fact that the importance of psychological factors (as opposed to illness entities) has been long recognized and despite the mass of evidence of the many studies that have related childhood experiences to the development of adult personality. From a treatment point of view, both psychiatric and social, it is

necessary to have some understanding of the internal resources which can be har-
nessed. The neglect of this area is the more surprising in the face of the widely differing
'opinions' regarding the diagnostic categories used by psychiatrists. This fact has been
discussed at length by Philip and McCulloch (1970). Philip (1969*a* and 1969*b*) has
made a most valuable contribution in an effort to redress this imbalance. He has
shown, among many other very interesting findings, that the patients who constituted the cohort he studied were more hostile than the normals or neurotics, especially
in their expression of extra-punitive attitudes. This finding is consonant with those of
McCulloch (1965) and of Kessel and McCulloch (1966), which showed that physical
violence towards their wives by male attempted suicides was very common, especially
among a group who had indulged in this type of behaviour on more than one occasion.
Philip (1969*a*) pointed out that, while attempted suicides are prone to 'act out' and to
be critical of other people to the point of being deluded, they nonetheless displayed
considerable self-criticism and guilt. He has also provided evidence that, compared
with normals, attempted suicides are somewhat anxious, very introverted and rather
lacking in social conscience. This finding agrees with the earlier study of Philip and
McCulloch (1968), and one can see all of these factors displayed in the case study of
Mrs. H. R. presented earlier in the chapter.

Cattell (1964) believed that anxiety was a disorganizing force or a symptom of disorganization rather than a drive or a motivating force, and this formulation is very
meaningful in the light of the evidence presented here regarding the clinical and social
findings about persons who 'act out' in a suicidal fashion. Philip's (1969*a*) findings
coupled with those of McCulloch and Philip (1967) regarding the high rates of various
types of social disorder in attempted suicide again suggest that some aberrations in
early child/parent relationships are involved. Philip (1969*a*) was careful to point out
that 'just as clinically there is no suicidal personality, so also is there no unique test
profile for persons who attempt suicide'. He pointed out that impulsiveness and poor
interpersonal relationships, high anxiety and hostility, though common in attempted
suicide, were not exclusive to it. Nevertheless, sufficient evidence exists to suggest that
there may be groups of people who may one day be identifiable as persons more prone
to suicidal behaviour than others.

SOCIAL DISORGANIZATION

As part of the Kessel (1965) study, the major precipitating factors for attempted
suicide in a series of 511 patients were examined and the table of his findings is reproduced here as Table 2.

It can be seen from Table 2 that not only are the items listed evidences of social
disorganization but they may also be evidence of the presence of, for some patients, an
unstable personality. Kessel's study offered further evidence of this disorganization by
showing that of the married patients in his series 85% of the men and 68% of the
women disclosed 'frequent hostility' with their partner and that the clinical assessment

TABLE 2

Major precipitating factors; percentages of approximately 165 males and 350 females (except for marital disharmony and forced separation, which are based on 68 married males and 147 married females) (from Kessel, 1965)

	Males	Females
Marital disharmony	68	60
Drinking problems	51	16
Financial difficulties	44	31
Unemployment	34	18
Kin disharmony	28	30
Isolation	15	
Crime	15	
Housing difficulties	14	19
Difficulties at work	14	
Love affairs going badly		16
Forced separation	12	

* More than one factor might be present. Factors occurring in less than 10% of cases have been omitted. They included bereavement, gambling and sexual problems.

of the 'state of the marriage' was 'poor' or 'bad' for 57% of the men and 43% of the women. Kessel also made the point that, where patients were single, relationships with key persons were equally bad (or worse) by showing that 70% of the men and 59% of the women got on badly with the principal figure in their life situation. 'This bad relationship with the key individual – spouse, other relative, or friend – was the dominant theme in the story for nearly every patient, whether narrated by himself or by an informant. More than any other factor it provided the setting for the self-poisoning act. Yet in many cases it but set the seal on a life pattern characterized by adverse circumstances – a bad work record, chronic debt, and constant changes of home, often the product of separations.' Kessel further suggested that this pattern of instability might be a repetition of parental experience. He based this on the finding that under the age of 15 years 28% of the patients in his series had had mother absent; 43% had had father absent; and 21% had had both parents absent. This finding follows very closely with that of Bruhn and McCulloch (1962). Even allowing for the findings of parental absence among 'normal' families shown by Munro (1969), the findings of the two studies quoted for attempted suicide for parental absence in childhood are extremely high. McCulloch (1965), in a follow-up study of Kessel's (1965) cohort, was concerned to investigate 'the social consequences of acts of deliberate self-poisoning'. He found that there were significant relationships between some of the demographic characteristics of the cohort and changes in their social state. The findings in this study were based on information gathered from 98.6% of the cohort four months after the act and from 99.6% of it after a period of one year. The results of the McCulloch (1965) study are presented as follows.

Demographic variables

For both sexes there was a statistically significant tendency for patients who were under 35 years old at the time of their self-poisoning to show more improvement socially than those from the older age groups. Patients with extant marriages were found to show improvement of their social state more often and deterioration of it less often than was the case for all other civil states. For men, social class appeared to have no bearing on subsequent social state, but women from social class three showed improvement more often than women in the other social classes and deterioration as frequently as women from social classes one and two but only half as frequently as women from the other two social classes. Patients whose work record had, at the time of their attempted suicide, been classified as 'fair' were found to have improved in their social state more often than those with better or worse work records. Patients who were not living in homes of their own at the time of their admission to hospital showed a worsening of their social state more often than those who had been living in homes of their own. Of the men in the cohort who did not have extant marriages, those who had been living with their parents or other relatives or friends showed more changes both for better and for worse, but manifested improvement in their social state more than twice as frequently as men who had been living alone. The follow-up findings for women did not reach the statistical significance of those for the men, but there was a definite trend for women who lived with their parents to show more frequent social improvement than other women from the Kessel (1965) cohort.

Clinical variables

Two of the variables used by Kessel (1965) – 'relationship with key person' and 'index of life endangerment' – showed no statistically significant relationship with observed changes in social state. Patients who had poisoned themselves with salicylates produced a greater proportion of patients whose subsequent social state changed for the better than patients who had used other drugs. Patients whose attempt was concerned with bad interpersonal relationships showed more social change (in either direction) than those whose motive for poisoning themselves had been more concerned with material things. For the most part, these subsequent changes were for the better. The social change of patients of both sexes who had changed in their mental state at the time of the follow-up visits ameliorated twice as frequently as the social state of those patients whose mental state had remained unchanged. For women, but not for men, there was a significant association between the classification 'character disorder' and changes in social state. Women who had been classified as 'psychopaths' deteriorated socially almost twice as frequently and improved socially only half as frequently as women who had been diagnosed as having some other form of character disorder or no character disorder at all.

Precipitating factors

Of the 11 factors listed in Table 2, which had been considered to have been factors which had 'precipitated' the act of self-poisoning, only two yielded statistically significant associations with subsequent change in social state. One of these, 'disharmony with kin', was associated with improvement in the social state of women but not of men, while the other, 'gambling', applied only to men and was associated with a much greater degree of social deterioration when it was present than when it was not. Work problems, unemployment, financial problems, bereavement, crime, alcohol, housing problems and sex problems, while having been associated frequently with the attempt, had no apparent relationship with subsequent social adjustment.

Subsequent changes in the patient's behaviour

On follow-up, when patients appeared to have altered their behaviour for the better, when they were more settled, contented, and better able to cope with everyday living, particularly the stresses which had been associated with the attempt, their social state had improved more often and deteriorated less often than that of patients whose behaviour had not changed in these ways. Also significant, though to a less striking extent, was the improvement in the behaviour of key persons in relation to the social state of patients without extant marriages.

Where a key person's behaviour, as it related to infidelity, pathological jealousy, drinking, gambling or getting into debt, changed for the better, the social state of the patients concerned improved twice as often and deteriorated less often than in the cases where the key person's behaviour had not shown any improvement in the period following the attempted suicide.

The manipulative aspects of attempted suicide are well known and have been well discussed by Stengel (1964) and others. However, the results of the author's follow-up study (McCulloch, 1965) indicate that, although change in the key person's behaviour was closely related to subsequent social change in the patient, the changes in the patient's own behaviour appeared to have the greatest influence on changes in social state. Improvement was usually found to be related to the fact that patients appeared to have found a new ability to discuss their problems with the key person in a more calm and constructive way. It appeared that successful manipulation took place when the patient rather than the key person changed his behaviour.

SOCIAL PROGNOSIS AND PREDICTIVE FACTORS

The prognosis of psychopaths and other character disorders, in terms of repeated acts of self-poisoning and subsequent completed acts of suicide, is not good (Kessel and McCulloch, 1966). Their chronic inability to maintain any improvement in their behaviour (McCulloch, 1965) is also reflected in the fact that of the 14% of Kessel's (1965) cohort who deteriorated socially between the two follow-up periods more than half were character-disordered.

Having made a previous attempt at suicide is perhaps the best single indicator of subsequent suicidal behaviour, whether such behaviour is fatal or not (Kessel and

McCulloch, 1966; McCulloch *et al.*, 1967; Philip and McCulloch, 1969). Kessel and McCulloch (1966) found that the patients most prone to repeat the act were those who, apart from having a prior history of attempted suicide, had been diagnosed as having a personality disorder, especially psychopathy, were dependent on alcohol or drugs, and had poor work records and unstable living conditions. Both socially and clinically these patients are difficult to treat and, despite increased understanding of the motivation for suicidal behaviour, the incidence of it continues to rise (Evans, 1967; Graham and Hitchins, 1967; Aitken *et al.*, 1969). When it is also realized that a very high proportion of patients – 15 % in one year and 25 % in three years – are readmitted to hospital following a further suicide attempt, the full realization of our inability to offer lasting treatment to those patients who behave in this way becomes painfully apparent, and any simple method of identifying 'high risk' patients must be of value. Glueck and Glueck (1950) and Mannheim and Wilkins (1955) have shown that a few factors relating to a person's past experience can be so combined that his future behaviour can be predicted. In the light of the evidence produced by McCulloch (1965), Kessel and Mc Culloch (1966), and McCulloch and Philip (in press), it seemed reasonable to suppose that patients who repeated their suicidal acts might be distinctive in some social aspects. Working from the follow-up study conducted by the author (McCulloch, 1965), Buglass and McCulloch, 1970, conducted a study designed to develop and validate scales which would predict future suicidal behaviour in a population who had already behaved in this fashion on at least one previous occasion. The scales were constructed separately for each sex. From the Kessel (1965) cohort it was verified that, after a period of three years, men and women showed markedly different correlates of repetition of suicidal behaviour. Only the four following items significantly discriminated male repeaters from non-repeaters: (1) diagnosis of alcoholism; (2) alcohol taken at the time of the act; (3) presence of violence in the relationship with a key individual; (4) for the widowed, divorced and separated, recent loss of partner, *i.e.*, within the preceding three months.

For women the following 11 items were found to be statistically significantly related to repetition of acts of suicidal behaviour: (1) previous psychiatric treatment; (2) current psychiatric treatment; (3) previous episode of attempted suicide; (4) diagnosis of psychopathy; (5) diagnosis of drug addiction; (6) four or more dwelling changes in the past five years; (7) poor or neutral relationship with their children; (8) fair, poor or bad work record (as opposed to excellent or good); (9) separation of six months or more from mother when under ten years old; (10) separation of six months or more from father when under ten years old; (11) presence of violence in the relationship with the key individual.

A scale for men was constructed by allocating one point for the presence of each of three items: (1) violence in key relationships; (2) diagnosis of alcoholism; (3) having taken alcohol at the time of the act. The fourth item was not included because it referred to a very small proportion of the men. There were nine items included in the scale for women: (1) previous attempted suicide; (2) previous psychiatric treatment;

(3) psychopathy; (4) drug addiction; (5) four or more dwelling changes in the past five years; (6) father absent when patient under ten years old; (7) mother absent when the patient was under ten years old; (8) poor work record; (9) violence in a key relationship. The item referring to the relationship with children was excluded since it could not be scored for the childless, and current psychiatric treatment had such a high degree of overlap with present psychiatric treatment that it also was omitted. A slightly shorter scale of seven items was also constructed for women by omitting items 8 and 9. Only 13% of the men who scored 0 on the three-point scale showed further suicidal behaviour within three years compared with over 50% of those who scored the maximum of three. For the women, there was a steady increase in the probability of repetition as the score increased. Women who scored 0 or 1 had a probability of under 10% of further suicidal behaviour, while those who scored four points or more had a one in two chance of repetition. For practical purposes the scales were simplified by dividing the scores into three sub-categories with a low, a medium, and a high risk of repetition. For men, these sub-categories were 0 = low, 1 or 2 = medium, and 3 = high. For women the sub-categories were divided in the following manner: 0 or 1 = low, 2 or 3 = medium, and 4, 5, 6 or 7 = high.

Because it is of more immediate clinical concern, the proportion of patients exhibiting suicidal behaviour within one year of their key admission was calculated using the same scales. Even within this shorter period it was found that the scales did distinguish between the low, medium, and high risk groups. It was also found that patients who killed themselves had similar risk scores to those who indulged in non-fatal suicidal behaviour, and the scale could not distinguish between these two groups.

There appears to be little doubt that the characteristics of patients who were admitted to the Poisoning Treatment Centre of the Royal Infirmary of Edinburgh during 1962–63 can be combined in such a way that predictions can be made about their subsequent suicidal behaviour, but, to be of practical use, predictive scales must be shown to be equally applicable to other groups. In order to test the predictive value of the scales created, they were validated on patients admitted to the Poisoning Treatment Centre during 1967 and followed up for a period of twelve months after their admission. Despite the very marked increase in the number of admissions to the Centre between the two periods of study, the proportion of repeaters remained remarkably constant. It was found that, for men, the scales had lost much of their predictive power but that those for women had remained predictive for the new cohort.

Many researchers who have studied suicidal behaviour are agreed that the influence of factors in the environment has a profound effect on the development of the personality of the person who behaves in this very dangerous and alarming manner. This does not mean that similar environmental influences have no effect on people who do not indulge in this kind of behaviour; it simply means that an effort has been made to identify a group of people who behave in a particular way. People who have behaved in a suicidal manner have come under scrutiny in an effort to find a way to prevent the act from occurring.

Kessel (1965) has shown that 41 % of the men and 64 % of the women in his study had a recognizable psychiatric illness. Other researchers in this field have shown similar figures and some have shown the sickness rates to be much higher among people who behave suicidally. By no means all of these persons have personalities which could be described as abnormal, and yet they too have attempted to take their own lives. It is necessary therefore to turn now to consider the social aspects of mental illness to try to find out if it is possible to consider the group of people who attempt suicide as a generic group. That is to say, is it possible to show some relationship between environmental influences and the genesis of mental illness which could explain the behaviour which is common to the group who are ill, the groups who have abnormalities of personality, and the group who, though they have attempted suicide, are considered to be 'normal'? It is possible that the behaviour of the last group can be understood completely in relation to faulty interpersonal relationships. Kessel (1965) suggested that for this group it was necessary to concentrate upon 'personal relationships in their social setting', and the author in his follow-up study (McCulloch, 1965) found that, among the group categorized by Kessel (1965) as having no psychiatric illness, social betterment after the act was very much dependent on the improvement of close interpersonal relationships.

SOCIOLOGICAL THEORIES OF MENTAL ILLNESS

Many social and sociological concepts have been used to explain the clinical aspects of mental disorder, and these have been outlined and discussed in the writings of Faris and Dunham (1939); Clausen and Kohn (1954); Jaco (1954); Dunham et al. (1966); Srole et al. (1962); Hollingshead and Redlich (1953); Hollingshead et al. (1954); Scott (1958); and many others. Whatever the psychiatric categories of illnesses used in the study of suicidal behaviour, there are sociological theories which can be offered in explanation of the illness and Schneider (1953) believed that these factors could be classified into a few categories. Mental disturbance, he believed, stemmed from: the individual's inability to meet role demands; membership of an under-priviliged group; forced abrupt transition from one social situation to another; disorganization of a social system; inability to attain social acceptance; subjective or objective mobility in the social class structure; incompatible values; and social isolation. There is a remarkable similarity between these categories and the list of precipitating factors shown in Table II.

From the facts and theories given thus far, there appears to be some doubt that mental illness *per se* can precipitate suicidal behaviour. Not all mentally ill persons do behave in this way. Equally, not all persons who attempt suicide are mentally ill. But all people who behave suicidally appear to have many social factors in common. It seems therefore that, if suicidal behaviour is to be fully understood, one must examine very carefully the social and developmental aspect of persons who behave in this way in addition to examining any mental illness which may also be manifested.

The reader may recall that the examination of these factors was very long delayed by a seeming insistence that suicidal behaviour could only be understood in terms of mental illness. Indeed, the study of suicidal behaviour in social terms is of comparatively recent origin. Scott (1958) has discussed many of the social aspects which have been outlined and has suggested that it appears likely that 'a reformulation of some of the macro-societal differences in micro-social terms will suggest genotypes which are not readily discernible at the grosser levels of empirical correlation. Even if these do not provide causal explanations for many of the psychological manifestations which accompany mental disorder, they may at least expand the field of enquiry in directions which could eventually yield more basic understanding of the nature of mental health and mental illness.' — And suicidal behaviour?

This chapter was begun with an apologia and perhaps should be ended with an apology. It is the author's belief that the reader might have been better able to follow the development of the argument presented in pursuit of a dynamic theory for suicidal behaviour had Schneider's (1953) classification of mental illness been used as an introduction. It was felt, however, that the information imparted would have greater impact if it could be shown that by approaching the subject from a clinical viewpoint, and following the emergent social and psychological leads, some substance for sociological theory would result.

REFERENCES

AITKEN, R. C. B., BUGLASS, D. and KREITMAN, N. (1969), The changing pattern of attempted suicide in Edinburgh 1962–67. *Brit. J. prev. soc. Med.,* 23, 2, 111–115.

BOWLBY, J. (1940), The influence of early environment. *Int. J. Psycho-Anal.,* 21, 154–178.

BOWLBY, J. (1956), *Maternal Care and Mental Health.* WHO, Geneva.

BOWLBY, J. (1960), Chapter in *Psychoanalytic Study of the Child.* Int. Univ. Press, New York.

BOWLBY, J. (1969), *Attachment and Loss.* Vol. I, Attachment. Hogarth Press, London.

BRIDGES, P. K. and KOLLER, K. M. (1966), Attempted suicides; a comparative study. *Comprehens. Psychiat.,* 7, 240–247.

British Medical Journal (1969), National Poisons Information Service: Fifth Annual Report for the year ended 31/12/68. *Brit. med. J.,* 3, 408.

BRUHN, J. G. and McCULLOCH, J. W. (1962), Parental deprivation among attempted suicides. *Brit. J. psychiat. soc. Work,* 6, 186.

BUGLASS, D. and McCULLOCH, J. W. (1970), Further suicidal behaviour: The development and validation of productive scales. *Brit. J. Psychiat.* 116, 483-491.

CASLER, L. (1961), Maternal deprivation: a critical review of the literature. *Monog. soc. res. Child Dev.,* 26, 2.

CATTELL, R. B. (1964), Psychological definition and measurement of anxiety. *J. Neuropsychiat.,* 5, 396–402.

CLARKE, A. D. B. and CLARKE, A. M. (1960), Some recent advances in the study of early deprivation. *J. Child Psychol.,* 1, 26.

CLAUSEN, J. and KOHN, M. (1954), The ecological approach in social psychiatry. *Amer. J. Sociol.,* 60, 140–151.

DUNHAM, H. W., PHILLIPS, P. and SRINIVASAN, B. (1966), A research note on diagnosed mental illness and social class. *Amer. sociol. Rev.,* 31 (2), 223–227.

DURKHEIM, E. (1897), *Le Suicide.* Alcan, Paris; Free Press, Glencoe, Ill.

EAST, W. N. (1913), On attempted suicide with an analysis of 1000 consecutive cases. *J. ment. Sci.,* 59, 428.

ELLIS, G. G., COMISH, K. A. and HEWER, R. L. (1966), Attempted suicide in Leicester. *Practitioner*, 196, 557–561.

EVANS, J. G. (1967), Deliberate self-poisoning in the Oxford area. *Brit. J. prev. soc. Med.*, 21, 97.

FARBEROW, N. L. and SHNEIDMAN, E. S. (1961), (Ed). *The Cry for Help*. McGraw-Hill, New York.

FARIS, R. E. L. and DUNHAM, H. W. (1939), *Mental Disorders in Urban Areas*. Univ. Chicago Press, Chicago.

FOULDS, G. A. (1965), *Personality and Personal Illness*. Tavistock, London.

FOULDS, G. A. (1967), Some differences between neurotics and character disorders. *Brit. J. soc. clin. Psychiol.*, 6, 52–99.

GLUECK, S. and GLUECK, E. (1950), *Unravelling Juvenile Delinquency*. Mass.

GRAHAM, J. D. P. and HITCHINS, R. A. N. (1967), Acute poisoning and its prevention. *Brit. J. prev. soc. Med.*, 21, 108.

HALBWACHS, M. (1930), *Les Causes du Suicide*. Alcan, Paris.

HOLLINGHEAD, A. B., Ellis, R. and KIRBY, E. (1964), Social mobility and mental illness. *Amer. soc. Rev.*, 19, 577–591.

HOLLINGSHEAD, A. B., and REDLICH, F. C. (1953), Social stratification and psychiatric disorders. *Amer. soc. Rev.*, 18, 163–169.

JACO, E. G. (1954), The social isolation hypothesis and schizophrenia. *Amer. soc. Rev.*, 19, 567–577.

KESSEL, N. (1965) Self-poisoning. *Brit. med. J.*, 2, 1265–1270; 1336–1340.

KESSEL, N. and GOSSMAN, G. (1961), Suicide in alcoholics. *Brit. med. J.*, 2, 1671.

KESSEL, N. and MCCULLOCH, J. W., (1966), Repeated acts of self-poisoning and self-injury. *Proc. roy. Soc. Med.*, 59, 89–92.

KESSEL, N., MCCULLOCH, J. W. and SIMPSON, E. (1963), Psychiatric service in a centre for the treatment of poisoning. *Brit. med. J.*, 2, 985.

KREITMAN, N., SMITH, P. and TAN, E. S. (1969), Attempted suicide in social networks. *Brit. J. prev. soc. Med.*, 23, 116–123.

LEESE, S. M. (1969), Suicide behaviour in twenty adolescents. *Brit. J. Psychiat.*, 115, 479–480.

MCCULLOCH, J. W. (1965), *The social consequences of acts of deliberate self-poisoning or self-injury*. Unpublished M. Sc. dissertation. Univ. Edin. Library.

MCCULLOCH, J. W., HENDERSON, A. S. and PHILIP, A. E. (1966), Psychiatric illness in Edinburgh teenagers. *Scot. med. J.*, 11, 277–281.

MCCULLOCH, J. W. and PHILIP, A. E. (1967), Social factors associated with attempted suicide: a review of the literature. *Brit. J. psychiat. soc. Work*, 9, 30–36.

MCCULLOCH, J. W. and PHILIP, A. E. (1967), Social variables in attempted suicide. *Acta psychiat. scand.*, 43, 341–346.

MCCULLOCH, J. W. and PHILIP, A. E. (1970), The social prognosis of persons who attempt suicide.

MCCULLOCH, J. W., PHILIP, A. E. and CARSTAIRS, G. M. (1967), The ecology of suicidal behaviour. *Brit. J. Psychiat.*, 113, 313–319.

MCDAVID, J. W. and HARARI, H. (1968), *Social Psychology*. Harper and Row, New York.

MANNHEIM, K. and WILKINS, L. (1955), *Prediction Method in Relation to Borstal Training*. HMSO, London.

MASARYK, T. G. (1882), *Der Selbstmord als sociale Massenerscheinung der modernen Zivilisation*. Vienna.

MENNINGER, K. A. (1938), *Man Against Himself*. Harrap, London.

MORSELLI, H. (1882), *Suicide; An Essay on Comparative Moral Statistics*. Appleton, New York.

MOSDZIEN, K. (1925), Beitrag zur Lösung des Selbstmordproblems. Ein Vergleich von Motiv mit pathol. anat. Befunden. *Deutsche Z. ges. gerichtl. Med.*, 6, 53.

MUNRO, A. (1969), The theretical importance of parental deprivation in the aetiology of psychiatric illness. *App. soc. Studies*, 1, 81–92.

PARKIN, D. and STENGEL, E. (1965), Incidence of suicidal attempts in an urban community. *Brit. med. J.*, 2, 133–138.

PHILIP, A. E. (1969a), The development and use of the hostility and direction of hostility questionnaire. *J. Psychosom. Res.* (In press).

PHILIP, A. E. (1969b), Personality characteristics of attempted suicides in Edinburgh. Paper read at the 5th International Conference for Suicide Prevention, London.

PHILIP, A. E. and MCCULLOCH, J. W. (1966), The use of social indices in psychiatric epidemiology. *Brit. J. prev. soc. Med.*, 20, 122–126.

PHILIP, A. E. and McCULLOCH, J. W. (1967), Social pathology and personality in attempted suicide. *Brit. J. Psychiat.*, 113, 1405–1406.

PHILIP, A. E. and McCULLOCH, J. W. (1968), Some psychological features of persons who have attempted suicide. *Brit. J. Psychiat.*, 114, 1299–1300.

PHILIP, A. E. and McCULLOCH, J. W. (1970), Test-retest characteristics of a group of attempted suicide patients. *J. consult. clin. Psychol.*, 34, 144.

SAINSBURY, P. and BARRACLOUGH, B. (1968), Differences between suicide rates. *Nature (Lond.)*, 220, 1252.

SCHEIER, I. H. and CATTELL, R. B. (1961), *Handbook for the Neuroticism Scale Questionnaire.* Institute for Personality and Ability Testing, Champaign, Ill.

SCHNEIDER, E. V. (1953), Sociological concepts and psychiatric research. *Interrelations between the Social Environment and Psychiatric Disorders.* Millbank Memorial Fund, New York.

SCLARE, A. B. and HAMILTON, C. M. (1963), Attempted suicide in Glasgow. *Brit. J. Psychiat.*, 109, 609–615.

SCOTT, W. A. (1958), Research definitions of mental health and mental illness. *Psychol. Bull.*, 55, 29–45.

SROLE, L., LANGER, T. S., MICHAEL, S. T., OPLER, M. K. and RENNIE, T. A. C. (1962), *Mental health in the metropolis: The Midtown Manhattan Study*, Vol. 1. McGraw-Hill, New York.

STELZNER, H. (1906), *Analyse von 200 Selbstmordfällen.* Karger, Basel.

STENGEL, E. and COOK, N. G. (1958), *Attempted Suicide.* Chapman and Hall, London.

STENGEL, E. (1964), *Suicide and Attempted Suicide.* Penguin, Harmondsworth.

WAGNER, A. (1864), *Die Gesetzmässigkeit in den scheinbar willkürlichen menschlichen Handlungen vom Standpunkt der Statistik.* Hamburg.

WHITLOCK, F. A. and SHAPIRA, K. (1967), Attempted suicide in Newcastle upon Tyne. *Brit. J. Psychiat.*, 113, 423–434.

ZMUC, M. (1968), Alcohol and suicide. *Alcoholism*, 4, 1.

20. *poisons information service and barbiturate poisoning*

H. L. Verhulst and J. J. Crotty

Sources from which information regarding poisons may be obtained are variously named throughout the world. In the United States and Canada they are described as Poison Control Centers; in Europe the term Poisons Reference Service, Poisons Information Center, Poisons Information Bureau or Poisons Information and Treatment Center are employed; in Australia, Poisons Information Service is the designation. Barbiturates are but one of the substances about which information may be sought; hence this chapter will not concentrate on barbiturates but will deal with information in general. The variation of polarity among the centers towards information or treatment makes adequate discussion of them difficult. However, despite the great variety of emphasis and experience, there are many common problems and some common solutions. Although this chapter relies heavily on the poison control activities in the United States, many of the problems can be shared and compared beneficially.

The 562 poison control centers in the United States, coordinated by their respective State Health Departments, virtually assure many variations in operational procedures. So far, the growth pattern and variability of operations have been healthy. This review furnishes an opportunity to re-examine poison control activities and perhaps improve their future development.

Europe, unlike the United States, has placed more emphasis on the planning of treatment centers to develop personnel and facilities to care for poisoned patients. There has been less endeavor to provide information on the very wide variety of toxic products. The very few established treatment centers are to be found in large hospitals, rich in clinical experience, and located in densely populated areas. Each country developed its own system of treatment and information but somewhat similar programs evolved, this process being hastened by the founding of the European Association of Poison Control Centers.

BACKGROUND

The rapid technological advances which occurred in the period after World War II resulted in the synthesis of a large number of new chemicals and a capacity to produce them. Many of these found their way into the formulas of medicine and of common household items – and many of these formulas had multiple trade names. A physician treating a patient who had ingested one of these products frequently found himself in a position where he could obtain no toxicity data. Often, even the manufacturer did not have this information.

In the United States, the pediatricians were the first medical specialists to fully appreciate the problem since it was chiefly children who were unknowingly experimenting with the wide variety of household products and medicines available in their homes. Therefore, in order to provide the information which the physician needed, and to learn more about the problem in general, the 'poison control center' was inaugurated. The first center established in the United States in 1953 saw its primary function to be the provision to physicians of ingredient and toxicity information on household products and medicines ingested by children, and to suggest treatment. Additionally it would keep records of the type of inquiries which were made to the center and assume the leadership in planning community education programs to prevent ingestion accidents among children (Verhulst and Cann, 1960). Sixteen centers had been established in major metropolitan areas by 1956. Most were established by the pediatric services of the children's centers in the area. New York City, the only exception, was placed in the City's Health Department. The operation of all the centers was fairly uniform. The chief of the pediatric service generally served as the director. The resident physicians staffed the service and answered requests for information. The hospital assisted in purchasing necessary texts, journals and special reference material. The descriptions of the activities of the early centers made it clear that the program was utilized mainly by physicians treating acute ingestions in children.

The poison control movement attracted much publicity with resultant popularity throughout the nation. Because of this, many local civic organizations, along with medical and paramedical groups, encouraged the establishment of a poison control center in their local hospitals. Unfortunately, in some instances the local hospital had insufficient personnel to perform the necessary functions. The community might have had better service had it concentrated on improving the emergency treatment facilities, and utilized a neighboring center in one of the larger medical centers for informational services.

Many European countries, in the light of American experience and perhaps influenced by better overall communications, have opted for severe restriction in the number of information centers. This restriction obtains in France; in the United Kingdom there are only four official centers; Switzerland has only one information center; there are, however, many in the Netherlands.

THE RECIPIENT OF INFORMATION

When considering the development of a poison information service, it is necessary that a determination be made as to the users of the program. The original concept was that the center would supply information to the physician for the recommended treatment of his patient. However, progressively more centers have adopted a policy of accepting calls from the general public. A review of 800 cases of ingestions reported to the Poison Control Center, Boston Children's Hospital (Robb *et al.*, 1963) demonstrated the desirability of having a source of information available to the public. In the study of 800 cases, it was determined that 36% required no treatment, 29% had home treatment recommended, and 31% were treated at the hospital; there were no data on the remaining 4%. With the shortage of physician manpower in most communities, a service which can handle 65% of the suspected emergencies by a telephone call is indeed worthwhile. Nor can we overlook the time and cost saved to the patients, many of whom might have had to travel considerable distances.

The common rebuttal to recommendations that poison control centers should take public calls is that the parent is not capable of treating a poisoning. This is certainly correct. It is seen in the above study and borne out in other surveys that, in many instances, the product ingested is not dangerous in the quantity taken. The center can inform the individual that no action is necessary – a poisoning has not occurred; or that poisoning has occurred, in which event the patient should then go immediately to his physician or nearest hospital for treatment. Under certain circumstances, first-aid instructions such as the use of an emetic or dilution should be recommended. The center should also caution against actions which are contra-indicated, such as the induction of vomiting when a lye preparation is involved. Unfortunately, a great emphasis has been placed on the need for quick action, often without stressing the need to obtain information as to what that action should be. The ready availability of accurate information can assure proper action in a minimum of time.

In some countries, however, the information available at the center has been provided in confidence by the manufacturer. Thus it is not available for dissemination to the public. This obtains in Britain, where the service will only give information to medically qualified persons, but in most European countries information is given directly to the public.

OPERATION

The type of personnel staffing a poison information center will vary in accordance with the users. The pharmacist and trained nursing staff have performed an excellent service in many centers where there is a high percentage of requests involving childhood accidents. They are capable of making the determination as to the hazard and supplying this information to the physician or parent. When treatment is necessary, a physician must be contacted. In some areas, trained non-professionals have performed an excellent service. These personnel are often likely to be permanent staff members who gain considerable knowledge from the great number of episodes in which they are involved. There must, however, always be a medical consultant on call to discuss the treatment for the poisoned patient with the physician requesting data. Ideally, a clinical toxicologist should be available, failing which there should be several consultants representing the various specialties of medicine, even though they may be called infrequently.

Operation of an efficient poison information center is not inexpensive. It requires staffing at all times, a system for reviewing current literature on new treatment, for filing pertinent information, and for an evaluation by professional staff of literature to determine selected and carefully reviewed references which can be cited when necessary. Specialists must be available to discuss clinical conditions if non-physicians are used during hours when the center receives minimal use. The information center can expect queries concerning possibilities of chronic poisoning even though the basic emphasis is placed on the acute type. A university medical center or a training hospital is best suited to conduct the activities of the poison information center. Indeed, they are mandatory when more than routine treatment is needed. Since the public benefits from the program participation by a governmental agency is necessary.

The poison control center concept has now been established throughout the world. The general expansion has almost paralleled the expansion within the 50 states of the United States. This has assured diverse types of operation. However, any program instituted should be appropriate to the needs of the community. The responsibility for the organization of the activity should be vested jointly in those governmental offices responsible for public health and in the medical profession of the community. Continuity of program personnel is probably the most important item for a successful center and this can best be fulfilled when continuous funding is assured. This is not always possible when the operation of the center is conducted on a voluntary basis.

THE OPTIMUM SERVICE

Few persons can retain an interest in a program if this program is utilized little or not at all. They quickly divert their talents to other activities. For this reason, it is desirable that an information center should service an area which can assure fairly constant requests for information. The benefits are twofold: the physician seeking information benefits from the center's expertise and the center personnel gain knowledge from discussion of the case. The input of information must include not only data gained from review of the written scientific literature but the clinical symptoms, dosage levels, and success of treatment obtained from actual cases. Where telephone communication is poor, as in some areas, the poison information center has rectified this situation through the use of short-wave radio communication.

Treatment of poisoning combines several equally important aspects. Perhaps the most essential ingredient is rapid, effective, initial treatment or first aid. Beyond this, the general treatment of the poisoned victim requires continuously available treatment encompassing knowledge of the substances ingested and the symptoms they might produce (Adams, 1963). The need for a bibliography is questionable when coping with the severely ill patient. This is not the time to sift and sort the pros and cons of a particular dialysis solution, for example. The evaluation of a mode of treatment must be a studied appraisal of information absorbed from the literature from day to day. The bibliography review and literature search must already have been done, and then tailored to the clinical condition of the patient.

EMERGENCY TREATMENT SERVICES

It is easy to visualize the continued growth of poison emergency treatment centers. Three essentials of such centers are: preparedness to institute appropriate immediate therapy; ability to direct the patient to a more definitive source of care when necessary; and a system to forward the preliminary epidemiologic data to those responsible for that phase of the control program. Improvement in the ready availability of information for the doctor in practice and for the emergency room staff makes possible immediate information on about 80% of ingested substances. The expense and technical knowledge necessary to provide the additional information around the clock strongly suggest that major information centers should be considered on a regional basis.

STORAGE AND RETRIEVAL OF INFORMATION

There has been much debate as to the type of retrieval system which should be used to obtain information. The use of automatic data-processing equipment for the retrieval of information is possible. Pilot programs are already being investigated in several nations of the world; they are, however, expensive to design and operate. While such programs are being developed and perfected, we must continue to distribute information. A manual file system can be assembled which will adequately serve most information centers. The material should be filed by the name by which a product is most commonly referred. In the United States, this is usually the trade name. A separate card with concise data for the immediate treatment should be developed for each formulation. The physician should not be expected to review data on four or five chemicals used in a formulation and attempt to make a judgment on the effects of the poisoning. Once the emergency treatment is administered, more detailed information should be available on all constituents in the formulation. We in the United States have produced our material on a 5″ × 8″ card which is easily filed and allows enough space for the data if we use both sides of the card. The major complaint received is that the card is removed from the file and not replaced.

The poison information center should be able to present a concise summary of the latest treatment or treatments as derived from current literature and evaluated by its professional staff. The center should not be considered a library, expected to have a bibliography of all articles on barbiturate poisoning, and to be able to furnish copies of such articles. The volume of medical literature has increased to a point where it is impossible for any one individual to review it all. It is necessary, therefore, that the information service arrange to receive input from members of the various specialties with different interests who read the specialty journals and can call an article to the attention of the center's staff. Some articles may add little to the existing literature but will serve to confirm what has been previously reported. The center personnel can gain additional information by requesting a clinical resumé on cases about which they are consulted when the case report would appear to have incomplete data. Such case reports are frequently not published. Many cases of poisoning will be routine and reports are of value mainly for preparing statistical tables on the incidence.

PROPAGANDA ON PREVENTION

Prevention of accidental poisoning in children would, of course, eliminate the need for treatment. A comprehensive three-year education project conducted in Charleston, South Carolina, demonstrated that through such a community-wide program, hospitalizations due to poisoning among children could be reduced (Maisel and Jenkins, 1964). The poison control center personnel should take an active part in developing community preventive programs. They are constantly aware of the products involved in poisoning. They know the seriousness of the poisonings. They are respected within the community, and their programs will be enhanced by appearing before civic groups; by supplying interesting case reports to the news media, illustrating the causes involved and techniques for prevention of accidental poisoning; and by appearing on radio and television.

TABLE 1

Country	Total enquiries 1968	Percentage of enquiries regarding barbiturates
Australia	7,655	25.3
Canada	38,900	2.8
Finland	1,444	2.2
Scotland	1,110	1.3
Switzerland	5,403	approx. 7.0
United States of America	60,021	2.5

THE INCIDENCE OF ENQUIRIES REGARDING BARBITURATES

The number of enquiries can in no way reflect the incidence of a particular form of poisoning. Also, at least two-thirds of episodes relate to ingestion by toddlers, who are much more likely to take substances other than barbiturates. However, the experience of the poison control centers in certain countries is noted in Table 1.

REFERENCES

ADAMS, W. C. (1963), Poison control centers: their purpose and operation. *Clin. Pharmacol. Ther.*, 4, No. 3, 293.
MAISEL, G. and JENKINS, M. (1964), Poison control is poison prevention. *J. S. C. med. Ass.*, 60, 354.
ROBB, G. L., ELWOOD, H. S. and HAGGERTY, R. J. (1963), Evaluation of a poison center. *Amer. J. publ. Hlth.*, 53, 1751.
VERHULST, H. L. and CANN, H. M. (1960), Poison control activities in the United States. *J. Amer. pharm. Ass.*, 21, 123.

21. the prevention of acute barbiturate poisoning

M. Govaerts-Lepicard

In countries where poison control programmes exist, prevention occupies a most important place. The epidemiological studies which follow should help to demonstrate the importance of these preventive measures. Clearly the admission of intoxication cases to hospitals, as well as the gathering of information from poison control centres or information services, can enable important details to be brought out. Information obtained about the victims and the circumstances of the poisonings helps to develop effective preventive programmes. Epidemiological studies are still more useful in dealing with special types of intoxication, such as that by the barbiturates.

EPIDEMIOLOGY OF BARBITURATE INTOXICATIONS

It is easy to determine the number of barbiturate intoxications as a proportion of all poisoning cases, but it is difficult to estimate their absolute number and very few studies give enough details to be of much value in prevention projects.

The following sources of data are the tools that the epidemiologist can use:

a. Reports of deaths and official statistics of mortality, despite their lack of precision and their evident limitations, certainly underestimate the figures. This is because all deaths, whether by poisoning or not, are insufficiently studied to allow of exact diagnosis, as Sunshine (1967) judiciously points out. It is also well known that, particularly in suicidal death, the doctor may be induced, out of respect for the relatives' feelings, to keep in the shade the true cause of death.

b. Thorough medico-legal investigations (Banciu and Droc, 1966; Eliakis et al., 1967) are undertaken in only a small number of cases and do not lay much stress on the circumstances relating to the fatal poisoning.

c. Hospital statistics in some countries only include intoxications severe enough to justify a short period in hospital. Theoretically this allows a history to be taken to bring out important epidemiological information, but unfortunately, except in wards specializing in clinical toxicology, the information usually collected is very inadequate.

d. The epidemiologist can analyse calls received by information centres to determine the incidence of inquiries regarding a particular agent. However, it must be recognized that the system of consultation by telephone does not permit a very thorough inquiry and it is to be regretted that much valuable information is not gathered, even if a system of inquiry by a follow-up letter is established. This accounts for the poverty of most information found in the literature. Nevertheless, hospitals and information centres can be valuable sources of information which qualitatively, if not quantitatively, are representative, provided some precautions are taken at the beginning of the inquiry. It is important to realize that every study of a prevention programme with epidemiological research in view requires precise information regarding the victims and the environment in which poisonings occur.

BARBITURATES IN POISONING STATISTICS

It is striking that, in spite of the important and constant increase in the number of non-barbituric hypnotics and tranquillizer drugs on the market, barbiturates maintain a privileged position in poisoning statistics, particularly as a means of attempted suicide.

Specialized adult hospital wards (Vedrine, 1965; Gaultier et al., 1968; Roche, 1968; Thys et al., 1969; and Matthew et al., 1969) mention 30–50% of patients as suffering from acute barbiturate poisoning. The rate is higher in hospitals where only very seriously ill patients are admitted. Curry (1965) reported that 10% of all acute medical admissions to hospitals in Great Britain were due to acute poisoning. In paediatric wards, the number of barbiturate poisonings is generally less significant; this is easy to understand as accidental poisoning is much less frequent than deliberate poisoning. However Gomez-Orozco and Santiago-Castanon (1966) stated that 12% of poisoning cases in children's wards were due to barbiturates, and Van Heyst (1966) showed that they are the second commonest product swallowed by children under ten.

Statistics of poison information centres, founded on inquiries or on the reports received, give very variable rates: in Finland, Visakorpi (1967) stated that sedatives and anti-epileptics accounted for 2.2% of cases reported; the National Clearinghouse for Poison Control Centres of the United States gave the figure for 1968 for barbiturates as 2.46% of all reports for adults and 0.41% for children under five. Canadian annual reports indicated that 5.01% of all enquiries regarding adult cases in 1963 were due to barbiturates and 3.70% in 1967; for children, the rates were respectively 1.47% in 1963 and 1.01% in 1967.

At the information centre of the Fernand Widal Hospital in Paris, barbiturates were concerned in 8% of all calls, and in the Belgian Poisons Information Centre the figure was 3.81%.

Certain comments can now be made: the importance of barbiturate intoxication among all poisoning is quantitatively limited, still more so if accidental poisoning is considered. On the other hand, ingestion of barbiturates remains one of the principal causes of hospitalization for poisoning, even among children in some countries (Wechselberg, 1967). Qualitatively, therefore, this group of drugs has evident importance. The chances of death following admission to hospital have become very slight due to expert treatment: for example, in Paris 2.5% of very serious cases result in death (Gaultier *et al.*, 1968) and in Edinburgh, 0.6% of all barbiturate poisonings (Matthew *et al.*, 1969). However, Banciu and Droc (1966) have shown that in Rumania, out of 2,175 medico-legal investigations, more than 50% of the fatal cases due to drugs were of barbiturate origin.

Severe intoxication, now very much less often fatal owing to the great improvement in general hospital care and the increasing number of specialized wards and qualified staffs, justifies a more extensive epidemiological study.

As we did not find in the literature sufficiently detailed information about the victims and the circumstances of the poisoning, we have undertaken a study directed towards the prevention of this specific form of poisoning. Since they are limited to one country, we recognize that our results will inevitably reflect local characteristics; however, it will be evident in the conclusions that some situations are not special to Belgium.

AN INQUIRY ABOUT THE CIRCUMSTANCES OF BARBITURATE INTOXICATIONS

This inquiry was held by the team of the Belgian Poison Control Centre during the year 1969. The material studied was taken from two series of cases.

The first are barbiturate poisonings arising from calls received at the Information Centre. It appeared very soon that the majority were suicide attempts and only a few were accidents, the victims in the latter case usually being children. That is the reason why we have associated with our inquiry the study of cases nursed in children's wards in Brussels and in Antwerp. At first we thought that the reason the number of calls received at the Information Centre was rather low lay in the fact that clinicians needed no information about this kind of intoxication. We were surprised to find only a small number of cases in the hospital wards; hence we extended our study for a longer period. At hospital it is easier to ask the family for all the desired details; on the other hand, the number of cases resulting from inquiries to the Information Centre is higher, and so the statistical study of circumstances is larger for that group.

ANALYSIS

The first study refers to 5,314 calls received at the Information Centre between 1 January 1969 and 31 August of the same year. Amongst these, 202 victims, representing 3.81%, had swallowed a barbiturate alone or with other products. It is perhaps useful to remember that drugs are incriminated in 48% of all calls. Two facts clearly emerge: firstly, most of the calls concerning barbiturate poisoning are due to suicide attempts (78.7%), which represent only 20% of all emergency calls and 37.5%

of calls for drug intoxication; secondly, accidents, which occur only among children, are few (14.3%) but a number proportionally high (7%) are due to therapeutic errors.

In suicide attempts, ethyl alcohol excepted, only drugs are associated with barbiturics in the case of polyvalent absorption.

About ten patent medicines in themselves account for a high number of calls. Thirty-three per cent of the cases are due to barbiturates taken alone, 46% to compound products with more than one component, 22% to more than two different drugs ingested at the same time. In more than 50% of the cases, the number of tablets, pills, or capsules ingested was high (1 or 2 tubes), suggesting that the victim had taken all he found. We have not been able to learn how often the potential suicide had hoarded a quantity of drugs prior to his attempt. A greater number of women than men (78% compared with 22%) tried to shorten their lives in this way.

The second study refers to four groups of children in paediatric wards. From 1950 to 1968, 59,442 children were admitted to the paediatric clinic of the Hôpital Universitaire Saint-Pierre in Brussels. Out of these 59,442 cases, about 1% (510 cases) were poisonings, and 61 cases (about 1% of all poisonings) had ingested a barbiturate. Amongst these 61 cases, 29 were accidents, 24 were overdoses or therapeutic errors and 8 were suicide attempts of teenagers aged between 10 and 15. Here also, the high number of therapeutic errors is surprising. The analysis of the circumstances showed that generally (18 cases out of 24) the parents wanted to quieten a nervous child, and had either given him several doses of a drug, or administered to an infant a dose suitable for an adult. Such parents are frequently mentally defective, psychologically disturbed, or alcoholics. They live in poor and inadequate homes such as caravans. Three cases were the fault of the chemist who sold the drug; one case was an overdose given to a child in an epileptic seizure in a special institution.

Accidents (29 out of 61 cases) occurred in circumstances similar to those indicated by calls to the Information Centre. However, more often the accident was the result of children being left alone or getting up at night to play while their parents were asleep; or children when playing together had given each other drugs which they had found in waste-baskets or out of doors. Frequently the drugs were found in waste-baskets or outside the home, and among these drugs Optalidon was found in 15 out of 29 cases. There is no clear association with the time of day, but accidents occurred mainly between 8 a.m. and 12 a.m., and 2 p.m. and 7 p.m. Seven of the eight suicide attempts by girls aged 11 to 15 were the result of serious family problems (divorced parents, alcoholism, father or mother under psychiatric supervision). One girl attempted suicide because of difficulties at school.

We have observed similar findings in the three other children's wards which participated in our inquiry:
- The rate of barbiturate intoxications among all hospitalizations for all causes is low: 1% or 2%.
- Therapeutic errors are not uncommon, often being the result of improper use, *e.g.*,

barbiturates given to cure influenza, asthma, or urinary troubles.
- Generally the drug involved is a compound used as an analgesic rather than as a hypnotic.
- Very often, the parents were not present and realized only when the first symptoms appeared that a drug had been ingested.

EPIDEMIOLOGICAL CONCLUSIONS

It must be noted that barbiturate poisoning is seldom an accident. Accidental ingestion practically never occurs in adults, and amongst children barbiturates are taken much less frequently than other drugs. Table 1 shows the percentages of the calls received by the Information Centre.

TABLE 1

	Suicides	Accidents	Therapeutic errors	Unknown
all ages – all products	15.8	72.9	3.5	7.8
all ages – barbiturates only	78.7	14.3	7	
children under four: calls for barbiturates only	0	82	18	
children under four: hospitalized for barbiturates only	0	61	39	

In spite of the increasing number of non-barbiturate hypnotics and tranquillizers, barbiturates are still preferred in suicide attempts: the desperate person expects death, certain but easy, while sleeping. People seem to be well informed of the dangers of these drugs, for they generally choose them for suicide attempts, but on the other hand store them more carefully to prevent accidents. The high number of accidents due to drugs not considered as barbiturates but rather as super-analgesics of polyvalent and common use, strengthens this notion further. But the frequency of therapeutic poisoning shows the ignorance about proper use of these drugs, mainly among poor people. They are particularly confused about the differences between hypnotics, sedatives, and analgesics. Only a few drugs are responsible for a large proportion of suicide attempts and accidents; we selected 30 main offenders among which no more than 10 were very often concerned.

We tried to find out if the container influenced the occurrence of accidents, but new containers (blister, strip, security caps) recently adopted by some manufacturers have made this part of the inquiry impossible to complete. Nevertheless, we have noticed that the barbiturate product most often encountered in children's overdoses is presented in pink sugar-coated tablets, packed in boxes of 25 which are easy to open. In a previous study we observed that pink or red sugar-coatings are the most attractive for children.

Generally, in contrast to what occurs with other products, the child who poisons himself with barbiturates is alone, does not find the drug by chance (as he might a bottle of cough-syrup forgotten on a table), but looks for it and finds it in the drawer of the bedside table, his mother's bag, or even in the family medicine-cabinet. The drug is 'in its place' but, unfortunately, within the child's reach; sometimes the child takes it out of the waste-basket.

The role of the socio-economic level and the psycho-affective climate of the home is obvious, and families with such problems have to be considered as a high risk group as regards preventive measures.

PREVENTION OF BARBITURATE POISONING

An episode of poisoning, voluntary or not, is the result of several factors, some of them essential, others only precipitating or aggravating. The *potential victim* must meet a *dangerous product* and have a *motivation* to absorb it. These three factors are essential. Precipitating or aggravating factors can be: surroundings and society, the family, the physician, the professional environment, sometimes the material setting in which the accident occurs (house, workroom, garden).

What are the importance and characteristics of these factors in the case of barbiturate poisoning?

THE VICTIM

THE VOLUNTARY VICTIM

We have seen that the victims are mainly: *a.* adults, voluntarily poisoned; *b.* children, poisoned by accident.

The adult or the teenager who takes barbiturates wants to focus on himself the interest of the community, which he thinks has become indifferent. He is similar to those who, aiming at the same effect, take other drugs in overdose. Generally, the feeling of loneliness in a world where they cannot any more find their place or the impression that their life is useless, induces the desperate to attempt suicide and in such a way to call for help.

Different studies and published works (Kessel, 1965; Graham and Hitchens, 1967; Gorceix and Zimbacca, 1968; World Health Organization, 1968) show that some groups, easily identified in society, are specially prone to attempting suicide: aged people, those mentally ill, drug addicts and particularly alcoholics, but also young adults and teenagers. We shall consider the characteristics of each of them, excluding the psychological aspect, which is in the field of mental health.

The aged

People in older age-groups, unoccupied, often isolated, frequently in poor financial conditions, have many reasons to think their lives are no longer useful. The feeling of being to some extent on the margin of the community can influence the fatal decision.

A statistical study made by the Belgian Poison Control Centre has shown that every year just before the Christmas and New Year festivities there is an increase of suicide cases amongst the aged. The solitude of their long winter evenings contrasts sharply with the preparation of feasts, exchange of gifts, bright shop windows and happy festivities of the community.

To prevent suicide at this level, socio-economic measures have to be promoted: to ensure to the older age-group an income sufficient to allow them to live in comfort and happiness; to organize medico-social supervision to deal with their individual problems; to limit their possible isolation by organizing a welfare programme of home visits, evening classes and clubs.

Children and adolescents

Children over nine and youngsters, mainly girls, living in broken homes or with inadequate or alcoholic families, are not uncommon candidates for suicide. Twenty-five per cent of all attempts at suicide and 14% of suicides by barbiturates alone or associated with other drugs, for which the Belgian Poison Control Centre has been consulted, are in the younger age-groups. Therefore barbiturates are not especially in favour in this age-group.

The teenager who attempts suicide is generally not, as Launay (1964) points out, mentally ill, but depressed or impulsive – a banal event such as bad results at school or a hurtful remark by an adult or a schoolfellow can give rise to the attempt. Such a cause is very difficult to prevent, as it is not at all specific. Sometimes the immediate reason, perhaps a disappointment in love, is more evident, but the act is still out of proportion.

Description by mass media of suicidal attempts perpetrated by celebrities or by other youngsters, can induce even slightly disturbed young people to imitate them. A special situation has recently been observed in the case of self-destruction by fire by a few French students, and that may be considered an imitative gesture.

Among children, attempted suicide is exceptional, but it can be motivated by wanting to play at being dead; it seems that the motivation is rarely real despair.

Early detection of a pathological environment in disturbed children, and the development of child guidance services and mental health clinics at universitities are the best preventive measures; and also the mass media ought to be more cautious about according publicity to acute poisoning so as to avoid the power of suggestion upon youth.

The mentally ill

It is not our purpose to analyse this particular group, as the psychiatrist has a dominant role in the case of these patients; it is well known, however, that they are particularly at risk regarding suicide attempts. Nevertheless, it is important to stress the danger of incautiously prescribed drugs which give opportunity for a suicide attempt. Psychiatric support for this group is especially important.

The drug-dependent and alcoholic

It is not surprising that many studies (World Health Organization, 1968) emphasize the high incidence of suicide attempts by alcoholics and those addicted to drugs. The reasons which lead to alcoholism and drug dependence have much in common with those which incite to suicide; on the other hand, alcoholism, like other addictions, induces mental disorders which can in themselves lead to suicidal attempts. Prescription of barbiturates to such patients should only be made when these two facts are kept very much in mind.

The current importance of drug addiction has urged many communities to look for the best way to combat it; some success has been achieved by the formation of medico-social clinics and treatment facilities.

The adult

If we consider adults as well as the other groups previously described, namely the aged, the teenagers, the mentally ill, alcoholics and drug addicts, then the entire population older than eight is included in the high-risk group. This is confirmed by statistics which show that voluntary intoxication, particularly that due to barbiturates, occurs at any age. Concerning the adult, special attention must be drawn to the period between 18 and 30 years of age, which has been thoroughly analysed in papers (Kessel, 1965; Vedrinne, 1965; Matthew, 1966; Graham and Hitchens, 1967; and Gorceix and Zimbacca, 1968). It is an important stage of life for young people, for they are confronted with the first responsibilities of independence, such as the necessity of earning a living, marriage, and professional adjustment.

Transition between this new and complete independence and the security previously provided by the home is frequently accompanied by conflicts, the intensity of which may overwhelm the capacity to adjust, thus leading to the suicide attempt. This behaviour is used as an escape valve; once again in these circumstances barbiturates and psychotropic drugs will tempt women especially.

All those committing or attempting suicide do not belong to high-risk groups. Under certain conditions, adults apparently of sound mental health can resort to this drastic measure, when they consider their situation as intolerable. Is there for such people any possibility of prevention? Many authors (Kessel, 1965; Vedrinne, 1965; Gorceix and Zimbacca, 1968) have pointed out that the candidate for suicide often reveals his intention before taking an overdose. Has this warning always registered and, if so, have effective preventive measures been taken? On most occasions probably not. It is vitally important that such warnings be taken seriously.

THE VICTIMS OF ACCIDENTAL POISONING

Accidental acute barbiturate intoxication in adults or adolescents is rare, and is principally due to a therapeutic error. The amount taken is usually small; the only case reported to the Belgian Poison Control Centre which could come under this category concerned a man aged 30 who had swallowed 25 Optalidon tablets to treat a dental abscess. Other such cases are essentially confusions, *e.g.* an anti-convulsant or a hypnotic taken to calm a headache, instead of acetyl-salicylic acid, or the result of impatience, *e.g.* five soporifics taken to induce sleep. Rarely are clinical features of acute poisoning evident in such instances. It is quite different with the child or infant who has been given doses suitable for adults. We noted in the epidemiological study the frequency of therapeutic accidents by barbiturates amongst children. To quieten a nervous child seems to be within many parents' competence and it is understandable that they should use sedatives; that they have used too large a dose of barbiturate is only a matter of ignorance. Statistics show that such mistakes generally occur among badly educated and poor people. Proper instruction of families by the physician who has prescribed the medicine is essential. Clearer wording and more easily understandable package inserts would certainly be an important measure towards safety. Nevertheless, it must be made clear that such mistakes are sometimes made by doctors, chemists and ancillary staff, perhaps with the exception of barbiturate poisoning caused by quasi-controlled overdosage in children with epileptic seizures. Stress must be laid on the absolute necessity, especially in infant care, of adhering exactly to the dosage for the particular age. However, it is accidental ingestion which is the most important barbiturate danger for the child under four. It has the characteristics of any accidental poisoning of young children (Govaerts-Lepicard, 1968). If a toddler swallows a barbiturate, it means that adults in his immediate environment have the drugs and let them get within the child's reach either out of carelessness, or, as is generally the case with analgesic compounds, out of ignorance of the danger.

From the preventive viewpoint, one can only repeat certain basic injunctions valid for all drugs. There is the necessity of proper storage. Children are mimics, and therefore a drug should never be taken in the presence of a child, especially if it is taken as a regular habit. For example, for a number of nights a 7-year-old child took a tablet from a tube of barbiturates which he managed to hide, in order to imitate his mother who each night took a contraceptive pill. The only real measure of security is through education, which will protect the child when he meets a circumstance unforeseen by the grown-ups who surround him. Too often parents call pills sweets in order to persuade the child to take them, thus making the two interchangeable in his mind.

THE PRODUCT

Although barbiturates have a well defined action they are included in many medications and prescriptions indicated for different purposes. The epidemiological study shows the importance of this distinction; analgesics containing barbiturates being incriminated as often as barbiturates prescribed for their hypnotic action.

The study done at the Belgian Poison Control Centre shows that several products, among which at least one contains barbiturates, are ingested in 21.78 % of the so-called barbiturate intoxications, barbiturates alone in 32.67%, and compound products in 45.54%. Other statistics (Gaultier *et al.*, 1968; Larcan *et al.*, 1969) stress also how often some brand of medicine is taken (*e.g.*, Optalidon).

Although the severity of poisoning by compound products is rather limited, the attention of users should be drawn to the real effects of their constituents, and the exact meaning of the term 'sedative' should be explained by the prescribing physician. However, irrespective of the type of barbiturate involved, it is rewarding to consider its shape and presentation.

THE APPEARANCE OF THE PRODUCT

The appearance of the product, whether it comes as tablets, sugar-coated pills, capsules or even suppositories (Arcadio *et al.*, 1967), is probably not very important to candidates for suicide. With children it is quite a different matter, for sugar-coated pills are more easily swallowed than tablets, and if they are coloured (pink, red, yellow) their similarity to sweets is attractive. This mode of presentation should be prohibited for all drugs likely to cause accidental poisoning. Moreover, large tablets and capsules, besides looking like sweets, are certainly more difficult to swallow. Whatever the appearance, a marking, as specific as possible for identification purposes, should be compulsory at manufacture. Such a marking would avoid searches, often long, when a few tablets are found, without any other information, at the bedside of the victim. Some poison control centres have established for identification purposes catalogues of tablets, capsules, etc., according to colours and sizes, corresponding to their national drug market. Beyond the fact that it is not easy to keep such a repository up to date, its establishment requires such labour that we hope that prompt, active and efficient help from the drug industry will be forthcoming on this particular point.

PACKAGING

During recent years the use of safety containers for pharmaceutic products has, fortunately, become of serious concern to the drug industry and also to physicians (Nathan, 1966; Done and Jung, 1968; Latham *et al.*, 1968).

Some years ago, safety caps were adopted by some manufacturers, principally on bottles of acetyl salicylic acid tablets for children. The ease with which children opened them, generally with their teeth, rendered them inadequate. More recently, a new process, based on a twisting manoeuvre difficult for young children, was introduced in Canada and the United States without consideration for the economical or commercial aspects. Recent studies (Done and Jung, 1968; Latham and Scherz, 1968) have shown the considerable interest in these caps, which could also be of use for products other than medicines. Their adoption for drug-containers is evidence of most important progress in prevention of accidental poisoning in children. Also important is the considerable improvement in safety achieved by individual packing of tablets and pills in strips or cellophane or plastic blisters from which the drug is extracted by pressure, one at a time. Even if it is rather easy for a child to obtain a single tablet out of such strips or blisters, the effort applied rapidly tires him, and the number of tablets removed and swallowed is small. This form of packaging represents a real advance in prevention, and it is simple and cheap.

Another important point in presentation of medicines is the total quantity of barbiturates available in one container. In some countries, it is permitted to sell without prescription small quantities of barbiturates (400 mg in Belgium). Obviously it is easy to collect a toxic dose of barbiturates by purchasing several containers in different shops. Another important measure consists in limiting even under prescription the total quantity of barbiturates in one container in order that it remains below a lethal dose, should the total contents be taken at the same time. Presently on the Belgian market some packings hold 10 grams of barbiturates.

LABELLING AND PACKAGE INSERT

Labelling of drug-containers varies in each country. Ideally, the name of the drug and the strength of each product should be clearly shown. Confusion would be avoided if a product had the same name in different countries and scientific reports, between poison control centres in particular, would thereby be much easier.

Sir Derrick Dunlop (1966) speaking for the British Committee on Safety of Drugs pointed out that the great difficulty lies in the labelling of prescribed medicines: 'The Committee on Safety of Drugs are very conscious that the adequacy of toxicity testing, clinical trials, and the monitoring of adverse reactions are not the only factors in the safe use of drugs. Patients, the general public, and particularly prescribing doctors in practice and in hospital have an important role to play. The Committee have always believed that it would conduce greatly to the safe use of drugs if their containers were labelled with the name of the medicine ordered, unless otherwise specified by the prescriber.'

Although the writing of elegant prescriptions is no longer fashionable, some doctors still like to include barbiturates in compositions specially adapted to their patients. Comments concerning the secrecy of the contents of a prescription have been made by the Committee on Safety of Drugs as follows: 'The suggestion that patients should usually be kept in ignorance of their treatment is quite inconsistent with contemporary medical thought. We realize, of course, that there are occasions when in the patient's interests it may be undesirable for him to know what drug he is being given. This is particularly the case when placebo or 'terminal drugs' are prescribed. Such contingencies, however, are covered by the qualification unless otherwise specified by the prescriber.'

Generally, a pamphlet describing indications, dosage and frequency of administration and sometimes side effects, together with precautions, is inserted in the container. This package insert is for the benefit of patients and is the best way to communicate useful information and thereby avoid therapeutic mistakes. However, a condition of basic importance is to realize that the material is for patients and is not to be considered as references for medical experts; using inserts in the latter way would limit their efficiency since the amount of the information given is considerably reduced (Chayet, 1967).

AVAILABILITY OF BARBITURATES

The physician plays a very important role in the availability of barbiturates, as in most countries they are obtainable only on prescription. When prescribing such medicines, it is highly desirable to keep in mind the importance of synergies and also to limit the total amount prescribed at one time. Also, as Matthew (1966) stressed, it is important to be sure that what is in fact required is a hypnotic for insomnia, for the insomnia may be due to depression. It may well be the depression which requires treatment and not the insomnia, and the prescription of a barbiturate provides the depressed patient with a ready means of attempting suicide. As insomnia is often a symptom of depression, great care is essential in the prescription of any drugs in this condition. Likewise, care must be exercised in the type of barbiturate prescribed, since medium- and short-acting preparations are likely to produce more serious effects in acute overdosage.

It is not always easy for the family doctor to control his patient's consumption of hypnotics for, if he refuses a prescription, the patient can of course apply to another practitioner. In rural areas where a patient could consult more than one physician but where there is only one chemist, the importance of the pharmacist's role has to be stressed. If the patient produces prescriptions for excessive amounts of hypnotics or sedatives the pharmacist should try to find out how and to whom the prescriptions have been given, and if in doubt should contact the physician. Most toxicologists have been tempted at one time or another to incorporate an emetic in hypnotic tablets in an attempt to induce vomiting when the quantity of hypnotic ingested is excessive. But if, for instance, ipecac were incorporated the ipecac itself might be absorbed, with all the dangers of ipecac poisoning. Further, there is a considerable risk of aspiration pneumonia and death if vomiting occurs in a semi-conscious patient. Research on this subject might prove to be of value.

REASONS, CIRCUMSTANCES AND ENVIRONMENT

It has not been possible to make as complete a survey of adult victims and their reasons as has been possible with accidental poisoning in the child. However, some preventive measures can be taken at this level in the field of social environment. In the case of deliberate poisoning the overdose is frequently taken as a last desperate attempt to change an intolerable way of life which cannot be endured any longer. Sometimes before the attempt the victim has visited his doctor, seeking help, but the overworked practitioner has perhaps not understood the *cri d'alarme*. Vedrinne (1965) mentions such cases. Of course, possibly the visit is made only with the aim of obtaining the prescription but, nevertheless, fundamentally the distress and the appeal are there. The help offered to the community by telephone services such as 'Samaritans' and 'Friends' shows the valuable influence of surroundings, even anonymous and impersonalized, on anxious or depressed patients.

Accidental poisoning in the young child also depends greatly on his environment. It is obviously not possible to influence the motives that incite a toddler to swallow a pill or tablet, for they are characteristics inherent in his development. Oral curiosity is normal, he is too young to have acquired the notion of danger, and he cannot read. Here environment can secure real protection. Never leave a medicine within a child's reach, *e.g.*, no barbiturates should be in the drawer of the night-table; teach as soon as possible the difference between sweets and medicines; watch the child closely and weave around him a protective network. These precautions will, however, only operate if adults acquire full awareness of the dangers.

Proper storage of drugs should be emphasized; the family doctor is probably best able to give advice. He should ensure that medicines are not left in the kitchen, in the bathroom, or in the mother's bag. The family medicine-chest, inaccessible to children, should be periodically inspected; any unused or unrequired drugs should be flushed down the lavatory. They should never be put in the rubbish-bin or in any place where a child might find them. Drugs should remain in their original containers and not kept in bottles bearing another label.

As Matthew (1966) suggests, in the course of his visits to the family, the doctor should check these few essential measures.

ORGANIZATION OF PREVENTION OF BARBITURATE ACCIDENTS

It is not easy, and probably not desirable, to isolate the prevention of barbiturate intoxication from that of other drugs or even from the problem of acute poisonings in general. That is why the measures and recommendations suggested must not be considered as particularly specific.

Programmes regarding prevention are quite frequently promoted by those who are most conscious of causes threatening public health. In addition, private centres giving help by telephone were created a few years ago; they are manned by volunteers of all social levels and persons saved by the organization itself may join as helpers. They offer the desperate useful support and friendly advice. Such centres should exist in every town.

Clergymen often strive to help hopeless persons but physicians are generally less prepared to offer the words of comfort that would be more useful than the prescription of medicine.

The new trend in medical education towards a better psychological and sociological approach to the total situation of the patient should be of great value in these particular cases. All private organizations interested in health education have a part to play in the prevention of poisoning. There are very few people, if any, who are not reached by the Red Cross, parent-teacher associations, child welfare clinics, environmental health committees, etc., so most people can be educated in the protection of the child against poisoning and the proper use of drugs and first-aid in cases of poisoning.

Pharmacists are in a key-position to control, help and educate. We have seen the role they must play in the particular case of prescribing barbiturates and other medicaments. It is desirable that they should strive still harder in social preventive action, as does the very active organization of the 'Comité d'Education Sanitaire et Sociale de la Pharmacie Française'.

THE ROLE OF EDUCATORS

In many countries, health education is not yet included in school programmes, and even if it exists, mostly it does not include instruction in the proper use of medicines and the safety measures already mentioned. Educators are generally ill prepared in these subjects, and therefore doctors should be willing and able to assist in this respect.

THE ROLE OF THE PHARMACEUTICAL INDUSTRY

We have seen that the pharmaceutical industry can make a very considerable contribution in the prevention of barbiturate poisoning. Containers, labelling instructions, package inserts, unit-doses – the whole problem of product presentation falls within their competence. Poison control centres for information and treatment can nevertheless very usefully focus the attention of producers on the special points it would be desirable to change or to improve, such as the maximum amount of barbiturate in every container and the systematic marking of pills, tablets, and capsules for identification. Joint commissions of personnel from poison control centres and from the pharmaceutical industry could make very useful contributions towards prevention.

THE ROLE OF POISONING TREATMENT CENTRES

Poisoning treatment centres have a very special position regarding prevention of poisoning. They can conceive plans and programmes based on the epidemiology and the natural history of the many types of intoxication they encounter. Consequently they must undertake propaganda in the community, motivate active groups of society, engage in discussions with the production and distribution industries and, not least, advise government departments. They must also cooperate with press and television to help in the diffusion of accurate information, neither sensational nor dramatized.

THE ROLE OF GOVERNMENTS

At the national as well as the international level, official rules and regulations attempt, in a changing scene, to ensure desirable protection of the health of the public. Still, these rules and regulations must be well advised, realistic, judicious and up-to-date. In the particular case of barbiturates certain suggestions have been made in this chapter, but the great complexity of regulations in different countries shows the urgency of international agreements aimed at combating poisoning by drugs.

REFERENCES

ANNUAL REPORT OF POISON CONTROL CENTRES (Canada, 1963). Poisonings by class of products and products reported by province (Table III).

ARCADIO, F., VINCENT, V. and PERROT, E. (1967), Intoxication par les suppositoires. *Bull. Méd. lég.*, 4, 259.

BANCIU, D. and DROC, I. (1966), Considérations sur les intoxications médico-légales en Roumanie. *Bull. Méd. lég.*, 6, 401.

BORBELY, F. (1968), Rapport médical sur l'activité du centre suisse d'information toxicologique. In: *Rapport Annuel du Centre d'Information Toxicologique.*

CENTRE D'INFORMATION TOXICOLOGIQUE DU CENTRE ANTI-POISONS DE PARIS (1966). *Bull. Méd. lég.*, 3, 203.

CHAYET, L. (1967), Power of the package insert. *New Engl. J. Med.*, 277, 1253.

CURRY, A. S. (1965), Systematic toxicological analysis. Symposium. *Identification of Drugs and Poisons*, p. 46. Pharm. Soc. Gt Britain. Unwin, Surrey.

DONE, A. K. and JUNG, A. L. (1968), A realistic approach to the prevention of childhood poisoning with special emphasis on aspirin. *Clin. Toxicol.*, 1, 63.

DUNLOP, D. (1966), Labelling of drugs. *Brit. med. J.*, 2, 361.

ELIAKIS, C., ELIAKIS, E. and COUTSELINIS, A. (1967), Les intoxications en Grèce pendant les années 1950–1966. *Bull. Méd. lég.*, 5, 24.

GAULTIER, M., FOURNIER, E., GERVAIS, P., EFTHYMIOU, M. L., BISMUTH, C., BODIN, F., CHRISTOFOROV, B., SICOT, C. and FREJAVILLE, J. P. (1968), Étude sur le travail du secteur de réanimation de la Clinique Toxicologique à l'Hôpital Fernand Widal, Paris Xe, pendant l'année 1967. *Bull. Méd. lég.*, 1, 21.

GOMEZ-OROZCO, L. and SANTIAGO-CASTANON, A. (1966), Analyse des cas d'intoxications chez l'enfant, observés à l'Hôpital Infantile du Méxique (1957–1962). *Bol. méd. Hosp. infant. (Méx.)*, 23, 477.

GOVAERTS-LEPICARD, M. (1968), Les intoxications accidentelles chez le jeune enfant. *Enfant (Brux.)*, 5, 357.

GORCEIX, A. and ZIMBACCA, N. (1968), Études sur le suicide. *Coll. Méd. Lég. Toxicol. Méd.*, Masson, Paris.

GRAHAM, J. D. P. and HITCHENS, R. A. N. (1967), Acute poisoning and its prevention. *Brit. J. prev. soc. Med.*, 21, 108.

KESSEL, N. (1965), Self-poisoning. *Brit. med. J.*, 2, 1265; 1336.

LARCAN, A., CALAMAI, M., LORENTZ, J. F., HELMER, J. and VOIRY, A. M. (1969), Les intoxications par Optalidon-statistique personelle. X Réunion Nationale de Toxicdogie Clinique.

LATHAM, G. H. and SCHERZ, R. G. (1968), Prevention of poisoning. *Lancet*, 1, 1252.

LAUNAY, C. and COL, C. (1964), Suicide et tentative de suicide chez l'enfant et l'adolescent. *Rev. Prat. (Paris)*, 14, 619.

Leading articles (1967), Barbiturate poisoning. *Lancet*, 1, 200.

Leading articles (1968), Treatment and prevention of poisoning. *Brit. med. J.*, 4, 787.

LESTER, D. (1969), The anti-suicide pill. *J. Amer. med. Ass.*, 208, 1908.

MATHE, P., BONSOM, R., CASTERA, J., JOUGLARD, J. and DUTHU, M. P. (1967), Activité du service de réanimation de l'Hôpital Sainte-Anne à Toulon, en pathologie toxique, de 1962 à 1966. Service du Docteur Mathé. *Bull. Méd. lég.*, 6, 348.

MATTHEW, H. (1966), Poisoning in the home by medicaments. *Brit. med. J.*, 2, 788.

MATTHEW, H., PROUDFOOT, A. T., BROWN, S. S. and AITKEN, R. C. B. (1969), Acute poisoning: organization and work-load of a treatment centre. *Brit. med. J.*, 3, 489.

NATHAN, T. (1966), A practical suggestion for poison control in the pediatric age group. Letters to the editor. *Pediatrics*, 38, 931.

National Clearinghouse for Poison Control Centers Bulletin (1969), Products most frequently ingested, 1968.

POISON CONTROL PROGRAM STATISTICS, 1967 (1969), Dept. Nat. Health and Welfare. Xème Réunion Nationale de Toxicologie Clinique, Strasbourg, France (1969). Rapports et communications.

RESNIK, H. L. P. (1969), Suicide prevention and niacin. *J. Amer. med. Ass.* 208, 2164.

ROCHE, L. (1968), Centre anti-poisons de Lyon – activité pendant l'année 1967. *Bull. Méd. lég.*, 1, 40.

SCHERZ, R. G. (1968), Childhood poisoning from medications: Three prevention programs that worked. *Military Med.*, 433, 911.

SUNSHINE, I. (1967), Problems of obtaining information on accidental ingestions and poisoning incidents. *J. clin. Pharm.*, 7, 61.

THYS, J. P., BOURGEOIS, M., CORNIL, A., FRANKEN, L. and DE COSTER, A. (1969), La réanimation dans les intoxications par les somnifères et les drogues psychotropes. Bilan de deux années d'activité. *Acta clin. belg.*, 24, 149.

VAN HEYST, A. N. P. (1966), Zeven jaren toxicologie. *Pharm. Weekbl.*, 101, 909.

VEDRINNE, J. (1965), L'intoxication aiguë volontaire. *Coll. Méd. Lég. Toxicol. Méd.*, Masson, Paris.

VISAKORPI, J. K. (1967), First five years' report of the poison control centre in Helsinki (1961–1966). *Suom. Lääk.-L.*, 22, 2241.

WECHSELBERG, K. (1967), Besonderheiten und Gesetzmässigkeiten kindlicher Vergiftungen in der Grossstadt. *Praxis*, 56, 110.

WORLD HEALTH ORGANIZATION (1968), Prevention of suicide. *Wld Hlth Org. techn. Publ. Hlth Pap.*, 35.

22. clinical toxicology for the medical school curriculum

E. G. Comstock

A physician who is knowledgeable in the general principles of the clinical management of acute intoxication is a fundamental necessity for the treatment of acute barbiturate poisoning. Such a physician assures the proper emergency care for such patients
by supervising an organized emergency room where all equipment and supplies are
ready for immediate use and where the emergency room staff is trained to administer
immediate, life-sustaining, supportive care. A standard routine provides that specimens of lavage or emesis fluid are collected and labeled properly, that pre-treatment
specimens of blood are obtained routinely and that the initial urine specimen is retained. The physician is alert to the commonly occurring complications of treatment.
He is aware of the multiplicity of other drugs and chemicals which may be ingested
with a barbiturate or must be considered in the differential diagnosis. A careful history
taken from the family records the pre-intoxication circumstances, past medical history
which may influence treatment, an estimate of time of ingestion, time found and by
whom, first-aid measures, and time of admission to the emergency room. The physician assures smooth transition of the patient from the emergency room to a medical
intensive care unit and he assures that proper psychiatric care is integrated with the
patient's awakening.

The absence of therapeutically-oriented training in toxicology during medical school
has resulted in a majority of practicing physicians having had no opportunity to gain
a well-rounded perspective concerning the treatment of the intoxicated patient. Opti-
mal circumstances for the treatment of acute barbiturate poisoning do not prevail,
and morbidity and mortality are increased needlessly.

Should the need for additional training in the management of acute intoxication be
realized by the physician in practice, it cannot be met, since therapeutically-oriented
training is not generally available in continuing education programs. Self-education
concerning the treatment of acute intoxication is fraught with hazards. Much of the
published literature consists of case reports accompanied by projections concerning
treatment which exceed the author's competence. Compilations of the fragmented,
inadequately documented, and sometimes erroneous literature attempt to handle the

treatment of the entire range of poisoning emergencies. These articles often manifest a rather shallow perspective and no effort by the author to verify the efficacy of the approaches to treatment that are cited. Such discussion perpetuates a number of fads which have emerged in recent years concerning the treatment of acute intoxication. In the absence of any general training or without extensive first-hand experience, the practicing physician cannot be expected to differentiate sound treatment from foolish.

In the emergency situation the physician may turn to any of a number of handbooks on the treatment of acute poisoning, many of which are compilations of the literature by physicians and scientists who lack any substantial personal experience with management of these patients. The general accord found among such texts is often mistaken for a consensus of authorities as to suitable treatment when, in fact, it represents reiteration of the original source.

The other 'training' resource for the physician during the acute emergency is the widely established network of poison information centers which has emerged in the United States. There has, however, been no control or standardization of the professional or technical capabilities of the poison information centers. Frequently, these centers are sponsored by professional and scientific organizations which lend to them an air of authenticity which may misrepresent their reliability. The poison information center movement has been poorly funded for the most part, and, consequently, the physician may obtain his information from relatively inexperienced house staff or even from a telephone answering-service. More often than not, the inquiring physician wishes to have a consultation rather than only information. It is only the pressure of circumstances surrounding the acute intoxication which drives the physician to accept this rather precarious route to consultation which professional ethics would prohibit under more leisurely circumstances.

The antidotal concept of therapy is one of the fads which is widely prevalent in the literature and in current medical practice. The frantic search for the 'antidote' may prevail, for instance, while the patient suffers terminal anoxia for lack of adequate respiratory support. In fact, there is an extremely small number of substances for which there exists a suitable antidote. Poisoning by these substances constitutes a very small fraction of acute poisonings. The concept of an antidote, however, is basically appealing and has been so widely promulgated that the conditioned reflex, 'antidote', upon the mentioning of poisoning will persist, unfortunately, for many years.

Another fundamentally appealing concept which finds very limited application in practice is the use of hemodialysis. The appeal of the idea of extracting the poison from the body by some machine is easily understood, but too frequently over-emphasized, while the simpler approaches which otherwise would be adequate are overlooked. The author has heard internists, who ordinarily practice impeccable medicine, comment that since the advent of hemodialysis all overdose patients are simply transferred to the medical center where the drug can be extracted. While some freely diffusible substances can be removed in large amounts by dialysis, the concept of dialysis should not prevail to the exclusion of rational medical treatment pending transfer of the patient to the dialysis unit. When the success of dialysis is evaluated, one should keep in mind that transfer of a patient to a more highly specialized medical staff and a better-equipped medical facility results in superior intensive medical care as a fringe benefit to extracorporeal dialysis.

The induction of vomiting with syrup of ipecac is another widely misunderstood concept. Immediate removal of an offending substance by the induction of vomiting is a procedure about which sweeping generalities have been made without definition of the population under discussion. An understandable appeal is achieved by the logic that a stomach full of poison might reasonably be emptied via the route of entry by the quasi-natural mechanism of induced emesis. The protagonists of this technique maintain that it is useful as a preventive measure, provided that syrup of ipecac is immediately available and that the clinical situation is one of accidental ingestion of potentially harmful substances which has been discovered almost immediately. It is advocated on the premise that the vomiting which ensues after ipecac administration to an asymptomatic child is so nearly a physiologic event that morbidity due to the ipecac is negligible compared with the possible advantage of early gastric emptying. A problem emerges, not from the initial protagonists, but from avid disciples who paraphrase the initial concept to read 'poisoning by ingestion should be treated by induction of vomiting'. The population initially under discussion has been significantly altered. Examination of the new population reveals that it is symptomatic. The original concept of induction of vomiting has been taken out of context and is now viewed as a method for treatment of poisoning rather than as a method for prevention of poisoning. Also, the population of poisoned patients now under discussion is not a pediatric population but is adult to the extent of 80–90%.

The recurring controversy over whether poisoning should be treated by induction of vomiting or be treated by lavage confirms by its persistence the general need for more adequate understanding of the principles of clinical toxicology.

Additional uncertainty persists concerning the induction of vomiting by any method because of the use of emesis rather than decontamination as the criterion of successful treatment.

Another fad which persists years beyond the time that it was advocated by anyone knowledgeable in clinical toxicology is the use of analeptic drugs for the treatment of sedative-drug-induced coma. How is the physician in practice to know that this approach is no longer advocated? It persists in the information distributed by the National Clearinghouse for Poison Control Centers. It is suggested by some pharmaceutical manufacturers in the section on 'Treatment of Overdose' of the package inserts, where it achieves pseudo-authenticity through review and approval for publication by the Food and Drug Administration.

In the published literature, cases may be used to illustrate an approach to treatment without mention of the manner in which a diagnosis was achieved, or the diagnosis may be based on history alone. The possibility of error in these cases is high as illustrated by a series of cases comparing the diagnosis based on history and clinical evaluation with the diagnosis by laboratory examination (Berman and Brown, 1970). Agreement occurs in less than 50% of the cases. Allowing validity for the primary diagnosis, there is confusion between clinical manifestations due to the toxic substance and those due to secondary processes such as dehydration, aspiration pneumonia, anoxemia, and iatrogenic respiratory alkalosis. The assessment of the clinical value of a method for treatment may be open to question. The efficacy of ipecac for decontamination of the gastrointestinal tract may be confused with its efficacy for induction of emesis. In some cases, the value of emesis may be demonstrated in a population where there is no assurance that an ingestion of any consequence has occurred. Treatment procedures applied late in the clinical course may be credited with a recovery which already is progressing.

Modern computer technology assures that all published information, irrespective of its validity, may be reduced to association phenomena and delivered in regimented columns for the benefit of anyone who might push the button.

It is to this mass, from which the experienced authority can extract the facts only with difficulty, that the practicing physician must turn to achieve an education concerning the clinical management of acute intoxication.

The time is long past due for the medical school faculty to assume a greater share of the responsibility for education of the physician concerning clinical toxicology.

A COURSE IN CLINICAL TOXICOLOGY

The term 'clinical toxicology' has been chosen to differentiate an area of clinical practice from its related basic science, toxicology. Clinical toxicology emphasizes the patient while classical toxicology emphasizes the poison. The role of clinical toxicology in the practice of medicine may be described as a bridge linking the basic science of toxicology to the front lines of medical practice. It must bring basic principles to bear on the intoxicated patient in therapeutically applicable terms. It must also recover the wealth of information potentially available from the circumstances of accidental and intentional intoxication and interpret this data with circumspect consideration for the pitfalls inherent in observations from clinical experience (Craver, 1969).

In order to discuss a training program, it is necessary to define the subject-matter of clinical toxicology. Clinical toxicology is concerned with the treatment of diseases caused by toxic substances of exogenous origin. These include: (1) accidental and intentional abuse of chemical substances, including therapeutic agents; (2) undesirable, excessive, and non-therapeutic drug effects; (3) injurious interactions of exogenous substances; (4) accidental exposure to toxic substances in the home and in industry; (5) intentional and inadvertent food additives and environmental pollutants; and (6) naturally occurring toxic hazards.

Multiple levels of training in clinical toxicology are required. There is need of a two-year training program for physicians interested in clinical toxicology as a medical specialty serving the medical profession and industry as a consultant, as an educator, and as an investigator. There is need for a definitive program in clinical toxicology during the medical curriculum at the undergraduate level and at the graduate level. Short-term intensive training programs for the physician in practice are required. Training programs should also be provided for emergency room nurses, emergency room technicians, and the medical intensive care nursing staff. The emphasis in the current discussion is on the undergraduate medical curriculum.

The basic course in clinical toxicology requires 18 – 24 hours. It should be presented during the years of clinical training. All of the principles presented should be emphasized by actual case discussion.

The actual mechanics of course presentation may vary a great deal depending upon the teaching methods with which the faculty are familiar. Since the patients under consideration do not lend themselves readily to a case presentation while they are showing symptoms, it is most essential that the lecture material be associated with first-hand experience in the emergency room. The individual experience of the student should be supplemented by weekly case-review or case-study sessions. Post-acute and continuing intensive care may easily be studied on the wards. The use of any of several programmed teaching machines may be worthwhile, since the teaching of sound principles of clinical judgment is the objective. These machines allow the sequential presentation of clinical circumstances which require that a judgment be made as to the choice of diagnostic and therapeutic procedures. The student may proceed at his own pace. Some have memory divices which recount errors and may be used to evaluate clinical judgment.

The course in clinical toxicology presents an ideal opportunity for the integration of clinical and basic sciences. Effort should be made to involve the basic science faculty of toxicology and pharmacology in the clinical rounds and case discussions (Comstock, 1968).

The question of the source for teaching faculty was partially answered during a teaching conference devoted to toxicology in 1969 by the American Society of Pharmacology and Experimental Therapeutics. Dr. Plaa summarized 77 replies to questionnaires submitted to the departments of pharmacology of various medical schools concerning the amount and type of training offered above and beyond the usual courses in pharmacology and therapeutics (Plaa, 1969). Eight per cent of the respondents offered no additional hours, 42% of the respondents offered between one and five additional hours, 42% offered between six and ten additional hours, and 7% offered twelve to twenty additional hours. Therefore, 91% of the respondents had one or more persons on their faculty with sufficient interest in toxicology to offer additional hours on the subject for the medical curriculum, and these individuals very probably would contribute to the faculty requirements for a course with a therapeutic orientation. While the number of hours devoted to toxicology might indicate that training is more universally available, the inadequacy of the existing training is indicated by the time during the medical school training when the courses were taught. Nine per cent of the respondents taught their toxicology course during the first year, 83% taught their course during the second year, and only 13% had any amount of toxicology instruction by the pharmacology department during the clinical years. These data reflect the abyss which tends to exist between many of the basic sciences and the related applied clinical areas. The course in clinical toxicology seems an ideal one to overcome the hesitancy which exists on the part of many instructors in basic science to become involved in actual clinical management and the slowness with which many clinicians accept their active participation. Teaching faculty for the clinical aspects of the course should present little problem. There are ordinarily one or more persons within each of the major clinical departments interested in problems related to clinical toxicology.

The general direction of the program should be under the department of medicine. Where there is a clinical pharmacology department, it should support a heavy commitment to the teaching responsibilities of the clinical toxicology course.

The department of anesthesiology should be second only to the department of medicine in a teaching program. The anesthesiologist is concerned with management of the airway complications which are the most common immediate cause of death. The pediatrician and the nephrologist should also be involved in the teaching program.

The following general goals should be achieved in an undergraduate training program in clinical toxicology: (1) understanding of the commonly used terminology; (2) an awareness of the professional and technical resources available to assist with acute intoxication and some appreciation for their relative reliability; (3) appreciation of the general concepts of the treatment of acute intoxication; (4) provision of specific guides for equipping and maintaining an adequate emergency treatment facility; and (5) understanding the role of intoxication in the differential diagnosis.

A topic outline of the proposed course is presented. This outline was first presented in 1967. It has been modified and expanded somewhat during the last three years (Comstock, 1968). The actual text of the course is somewhat experimental and has still to be shaped by information on the results of its use. The contributions of other authors of this monograph very likely will be directly applicable as subject-matter within the outline.

TOPIC OUTLINE FOR COURSE IN CLINICAL TOXICOLOGY

I. INTRODUCTION

A. *Definitions*
Clinical toxicology, intoxication, minimum lethal dose, LD_{50}, etc.

B. *Scientific and professional information resources*
1. Cautionary labeling
2. Local and regional poison information centers

    3. Inserted material in drug packages
    4. Chemical and pharmaceutical manufacturers
    5. Drug information centers
    6. Private and governmental service organizations
    7. Other professional specialties
    8. Bibliography of recent texts and review papers
    9. Relative reliability of above resources

  C. *Poison information versus consultation services*

II. EPIDEMIOLOGY

  A. *Accidental*
    1. Home
    2. Industry
    3. Disasters of transport

  B. *Suicidal*
    1. Intentional
    2. Unintentional
    3. Lethality *versus* intentionality
    4. Psychopathology in self-inflicted injury

  C. *Homicidal*

  D. *Iatrogenic*
    1. Multiple physicians
    2. Multiple prescriptions
    3. Inadvertent prescription errors
    4. Errors in compounding and dispensing
    5. Errors in administration
    6. Quantity

  E. *Adverse drug reactions*
    1. Side effects
    2. Interactions
    3. Hypersensitivity
      a. genetic
      b. acquired

  F. *Abuse*
    1. Legitimate drugs
    2. Illegitimate drugs
    3. Other substances

III. CLINICAL DIAGNOSIS OF POISONING

  A. *Diagnostic criteria and their relative reliability*

  B. *Clinical diagnosis*
    1. History
      a. past history and pre-existing illness
      b. current drug therapy and drug-use history (emphasis on need for maintenance therapy or possible withdrawal reactions)
      c. physicians seen and prescriptions received over the past year, particularly where injury may have been intentional

    d. employment history, especially recent job changes

    e. avocations and unusual activities

    f. changes in attitudes or personal habits

2. Present illness

    a. time last known to be well

    b. time of onset and nature of first symptoms

    c. activities immediately prior to onset

    d. environmental survey for possible containers of toxic substances and clues to route of contamination, *i.e.*, toxic or asphyxiant gases

3. Physical examination; points of special emphasis (note time)

    a. voluntary or involuntary activity

    b. odor

    c. state of consciousness

    d. skin: stains, burns, contaminating oils, trauma, puncture wounds, capillary beds, sweating

    e. head: hair distribution, scalp lesions, trauma

    f. eyes: movement, pupil size and reactions, reflexes, fundi, chemical damage to mucous membranes or cornea

    g. mouth: stains, burns, irritation, coagulation necrosis, foreign bodies, trauma to mucous membranes

    h. chest: respiratory rate, pattern, excursion, auscultatory findings

    i. heart: rate, rhythm, valve sounds, murmurs

    j. abdomen: distention, bowel sounds, tenderness, palpable organs

    k. genitalia and rectum: excoriation, irritation, foreign bodies

    l. muscles: tone, tics, fasciculation, paresis, paralysis, muscle-mass loss

    m. neurological: orientation, hallucinations, sensory perception, motor disturbances, tremors, convulsive activity, normal and pathological reflexes, depth of coma

C. *Instrumental methods*

    1. Electrocardiograph

    2. Electrocephalograph

    3. Electromyograph

    4. X-rays

        a. radio-opaque substances

        b. stomach contents

        c. chest

IV. LABORATORY DIAGNOSIS

A. *Routine (conventional) laboratory examination*

pointing out procedures with toxicologic implications

    1. Lumbar puncture: pressure, gross appearance, cell count, chemistries

    2. Blood chemistries: electrolytes, enzymes on admission and after 24 hours

    3. Urine: gross appearance, microscopic morphology, chemical examination

B. *Analytical toxicology*

chemical identification of the toxic substance or its metabolites

    1. The original material

    2. Emesis or lavage fluid

    3. Blood specimens

    4. Urine specimens

    5. Stool specimens

    6. Skin washings

    7. Fat biopsy

    8. Expired air

    9. Other specimens

C. *Rapid methods for chemical diagnosis of poisoning in the emergency room*
(numerous relatively simple laboratory methods have been developed for detection of toxic substances in body fluids within one hour *(Manual of Rapid Procedures* should be provided)

D. *Pitfalls in the diagnosis of poisoning*
(as illustrated by case presentation)

E. *Multiple etiology*
(discussion of hazards involved when thorough laboratory studies are not performed, with case presentation illustrating misinterpretations which result)

F. *Interpretations*
('normal values', 'lethal level')

V. PRINCIPLES OF THE TREATMENT OF POISONING

A. *Decontamination*
  1. Clothing
  2. Hair, skin, fingernails, eyes, mouth
  3. Gastrointestinal tract
     a. induction of vomiting: how, when, for what
     b. gastric lavage: how, after how long, for what
     c. purgation: with what, for what, when

B. *Prevention of absorption*
  1. Immiscible phase
  2. Adsorbants: activated charcoal, etc.
  3. Formation of insoluble derivatives
  4. Reaction with a fixed ion, ion-exchange resins

C. *Neutralization*
  1. Acids
  2. Bases

D. *Increase in rate of excretion*
  1. Diuresis: chemical, osmotic, pH control
  2. Enteroenteric, enterohepatic circulation, interruption by binding materials in the gut
  3. Dialysis
     a. peritoneal
     b. extracorporeal
        1) lipid
        2) aqueous
        3) other: charcoal column
  4. Ionic trapping
  5. Conversion to a more readily-excreted form

E. *Prevention of the formation of a more toxic derivative*
  (*i.e.*, methanol treated with ethanol)

F. *Removal of dependence on a sensitive system*
  (*i.e.*, hyperbaric therapy for methemoglobinemia)

G. *Blocking the sensitivity of an end organ*
  (*i.e.*, atropine block of hypercholinergic crisis by stabilizing the polarized cell membrane)

H. *Reversal of enzyme inhibition*
  (*i.e.*, proto-PAM)

    I. *Conversion to less toxic form*

    J. *Non-specific*
       1. Supporting vital function
       2. Awareness of delayed effects and sequelae; how long should a patient be observed when he is asymptomatic

VI. CURRENT PRACTICES IN CLINICAL TOXICOLOGY

    A. *First-aid and patient transportation*
       1. Mobile life support systems
       2. Air *versus* surface transport

    B. *Emergency room organization*
       1. Equipment
       2. Formulary
       3. Standard orders for emergency life-support procedures

    C. *The first ten minutes* (significance of care)

    D. *Supportive care for drug-induced coma*
       1. The management of coma:
         a. determining and monitoring the depth of coma
         b. respiratory support
           1) airway
             a. oropharyngeal
             b. intratracheal intubation
             c. tracheotomy
           2) intermittent positive pressure respiration:
             a. mouth-to-mouth
             b. face-mask and bag
             c. anesthesia machines
             d. automatic positive pressure respirators
           3) inhalation therapy:
             a. choice of gases
             b. aerosol and mist therapy
             c. monitoring blood gases
           4) routine maintenance of the respiratory tract during prolonged coma

         c. support of blood pressure
            1) intravenous access
            2) central venous pressure
            3) choice of intravenous fluids
            4) use and misuse of central nervous system stimulants

         d. fluid and electrolyte balance in prolonged coma
          e. renal function and maintenance of urinary output
          f. nursing care during prolonged coma
       2. Differential diagnosis of coma

    E. *Clinical management of intoxication due to individual substances or groups of substances*

DISCUSSION OF COURSE

The physician treats the patient, not the poison.

    The above statement is axiomatic. The usual and ordinary clinical skills of the well-trained physician when they are applied methodically as required by the symptomatic manifestations of the acutely intoxicated patient will result in a very favorable recovery rate. Even intoxication from such highly toxic substances as some of the alkyl phosphate ester anticholinesterase insecticides will be treated reasonably if the clinical syndrome is viewed as a hypercholinergic crisis. In the absence of any specific information, the use of the most commonly available anticholinergic agent, atropine, is derived rationally from clinical manifestations alone.

For clinical purposes, all toxic substances may be divided into two groups: those producing an illness for which no specific treatment is known, and those producing, an illness for which there is a specific treatment.

The vast majority of substances fall into the first category, for which sound symptomatic medical care is the only approach. Only poisoning for which a specific treatment exists needs to be singled out from the tens of thousands of potentially toxic substances. Discussion of these substances is further simplified by classification of the type of treatment or therapeutic agents. Then the etiologic agents for which the treatment is appropriate may be appended. Section V, Principles of treatment of poisoning offers an outline of modalities of treatment.

Emergency room organization

By the time the course is completed, the student should be in a position to set up a minimally adequate emergency room facility for the treatment of the commonly occurring intoxications. An inventory of emergency room equipment should be presented in printed form, for handing to an emergency room supervisor. A formulary of drugs used in the treatment of poisoning should also be available in printed form. There are relatively few toxic substances for which really effective therapeutic agents are available. Failure of an emergency room treatment facility to have these few pharmacologic agents available for emergency therapy is indefensible. Standing orders are needed for immediate use by emergency room personnel without further medical authorization in the event of compromise of vital functions. Provisions should be made for regular in-service training programs of emergency room personnel so that routine treatment of intoxicated patients is, in fact, routine.

Psychiatric aspects

The psychiatric aspects of acute intoxication are overlooked frequently during the rush for immediate medical care. In the experience of the author, more than 80% of the acute intoxications of clinical consequence are self-inflicted. Psychosocial factors attendant on self-inflicted poisoning have been a big deterrent to adequate care for the acutely intoxicated patient. Such patients are frequently antagonistic and uncooperative. They are viewed as psychologically, economically, and socially undesirable in the minds of many physicians and their medical staff. These patients are seen as malingerers who deserve punishment rather than treatment. All too frequently the attitude is 'treat them rough' so that the severity of the treatment may constitute a deterrent to repetition of the self-inflicted intoxication. This may be self-defeating for two reasons: (1) in the suicidal gesture where the fundamental purpose is to achieve a manipulative advantage in interpersonal relationship, the more severe the treatment the more effectively the episode serves the patient's purposes; and (2) over-aggressive treatment may convert the primary intoxication of low medical lethality into a significant illness due to complications such as aspiration pneumonia. In other cases, the apathy of the medical staff toward these patients may result in inadequate care. Neglect of the self-inflicted poisoning is sometimes tolerated by the medical community on the basis that the patient had attained his purposes, i.e., self-annihilation. The death review committee policies of many hospitals provide that 24 to 48 hours of hospital residence are necessary before a case will come up for review. As a result, the treatment of the acutely intoxicated patient where death has occurred in less than 24 hours is rarely subject to scrutiny. The psychological attitude toward the suicidal patient must be properly oriented during the course.

Treatment of the acute intoxication is only a form of first-aid when significant psychopathology exists. Recovery from the acute episode leaves the patient with all of the psychiatric and social problems which precipitated the episode with the addition, in many instances, of a greater economic burden. It is essential that psychiatric care is initiated at the earliest possible time that return to consciousness will allow.

When assessing the prognosis of the suicidal patient, the severity of acute medical impairment cannot be used as a measure of psychopathology. Often the manipulative patient is only a poor pharmacist who leads himself to a life-threatening acute illness by accident. On the other hand, many of the suicidal attempts appearing on the surface to be inconsequential issue from individuals with dramatic psychopathology which has a poor long-term prognosis. Ingestion of noxious substances, like strong caustics and carbon disulfide or formaldehyde, would be considered by a patient only during an acute psychotic episode.

Significance of diagnostic errors

The proper diagnosis is no less significant in intoxication than in any other aspect of medical practice. However, a satisfactory clinical outcome will be obtained by the proper application of supportive therapy alone in the vast majority of instances of acute intoxication. Therefore, failure to achieve a specific diagnosis among substances for which there is no specific treatment is of little clinical consequence. Failure to recognize, however, the less frequently occurring intoxications for which specific therapy is available – for example, the alkyl phosphate ester insecticides – may result in needless morbidity and mortality. This diagnostic effort, however, should not be allowed to interfere with proper intensive supportive care since discovery of a specific antidote is of little value if inattention to the patient has resulted in terminal anoxia as the price of discovery.

The far-reaching consequences of diagnostic errors as they relate to the state of the art of clinical toxicology are less commonly appreciated (Comstock, 1970). While errors in diagnosis within groups of substances for which there is no specific treatment may not influence significantly the clinical outcome in the presence of adequate supportive care, the significance of these errors in terms of conclusions to be drawn from the clinical course may be very great. All published reports should contain an estimate of reliability of the diagnosis. Failure to establish the diagnosis contributes heavily to the inadequacy of the accumulated medical literature concerning intoxication. Closely related is the failure to differentiate between primary and secondary causes of clinical signs and symptoms, resulting in the assignment of toxic actions to substances in the absence of any direct causal relationship. An illustration is that of a sedative-drug-intoxicated patient with aspiration pneumonia, respiratory depression, and anoxemia, who, after a period of positive pressure respiration, develops a major cardiac arrhythmia. The arrhythmia then is attributed to the primary toxic substance and the literature now contains the statement that this substance has the generation of cardiac arrhythmia as a toxic effect.

While many of those who will be trained in this curriculum will never publish, emphasis of the significance of diagnostic errors must be strong. In the current age of computer technology, virtually every discharged diagnosis has a chance of turning up in a computer. The usefulness of the accumulated data is only as good as the validity of the diagnosis in the individual case.

Rapid method for the diagnosis of acute intoxication

Encouragement should be given to the installation of bedside chemical techniques for the identification of common toxic substances. The conventional technology of analytical toxicology makes it impossible to use the laboratory to best advantage in the vast majority of clinical situations. Since it is inconceivable that the present technology can be expanded sufficiently within the foreseeable future, the emphasis must now be placed on the development of analytical techniques which are compatible with the ordinarily available clinical skills and clinical diagnostic equipment. Only in this way will analytical toxicology become available to the clinician as a practical tool in the treatment of acute intoxication.

Emergency room experience

Practical experience with the management of poisoning can be achieved only in the emergency room and during the subsequent hours of continuous attendance in the intensive care unit. The basic organization to provide practical experience in the treatment of poisoning is the poison team to which members of the house staff are assigned. The chief should be an individual on 24-hour call. During this assignment, the physician will become familiar with any special supplies or equipment used in the treatment of poisoning. He will be responsible for the continuous state of readiness of the poison room. The poison team should include an assistant from the intern staff; on-call residents in surgery, pediatrics, anesthesiology, and neurology; and follow-up members from physical medicine and psychiatry. Medical students assigned to this team can provide a great deal of practical assistance in clinical management. Assignment of responsibility among the team members for care of the varied needs of the acutely poisoned patient should provide for maximally effective use of resources both for treatment and for training. The poison team must be supported by the consulting staff, on whom they may call as special problems arise.

CONCLUSION

An urgent need exists for the inclusion of therapeutically-oriented training in clinical toxicology in the medical curriculum. The physician should be oriented to treat the patient first, then the poison.

REFERENCES

BERMAN, E. and BROWN, R. (1970), Significance of drug levels in biological fluids in pediatric poisoning. *Proc. Clin. Tox. Bull.* 1/1, 4.
COMSTOCK, E. G. (1968), The treatment of poisoning: a program for the medical curriculum. *Clin. Tox.* 1/1, 49.
COMSTOCK, E. G. (1970), Significance of diagnostic errors in clinical toxicology. *Clin. Tox.* (to be published).
CRAVER, B. (1969), Clinical investigation of the poisoned patient. In: *Proceedings of the 1968 Annual Meeting of the American Academy of Clinical Toxiology, 8.* American Academy of Clinical Toxicology, Houston.
PLAA, G. L. (1969), Current teaching practices. *Amer. Soc. Pharmacol. Exp. Ther. Teach. Inst. (Pittsburgh)* (in press).

23. the post-mortem findings in acute barbiturate poisoning and their interpretation

F. E. Camps

There is a striking lack of information about the post-mortem findings in acute barbiturate poisoning. This is largely because inadequate facilities have resulted in insufficient chemical analyses. Another factor lies in the approach of the pathologist to each case whereby he has accepted the dictum of an eminent forensic pathologist that all that the coroner or fiscal wishes to know is the cause of death. Forensic pathologists without clinical training tend to accept the obvious and, in cases of poisoning where the truth *can* be established, this is not always correct without proper and accurate analysis. For example, it has been pointed out that it is frequently the missing capsule which is the 'culprit', and not necessarily the one which is found in a container. The relevance of this is obvious when the question of treatment is urgent, because the method to be adopted may depend upon such facts as the type of barbiturate, whether other drugs have also been ingested and, perhaps more significantly, whether alcohol has also been taken.

It is proposed to discuss the post-mortem findings in relation to the different types of barbiturate poisoning – the mode of death and the chemical investigation, hoping thereby to assist clinicians in their treatment, and to aid lawyers in their interpretation of the differentiation between suicide and accident. At the same time, it may be asking too much to decide whether an overdose was ingested with intent of self-destruction or as a manipulative gesture to secure redress of an intolerable situation.

Before discussing the post-mortem findings and their interpretation, it is only proper to record that examination of the cases which are dealt with by the Department of Forensic Medicine, The London Hospital Medical College, fully substantiates the view that, if a patient suffering from acute barbiturate poisoning reaches a special hospital poisoning unit alive, there is a very high probability of survival.

It is essential to consider the possibility of acute poisoning in all cases of unexpected death. This applies to sudden collapse, for this mode of death can, surprisingly enough, occur with massive overdosage and underlines the importance of establishing the state of absorption. So, too, although homicide from barbiturate poisoning is *apparently* rare, it must not be forgotten that an overdose of a drug which is normally prescribed is easy to give to an ill person. Murder by barbiturate poisoning has been recorded – perhaps the most interesting case was that of Armstrong, who was convicted of killing his child by administering Seconal capsules. Close scrutiny of the case suggests that it was the capsule rather than the drug contained which killed the child, as it had not been weaned.

In most deaths from barbiturate poisoning, there will be clinical cyanosis of the lips and extremities, sometimes with pressure whitening due to obstruction of the external air passages by the face in a pillow, or deep congestion from posture (the head hanging downwards). This congestion may well also produce skin petechial haemorrhages and similar appearances in the scalp on reflection. The appearances of the internal organs will vary according to the rapidity of death and hence the degree of asphyxial congestion. The brain is usually swollen, with oedema of the meninges and accentuation of the cut ends of the vessels. The chemical changes in the brain are still under investigation (Shaw *et al.*, 1967). There may be a watery oedema of the glottis and in many cases there is excess of lymphoid tissue at the root of the tongue which will contribute to obstruction of the airway. The lungs are usually plum-coloured and show loss of aeration with some oedema and collapse. This appearance is similar to the findings seen in ventricular fibrillation and may well have been ascribed to primary myocardial ischaemia in the absence of analysis and the all too common presence of narrowing of the coronary arteries. Petechial haemorrhages are usually present in the pleural and pericardial surfaces. Apart from various pathological vascular changes which will be found in the population, the right side of the heart may be dilated with dark blood. In many cases, the aorta may be hypoplastic with minimal atheroma below the age of 40 years. The findings may be summarized at this stage as those of generalized congestion and, as many such deaths occur in females in the premenstrual phase, there may be haemorrhage into the corpus luteum.

The diagnostic features can be seen in the oesophagus and stomach and these will depend upon the type of barbiturate and the rapidity of death. The presence of undigested food in the stomach is *not* a contra-indication to barbiturate poisoning, but the presence of gelatinous material in the oesophagus with white powdery material and corrosion is a strong presumption of an overdose. Sometimes the colour (red or blue) derived from the capsule may give an indication of its nature. The stomach itself is the most revealing source of information. In large doses of intermediate- or short-acting barbiturates, there may be impaction at the pylorus with gross ulceration or areas of corrosion with adherent granules. The remaining mucosa show irritation. This is due to the fact that the pH is strongly alkaline. With the intermediate- and long-acting drugs, there may be no irritation, but butobarbitone may result in some pink discolouration. There may be irritation of the duodenal mucosa whilst in most cases the stomach will have lost its tone. The liver may show fatty changes as an indication of alcoholism. The spleen shows no specific changes but the kidneys are congested. This is the picture usually found in the acute type of poisoning with death within an hour, but it must be stressed that absorption is not always a continuous process and that irritation may cause pylorospasm and shock or coma cause loss of stomach tone. In such events relaxation of spasm or return of tone may lead to further absorption.

The barbiturates now usually prescribed rarely allow survival sufficiently long for bronchopneumonia to be established but, in the days of sodium barbitone and phenobarbitone, bronchopneumonia was a common terminal finding. However, routine examination of the lungs in acute poisoning does show changes at a surprisingly early stage, an observation which may have been unrecorded because of failure to utilize routine histology on such cases.

It must be obvious from the appearances described that the only specific naked-eye findings are in the oesophagus, stomach, and duodenum, hence the importance of chemical analysis is underlined. Proper collection of material at the time of examination is therefore vital.

The choice of material is *not* empirical but is based on knowledge of the pharmacology and fate of the various drugs after ingestion:

1.   The whole contents of the stomach with measurement of the volume, from which can be established; the identity of the drug(s) and presence of alcohol; the quantitative estimation and hence the amount still in the stomach.

2.   The peripheral blood from the vessels of the arms or legs; a volume of at least 10 ml must be collected. From this can be established the identity of the drugs and quantitative estimation.

3.   The liver blood obtained by slicing the liver (admittedly this is a mixture of portal and systemic blood and bile but it is of considerable value) for identity and quantitative estimation.

4.   Bile.

5.   Urine: total volume; pH;identification of presence of protein; glucose; ketone bodies and drugs.

In addition, alcohol estimations should be carried out on the peripheral blood and urine. It is also our standard procedure to examine the urine for salicylates and, if positive, perform a quantitative examination on the blood.

INTERPRETATION

From this information it is frequently possible to elicit information which is of assistance in establishing not only the true cause of death but the circumstances leading up to it. A brief summary is recorded below:

1.   The identification of the drugs.

2.   If the peripheral quantity is less than the liver quantity and there is still drug present in the stomach, then death has occurred before peak absorption *and* is probably rapid.

3.   If peripheral blood quantity is higher than liver quantity and there is only a small stomach residue, then peak absorption has probably occurred and death has been delayed.

TABLE 1

Acute barbiturate poisoning. Analytical results in some fatalities. Case 7 is an example of mixed alcohol poisoning; Case 8 was mistaken for barbiturate poisoning.

Case	Age	Barbiturate	Barbiturate					Ethanol		
			Peripheral blood (mg/100 ml)	Liver blood (mg/100 ml)	Urine (mg/100 ml)	Stomach contents (mg/100 ml)	(vol) (ml)	Blood (mg/100 ml)	Urine (mg/100 ml)	
(1) D.G.	41 M	Pentobarbitone	2.84	3.7	9.26	190	227	Nil	Nil	Died in bed (rapid)
(2) J.S.	42 M	Amylobarbitone	0.5	0.96	2.9	73.6	150	Nil	Nil	No nitrazepam
(3) F.P.	34 M	Short-acting (Secobarbitone)	0.4	1.0	0.9	95	114	150	204	Gastrectomy, alcohol and barbiturate (obstructed airway)
(4) G.J.	54 M	Amylobarbitone	1.3	9.4	0.3	267	250	Nil	Nil	Died in bed (very rapid)
(5) A.H.D.C.	58 M	Phenobarbitone	15.6	21.6	31.2	103	28.4	78	65	Phenobarbitone intoxication with added pentobarbitone
(6) J.G.	43 M	Tuinal	1.93	3.4	13.8	20	114	Nil	Nil	Late effect with posture
(7) J.W.	35 M	Mixed alcohol	—	—	—	153	200	129	164 Methanol)	Mixed alcohol
						115	200	126	224 Ethanol)	
(8) J.L.	60+ F	Glutethimide	16.25	—	—	2.25 g	114	Nil	Nil	Mistaken for barbiturate
(9) G.A.	68 M	Butobarbitone	9.85	—	8.5	2.9 g	100	Nil	Nil	urate
						48.0 g (oesophagus)	5 g			

4. If the quantity in the peripheral blood is higher than in the liver blood or the amount in the liver blood is low while there still remains a large quantity in the stomach, then absorption has ceased before death.

5. If the peripheral blood shows a higher quantity of one drug than another (if more than one drug is present) and there is a mixture of more than one drug in the stomach, it is probable that a second ingestion took place.

6. The amount of alcohol in peripheral blood, urine and stomach contents may be of assistance in deciding whether the person was intoxicated prior to taking the drug.

7. The presence and quantity of alcohol may give an indication of its contribution to a fatal termination.

8. The presence of other drugs may also be of significance.

CONCLUSIONS

1. A proper post-mortem examination must include chemical analysis if it is to be of any value.

2. The analytical procedures are of little value if inadequate by reason of limited sampling.

3. Statements of so-called 'fatal' doses must be taken in relation to other factors such as natural disease, obstructed airway, type of drug, rapidity of absorption, habituation to the drug, and the presence of other factors.

4. There appears to be some evidence in favour of gastric lavage, especially with the slow-acting barbiturates and proper evaluation of fatal cases may be of assistance in clinical treatment.

5. Proper investigation and evaluation of fatal cases may assist in factual evaluation of the difference between deliberate and accidental death and thus with the problem of insurance payment.

REFERENCE

SHAW, D. M., CAMPS, F. E. and ECCLESTON, E. G. (1967), 5-Hydroxytryptamine in the hind-brain of depressive suicides. *Brit. J. Psychiat.*, 113, 505.

subject index

index of contributors